Series editor
Wilfred Yeo
BMedSci, MB, ChB, MD, MRCP
Senior Lecturer in Medicine,
Medicine/Clinical
Pharmacology and
Therapeutics,
University of
Sheffield

Gastroenterology

Emma Lam
BSc (Hons), MB ChB, MRCP (UK)
Specialist Registrar
Llandough Hospital
Cardiff

Martin Lombard
MD, MSc, FRCPI, FRCP (Lond)
Consultant Physician and
Gastroenterologist
Royal Liverpool University
Hospital,
and
Senior Lecturer in Medicine,
University of Liverpool,
Liverpool

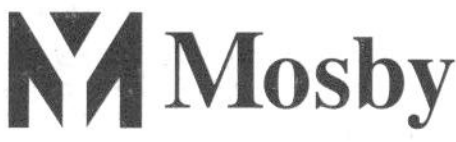

London Edinburgh New York Philadelphia Sydney Toronto

Editor	**Louise Crowe**
Development Editor	**Linda Horrell**
Senior Project Manager	**Jane Tozer**
Project Manager	**Jane Tozer/Lindy van den Berghe**
Designer	**Greg Smith**
Layout	**Jim Evoy**
Illustration Management	**Mike Saiz**
Illustrators	**Rob Dean**
	Marion Tasker
	Jenni Miller
Cover Design	**Greg Smith**
Index	**Janine Ross**

ISBN 0 7234 3153 1

Published in 1999 by Mosby, an imprint of Harcourt Brace and Company Limited.

Text set in Crash Course—VAG Light; captions in Crash Course—VAG Thin.

Cataloguing in Publication Data
Catalogue records for this book are available from the British Library and the US Library of Congress.

Preface

Having recently been through the system of medical school and MRCP (and revising at my desk until the early hours of the morning) I know what an enormous help a concise and well illustrated text can be! This book is primarily aimed at undergraduates who are revising for their exams, but it can serve as an aide-mémoire for house officers and other medically related professionals. Those preparing for MRCP will also find it useful as an overview of gastroenterology. However you use it, enjoy it—if only this book had been around when I was doing my exams!

Emma Lam

Despite their best intentions and notice of timetables, all students find that exams come too soon. *Crash Course* is written by people who've been there for people who are getting there! The clinical series is largely written by young doctors in training who have recently passed their exams and who know what you need to know to pass and excel in your exam. This book on gastroenterology tells you that, but I hope is comprehensive enough to give you even more—a good grounding in gastroenterology. It may therefore prove useful as a brief reference for forgotten facts even for those not doing exams. It doesn't pretend to give all of the detail required to practice gastroenterology, but should be used as a primer for those starting out in a career in gastroenterology and as a crash course for those coming up to examinations. The illustrations in this book pack in thousands more words than we could in the text and I hope you will enjoy learning from them.

Martin Lombard

Preface

So you have an exam in medicine and you don't know where to start? The answer is easy—start with *Crash Course*. Medicine is fun to learn if you can bring it to life with patients who need their problems solving. Conventional medical textbooks are written back-to-front, starting with the diagnosis and then describing the disease. This is because medicine evolved by careful observations and descriptions of individual diseases for which, until this century, there was no treatment. Modern medicine is about problem solving, learning methods to find the right path through the differential diagnosis, and offering treatment promptly.

This series of books has been designed to help you solve common medical problems by starting with the patient and extracting the salient points in the history, examination, and investigations. Part II gives you essential information on the physical examination and investigations as seen through the eyes of practising doctors in their specialty. Once the diagnosis is made, you can refer to Part III to confirm that the diagnosis is correct and get advice regarding treatment.

Throughout the series we have included informative diagrams and hints and tips boxes to simplify your learning. The books are meant as revision tools, but are comprehensive, accurate, and well balanced and should enable you to learn each subject well. To check that you did learn something from the book (rather than just flashing it in front of your eyes!), we have added a self-assessment section in the usual format of most medical exams—multiple-choice and short-answer questions (with answers), and patient management problems for self-directed learning. Good luck!

Wilf Yeo
Series Editor (Clinical)

Contents

Contents

Acknowledgements

Grateful thanks to the following at Royal Liverpool University hospital for their helpful contributions and comments to this book: Dr Conall Garvey, Consultant Radiologist for all of the radiology pictures; Dr Fiona Campbell, Consultant Pathologist for all of the histology photomicrographs, and Tracy Norris for the graphs of oesophageal manometry and pH. We each would also like to thank our mentors and students respectively for all that they have taught us.

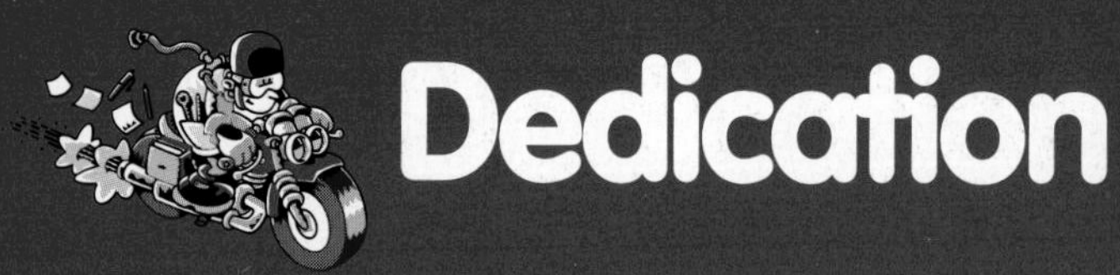

Dedication

Dedicated to the memory of my father.

E.L.

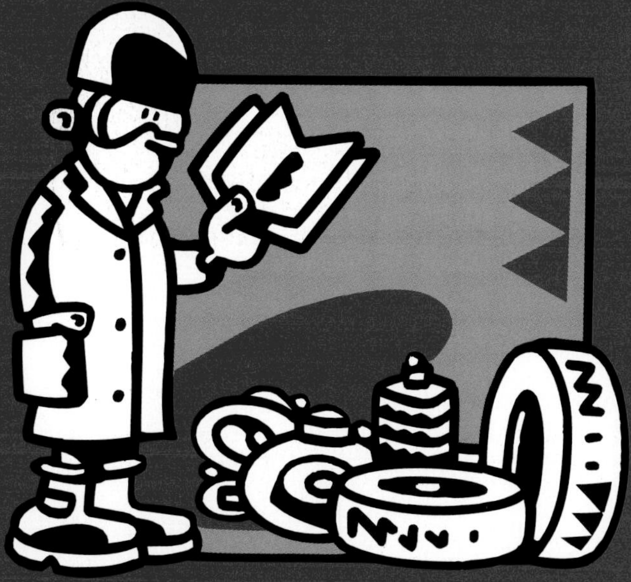

THE PATIENT PRESENTS WITH...

1. Indigestion

'Indigestion' encompasses a vast number of symptoms representing upper digestive problems with which a patient may present. These include:

- Heartburn.
- Fullness.
- Early satiety.
- Upper abdominal pain or ache.
- Flatulence.
- Hiccups.
- Belching.

The generic term that is useful to describe this constellation of symptoms is dyspepsia.

Dyspepsia:

- Is very common and occurs in up to 10% of the adult population. At least half of these 10% seek advice from their family doctor.
- Accounts for 40% of referrals to gastroenterology units.

Dysphagia, or difficulty in swallowing, is dealt with separately.

HISTORY OF THE PATIENT WITH INDIGESTION

When taking a history from a patient with dyspepsia, it is useful to classify the problem according to the group of symptoms present, although this does not always correlate with the pathology. Dyspepsia is characterized as:

- 'Reflux-like', if heartburn or chest pain predominate.
- 'Ulcer-like', if the characteristics convey the impression of peptic ulcer disease. This is confirmed by the presence of *Helicobacter pylori* in the gastric antrum (see Chapter 19).
- 'Non-ulcer dyspepsia', this describes similar symptoms in the absence of *H. pylori*.

History of heartburn

Heartburn is the key to differentiating reflux-like dyspepsia from other forms. It is described as a burning sensation which the patient locates retrosternally (behind the sternum). It is a diffuse and poorly localized sensation, typically worse on lying and leaning forward.

Excess saliva

'Waterbrash' is a specific phenomenon which the patient will describe as a flood of saliva in the mouth. Excess saliva is produced in the mouth and pharynx as a reflex response to acid in the lower oesophagus.

Chest pain

This is a common feature of gastro-oesophageal reflux.

Pain due to heartburn often radiates between the shoulder blades. Oesophageal spasm more commonly causes chest pain, which occurs after a meal but can arise spontaneously. The pain is:

- Typically over the sternum.
- Often severe.
- Sometimes described as 'something squeezing my inside'.

This pain is often confused with cardiac chest pain and, more confusingly, nitrates will relieve both spasm and

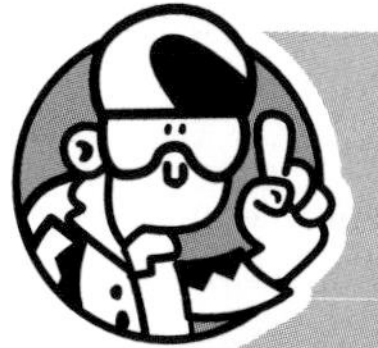

Oesophageal spasm tends not to be exercise-related. However, radiation of the pain to the jaw and left shoulder/arm can occur in severe cases, similar to cardiac pain. Change in severity of the pain in relation to body position is a helpful clue, since reflux symptoms will worsen when lying flat (e.g. in bed) or stooping forward (i.e. to pick something off the floor), and can be relieved when the patient sits or stands upright. Nausea or vomiting is unusual with reflux, but not uncommon with myocardial infarction.

angina, making it a diagnostic conundrum.

Other common causes of oesophageal spasm are:

- Underlying acid reflux.
- Achalasia.

A history of either condition should raise suspicion in someone presenting with atypical chest pain.

Other causes of chest pain are usually easy to differentiate. Pain due to pulmonary disease is more often sharp or stabbing like a knife-cut, and is referred to as pleuritic. It is worse when breathing deeply, which does not have an effect on oesophageal pain.

Nocturnal cough/asthma

Some patients with severe acid reflux do not complain of heartburn or chest pain, but develop cough or wheeze during the night when they are lying flat. They often lack symptoms during the daytime. Characteristically, they will demonstrate a 'morning dip' in their peak-flow recordings (Fig. 1.1). The bronchospasm is thought to be due to microaspiration of acid, but a vagal reflex may also be involved because experimentally, oesophageal acid-induced bronchospasm is ablated by vagotomy.

Asthmatics have a higher than average prevalence of heartburn. Increased intra-abdominal pressure may play a role, but some drugs such as theophylline also lower the sphincter tone.

Aggravating and risk factors for reflux

The most important risk factor is increased intra-abdominal pressure (Fig. 1.2) which can 'squeeze' the stomach contents upwards and, ultimately, squeeze the stomach itself through the hiatus in the diaphragm (hiatus hernia).

Ask about lifestyle habits and medication as:

- Stooping and bending (occupation or sport) aggravate the problem.
- Certain foods, especially those with a high fat content or that are spicy, often aggravate the problem.
- Alcohol ingestion can result in increased acid output, delayed gastric emptying, and gastritis.
- Cigarettes often make reflux symptoms worse: nicotine causes smooth muscle relaxation in the lower oesophageal sphincter.
- Non-steroidal anti-inflammatory drug (NSAID) ingestion can interfere with prostaglandin cytoprotection.
- Caffeine and theophylline cause relaxation of the lower oesophageal sphincter.
- Neuroleptic drugs have an anticholinergic action which also lowers oesophageal tone.

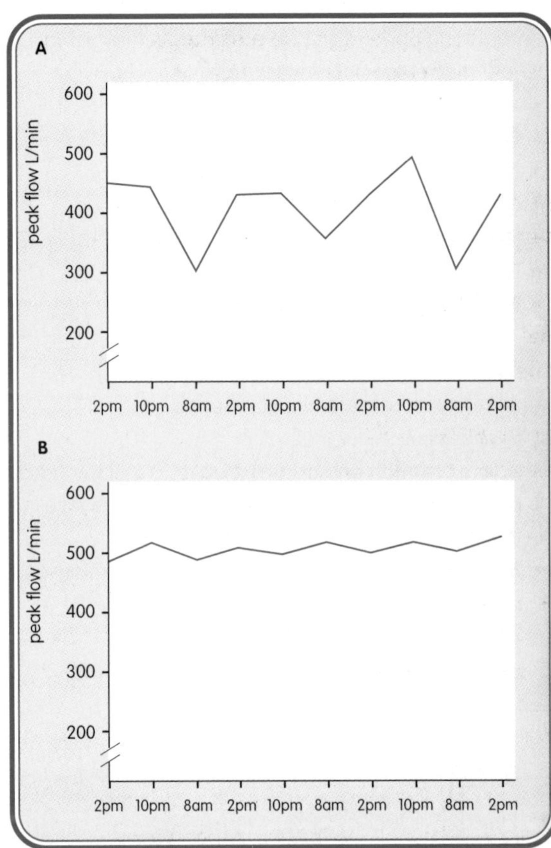

Fig. 1.1 (A) Peak flow measurement in an asthmatic demonstrating 'morning dip' due to acid reflux. (B) This was ablated when the patient took antisecretory medication before going to bed.

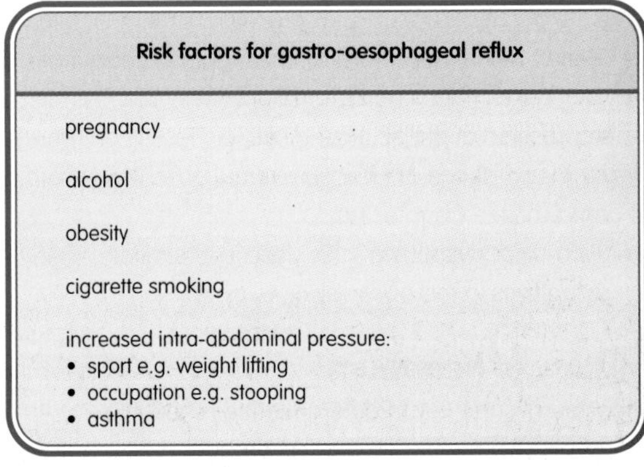

Risk factors for gastro-oesophageal reflux

pregnancy

alcohol

obesity

cigarette smoking

increased intra-abdominal pressure:
- sport e.g. weight lifting
- occupation e.g. stooping
- asthma

Fig. 1.2 Risk factors for gastro-oesophageal reflux

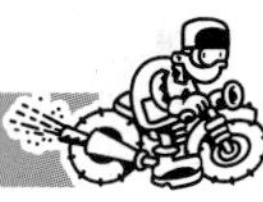

A long history of heartburn followed by difficulty in swallowing (dysphagia), but improvement in the heartburn may herald a fibrotic stricture in the lower oesophagus.

Most patients that present with heartburn/reflux symptoms will have tried antacids at some point; these will often provide some form of relief.

All of these dyspeptic symptoms constitute 'gastro-oesophageal reflux disease' sometimes abbreviated as GORD.

Epigastric pain

Epigastric pain is not a feature of GORD, but characterizes dyspepsia as 'ulcer-like'. It is a very common presenting complaint, but:

- The history is often vague.
- Sometimes patients have difficulty ascribing the term 'pain' to what they feel. The pain is often described as 'gnawing' or a dull ache which never goes away.

Pain due to:

- Peptic ulcer disease is occasionally more easily localized. The patient may point to a spot with one finger, although this is not a reliable sign.
- A gastric ulcer is often worse immediately after eating.

Duodenal ulcer pain is:

- Commonly relieved by antacids.
- Worse at night or in the fasted state, so the patient will often eat or drink milk before going to bed at night.

A family history is common. Find out about lifestyle habits such as smoking and drinking; these are important because they may contribute to gastritis.

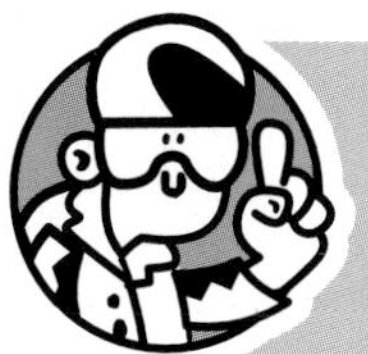

Peptic ulcers associated with NSAID use are usually painless and often present with occult bleeding.

Medication such as NSAIDs can also cause gastritis, erosions, and ulcers.

Epigastric pain presenting with weight loss may indicate gastric carcinoma and warrants urgent investigation.

Flatulence, belching, bloating, early satiety

These symptoms are characteristically more vague. The term 'non-ulcer dyspepsia' is used to account for symptoms that occur in the absence of demonstrable acid reflux or Helicobacter-related disease (duodenal and gastric ulcer; duodenitis and gastritis).

Non-ulcer dyspepsia and peptic ulcer pain can be difficult to differentiate from other causes of acute and chronic abdominal pain, discussed in Chapters 3 and 4. Non-ulcer dyspepsia is thought to be due to abnormal motility or abnormal sensitivity of the upper GI structures to distension.

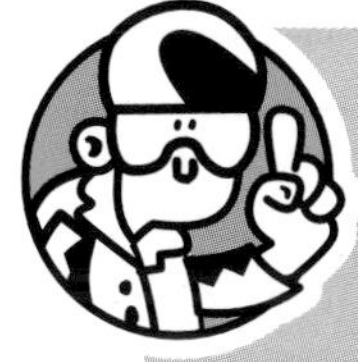

Weight loss or anaemia is never due to dyspepsia alone. The presence of vomiting more typically occurs with other causes of abdominal pain.

EXAMINING THE PATIENT WITH INDIGESTION

Check for:

- Obesity or pregnancy—these may support a diagnosis of GORD.
- More subtle signs, such as tar staining on fingers and features of iron deficiency anaemia—these may also be consistent with GORD but not exclusively so.
- Chronic GI blood loss and iron deficiency—these may be caused by ulceration of the oesophageal mucosa and may indicate chronic severe acid reflux.
- Tooth erosion by acid—this may be a sign of very severe reflux.

Often, physical examination is normal for patients with reflux disease. Examination is also unremarkable in the case of oesophageal spasm.

Cardiac pain can sometimes be very difficult to differentiate from the pain of GORD and associated spasm. Features that may predispose to ischaemic heart disease should be looked for, such as:

- Tar staining on the fingers.
- Obesity.
- Hypercholesterolaemia, xanthomas.

Tenderness on deep palpation may indicate that the patient has 'ulcer-like' dyspepsia due to gastritis or ulcer disease. Careful examination is important to exclude other causes of abdominal pain.

INVESTIGATING INDIGESTION

An algorithm for the investigation of the patient with indigestion is shown in Fig. 1.3.

In the majority of cases of reflux, the symptoms are mild and the diagnosis can often be made clinically and appropriate treatment commenced. More symptomatic cases may require investigation to exclude or confirm underlying oesophagitis. Any 'ALARMS' symptoms are an indication for urgent referral and investigation.

Upper GI malignancy can also present with these symptoms, and therefore patients over 45 years of age with dyspeptic symptoms will generally require investigation.

There is not yet universal agreement on the place of *Helicobacter* testing in the investigation of patients with dyspepsia.

Investigations to consider are discussed below.

Full blood count

A full blood count may be performed to exclude underlying anaemia. Microcytic anaemia is common with severe oesophagitis but rare in ulcer disease. Plummer–Vinson syndrome comprises anaemia associated with oesophageal web.

ALARMS symptoms in dyspepsia:

- **Anaemia.**
- **Loss of weight.**
- **Anorexia.**
- **Refractory to anti-secretory medication.**
- **Melaena.**
- **Swallowing problems.**

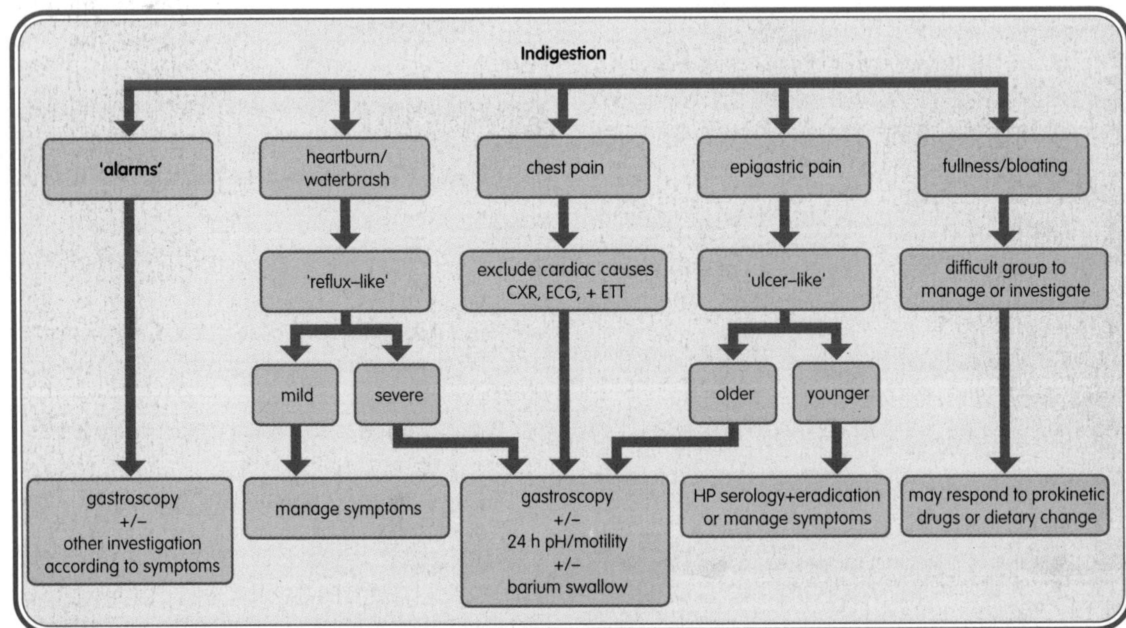

Fig. 1.3 Algorithm for the investigation of patients with dyspepsia. (CXR, chest X-ray; ECG, electrocardiography; ETT, exercise tolerance test; HP, *Helicobacter pylori*.)

Electrocardiography

Electrocardiography is particularly useful for patients with atypical sounding pain that may be due to oesophageal spasm or angina pectoris. However, non-specific T-wave changes can occur with reflux. An exercise tolerance test may be necessary to differentiate between oesophageal and cardiac pain.

Occasionally other investigations such as a thallium scan and coronary angiography are necessary to discriminate between cardiac and oesophageal symptoms.

Chest X-ray

A chest X-ray may demonstrate a hiatus hernia behind the cardiac shadow (Fig. 1.4).

Barium swallow

Barium swallow or scintigraphy is useful in demonstrating reflux. It can give rise to a 'corkscrew' appearance during an attack of spasm, and this is usually diagnostic (Fig. 1.5).

Oesophageal motility studies

These may be required to demonstrate the diffuse contraction and reduced peristalsis during a provoked attack. Pressures in the oesophagus can be exceedingly high, and the term 'nutcracker oesophagus' has been coined for these cases.

pH monitoring

pH monitoring is usually reserved for patients whose symptoms are more marked than expected from the endoscopic findings.

Breath tests

Breath tests have been devised to detect the presence of *Helicobacter pylori* without the requirement of endoscopy and biopsy (see Chapter 7).

Serology

Serology may be used to identify past infection with *Helicobacter pylori*.

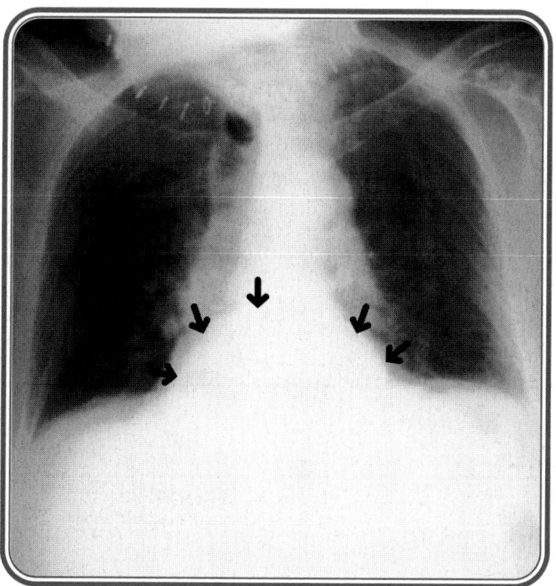

Fig. 1.4 Chest X-ray showing a hiatus hernia behind the cardiac shadow. (Incidentally shown on this X-ray are surgical staples around the neck following operative dissection.)

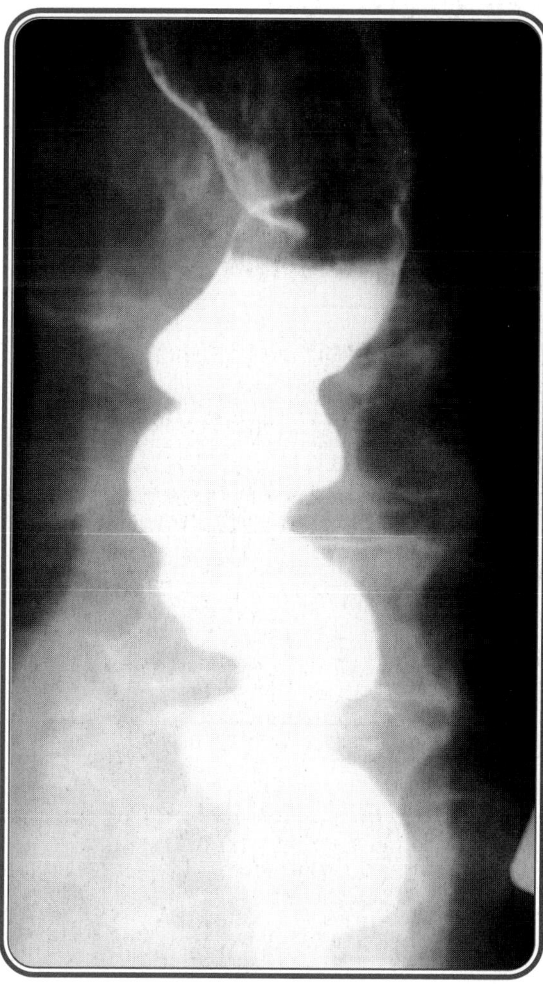

Fig. 1.5 Barium swallow demonstration of 'corkscrew' oesophagus caused by oesophageal spasm.

Endoscopy

Endoscopy is useful for the assessment of the presence, extent and severity of oesophagitis. It may also be used to identify:

- Hiatus hernia—this may be noted on endoscopy but itself is not diagnostic of acid reflux because it is often a coincidental finding, especially in elderly people.
- Ulcer disease and gastritis—biopsies can be taken to differentiate each type and also to look for the presence of *Helicobacter pylori*.

Barium meal

This is an alternative for patients for whom endoscopy may be difficult. It may demonstrate ulcer disease or malignancy.

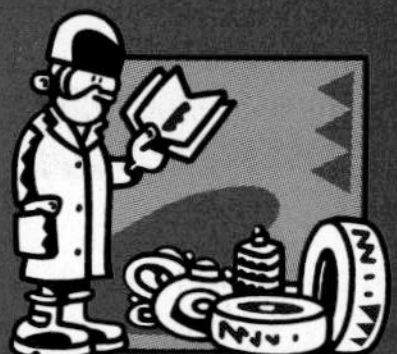

2. Swallowing Problems

DIFFERENTIAL DIAGNOSIS

The patient will usually complain of difficulty swallowing or the sensation of food sticking as it goes down (dysphagia). Difficulty with the passage of food typically begins with solids like bread or meat, followed by liquids if the condition is progressive. The condition is usually painless and is due to a narrowing of the oesophageal lumen.

The differential diagnosis therefore includes in order of importance:

- Oesophageal carcinoma.
- Achalasia.
- Benign oesophageal stricture.
- Oesophagitis.
- Oesophageal spasm.
- Failure of peristalsis due to other reasons, e.g. scleroderma.
- Oesophageal pouch or diverticulum.
- Oesophageal web.
- Incarcerated hiatus hernia.
- Foreign body obstruction.

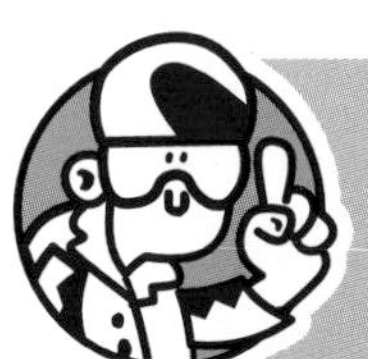

Dysphagia is often unnoticed or even denied by patients until it becomes troublesome. They may also relieve their distress by changing posture, belching regurgitation of food, or by taking a drink.

HISTORY OF THE PATIENT WITH SWALLOWING PROBLEMS

Taking a careful history of the presenting complaint is the key to sorting out the differential diagnosis. Important features to ask about are discussed below.

Duration of symptoms

A long or intermittent history, usually accompanied by manoeuvres to relieve the symptom, often indicates anatomical or mechanical obstruction due to:

- Pouch.
- Diverticulum.
- Webs.
- Incarcerated hernia.

The first three are more common in younger adults; the last in elderly people.

Level at which dysphagia occurs

Ask at what level dysphagia occurs as:

- High-level dysphagia can be due to cricopharyngeal spasm, a contraction of the cricopharyneus muscle and inferior constrictors, which is closely associated with pharyngeal pouch.
- Low-level dysphagia is more common with peptic strictures.
- Carcinoma occurs at all levels (Fig. 2.1).

Weight loss

Minor weight loss is common because patients may have modified their diet to cope with dysphagia. Significant weight loss is an ominous sign and almost always indicates carcinoma.

History of heartburn

A history of heartburn preceding the dysphagia is highly suggestive of benign oesophageal stricture, and preventing further reflux.

Reflux

Reflux and dysphagia occurring together suggest achalasia, a condition in which there is uncoordinated oesophageal peristalsis and failure to relax the lower oesophageal sphincter. This tends to present in early adulthood with chest pain, occurring due to oesophageal spasm, which can be mistaken for cardiac pain. Sublingual nitrates, the standard medication for angina pectoris, relieve the chest pain caused by oesophageal spasm, because they cause smooth muscle relaxation.

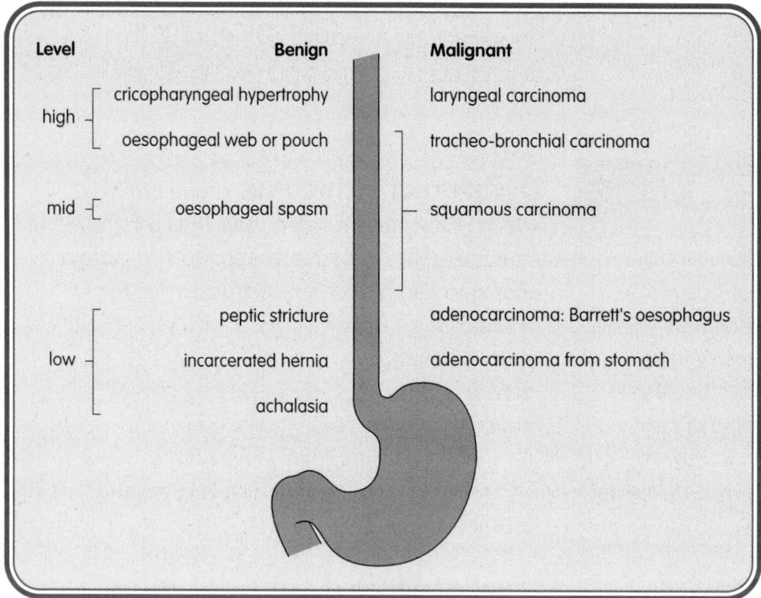

Fig. 2.1 Sites at which oesophageal lesions cause dysphagia. The patient will often describe the level of obstruction as high, mid-chest, or lower chest but this does not reliably correlate with site or nature of pathology.

Regurgitation of food

This is common if pouches are present. It differs from vomiting in that:

- There is an absence of nausea.
- Only small boluses are regurgitated back into the mouth and are often swallowed immediately.

Fluids are often more problematic than solids. Occasionally, dysphagia may be present because of obstruction by the pouch itself, but this is usually intermittent.

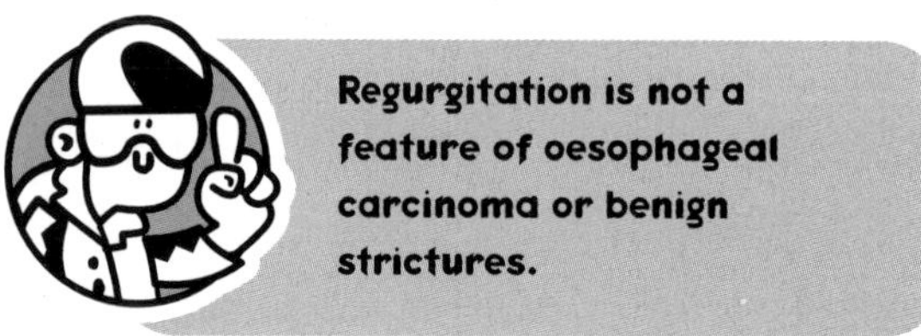

Recurrent pulmonary infections

Recurrent pulmonary infections resulting from aspiration can be due to:

- Achalasia.
- Pouches.
- Diverticula.

Progression of dysphagia

Progression is marked by the patient finding difficulty with food of a sloppy or liquid consistency as well as solids. This may be of relatively short duration (weeks or months) and is an ominous development, most often occurring in oesophageal carcinoma.

Pain with dysphagia

Pain on swallowing is termed odynophagia and may or may not be accompanied by dysphagia. Odynophagia may be caused by:

- Infection with *Candida*—this is the most common cause, and may result from underlying immunosuppression, e.g. steroid treatments, diabetes, malignancy, or immunodeficiency. Herpes and cytomegalovirus (CMV) infection of the oesophagus are more likely to be found in people infected with the human immunodeficiency virus (HIV).
- Impaction of a foreign body—this may cause dysphagia and will usually have an obvious history, e.g. fish bones represent the most common cause.

Pain between the shoulder blades in association with heartburn usually signifies oesophagitis.

A 'lump' in the throat can be due to pharyngitis, but is also a presentation of globus hystericus. Globus is a functional disorder that usually affects young females.

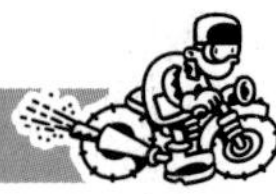

True dysphagia of solids followed by difficulty with liquids is absent. A history of depression and/or anxiety is apparent in most cases, and it is important to establish the root of the patient's concern in order to allay unfounded fears, e.g. 'My father died of throat cancer, etc...'.

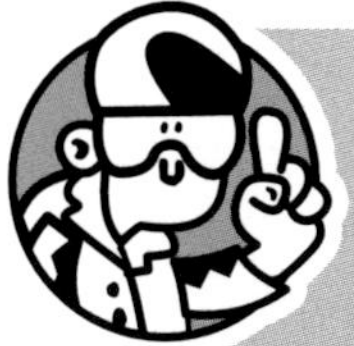

The diagnosis of globus should not be accepted without investigation and exclusion of more common or more sinister causes of dysphagia.

Important past medical history

Find out about the patient's past medical history, particularly:

- Risk factors for carcinoma—these include Barrett's oesophagitis, tylosis, and smoking.
- Chronic systemic diseases —neuromuscular disorders such as motor neuron disease, myasthenia gravis, and mytonia dystrophica are associated with disordered peristalsis.
- Collagen vascular disease, for example, scleroderma, which can interfere with the elasticity of the oesophagus and impair peristalsis.

EXAMINING THE PATIENT WITH SWALLOWING PROBLEMS

Look out for:

- Weight loss—if marked, should give cause for concern; patients with carcinoma are often cachectic. A healthy, well-nourished patient with a history of dysphagia usually indicates a benign aetiology, but not always so.
- Anaemia—sometimes manifested by pallor, can occur with oesophagitis and classically has been a feature associated with oesophageal web (Plummer–Vinson or Paterson–Kelly syndrome). It is more common with malignant disease.
- Systemic features such as clubbing, tylosis (thickening of the palms of the hand and soles of the feet), supraclavicular lymph nodes, and hepatomegaly are suggestive of malignant disease in the context of dysphagia.
- A gastric mass—may be palpable if the tumour extends into the cardia, but there are no clinical signs that are specific for oesophageal carcinoma.

INVESTIGATING SWALLOWING PROBLEMS

It is imperative to investigate any patient who presents with dysphagia. A summary algorithm is shown in Fig. 2.2.

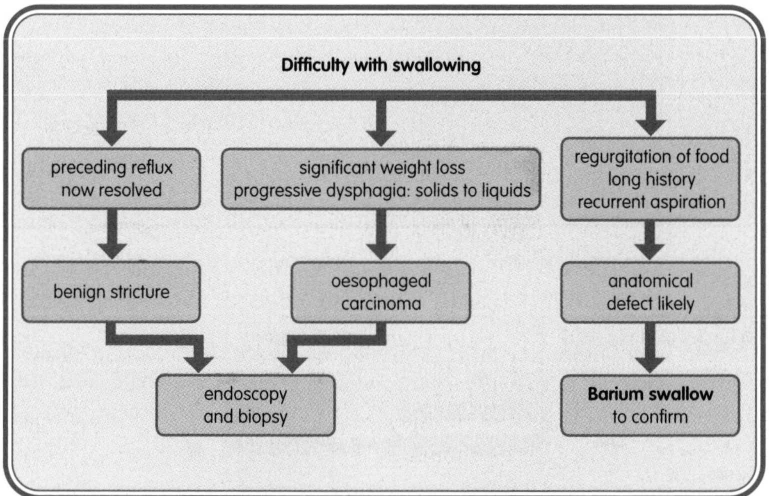

Fig. 2.2 Algorithm for the investigation of a patient with difficulty in swallowing.

Full blood count and biochemistry

Full blood count and biochemistry should be performed to assess anaemia and, in severe cases, dehydration. Blood tests such as serum glucose and thyroid function test will exclude other causes of weight loss such as diabetes and thyrotoxicosis. Occasionally, a retrosternal goitre may cause dysphagia.

When endoscopy is negative and dysphagia persists or is high level, a barium swallow should always be done as well.

Endoscopy

Endoscopy and biopsy are the investigations of choice for most patients with a history of dysphagia because not only can they confirm a malignant lesion, they will also differentiate between a benign stricture due to reflux and a malignant stricture.

Laryngoscopy

Indirect or direct laryngoscopy may be necessary to investigate high dysphagia.

Barium swallow

Barium swallow can be undertaken for patients who cannot tolerate endoscopy for whatever reason, but appearances between benign and malignant strictures can be difficult to interpret. Generally:

- Benign strictures are smooth and tapering.
- Malignant strictures are irregular and 'shouldered' (Fig. 2.3).

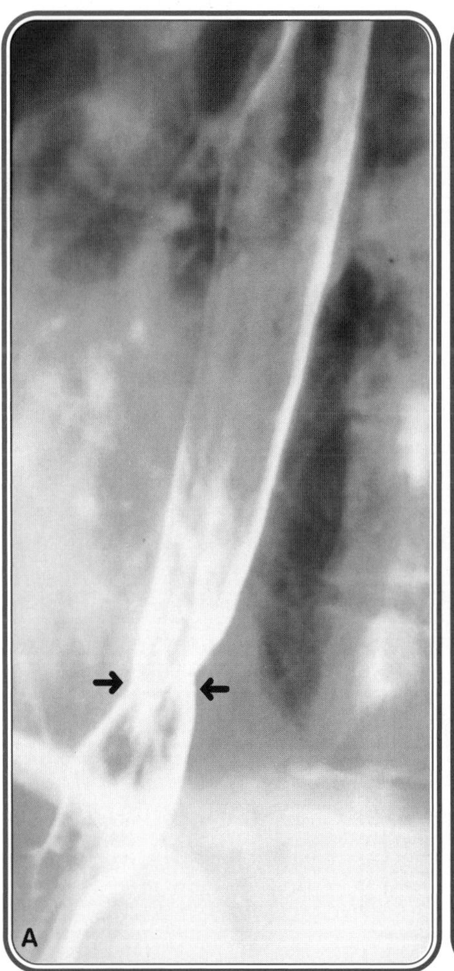

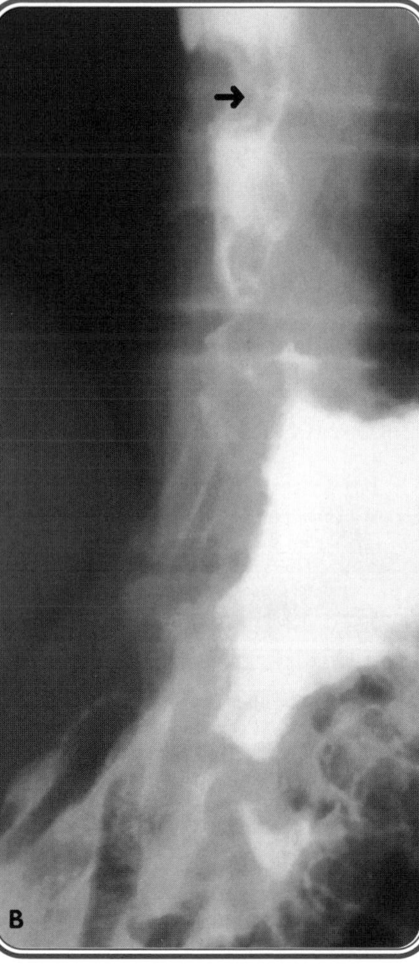

Fig. 2.3 (A) Barium swallow showing smooth tapering stricture of benign oesophageal type (arrows), and (B) the 'shouldered' appearance of malignant stricture (arrow) due to infiltration of the oesophagus from adenocarcinoma of the stomach cardia.

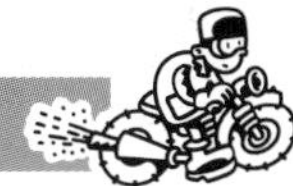

Barium swallow is very useful in demonstrating anatomical anomalies such as:

- Pouches, usually high in the midline, caused by a defect in the overlapping muscle layers.
- Diverticula—usually small and associated with disordered peristalsis.
- Webs can be high at the cricopharyngeus or lower down the oesophagus.
- A Schatzki ring is a fibromuscular attachment originating from the diaphragm usually associated with a small hiatus hernia.

Barium swallow can be diagnostic of achalasia with the typical appearance of:

- A dilated oesophagus with no peristalsis.
- A narrowed lower oesophagus (bird's beak appearance) due to the failure of the lower oesophageal sphincter to relax (see Fig 18.5).

Achalasia is often missed at endoscopy.

Oesophageal motility studies

These are useful to confirm spasm or achalasia. Twenty-four hour oesophageal pH is useful to confirm acid reflux (see Figs 17.9 and 17.10).

Chest X-ray

A chest X-ray, often forgotten, provides useful information about patients with swallowing problems, especially those who present with pneumonia. A dilated oesophagus can be seen as a double cardiac shadow with a fluid level behind the heart.

Other investigations

Occasionally, the cause of dysphagia may be difficult to find.

Bronchoscopy or a computed tomography (CT) scan may be required if tracheobronchial carcinoma is suspected.

Patients found to have a malignant stricture will need to be assessed for surgical resection.

Metastatic spread to the liver should be excluded by abdominal ultrasound.

In some centres, CT of the thorax is performed to assess local lymph node spread. However, most patients tend to be elderly and present late to the clinician; in most of these cases, palliative treatment is the only suitable option.

3. Acute Abdominal Pain

Acute abdominal pain is a common presentation in clinical medicine and often the most difficult to deal with. It usually refers to pain of sudden onset and a duration of less than 48 hours.

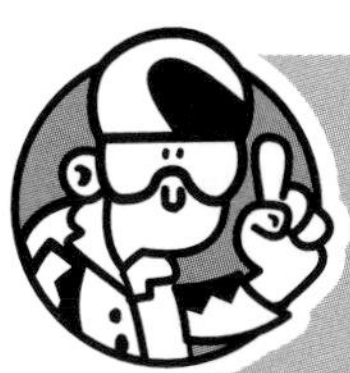

It is important to organize management (e.g. intravenous access, analgesia, etc.) at the same time as attempting to make a diagnosis.

The differential diagnosis of acute abdominal pain includes:

- Acute peptic ulceration.
- Biliary colic.
- Acute cholecystitis.
- Acute pancreatitis.
- Acute appendicitis.
- Acute diverticulitis.
- Perforation of abdominal viscus.
- Bowel obstruction.
- Acute renal colic or acute urinary retention.
- Acute infarction of bowel, spleen, or kidney.
- Myocardial infarction occasionally presents with acute abdominal pain.
- Acute hepatic vein thrombosis (Budd–Chiari syndrome).
- Metabolic causes: diabetic ketoacidosis, Addison's disease, acute intermittent porphyria.
- Gynaecological causes: ectopic pregnancy, acute salpingitis, ovarian cyst rupture.

HISTORY OF THE PATIENT WITH ACUTE ABDOMINAL PAIN

A good history is vital in helping to discern the cause of acute abdominal pain. The following points should be considered.

Site of pain

The site or seat of pain gives the most important clue to its cause (see Fig. 14.1). Epigastric pain is suggestive of:

- Peptic ulcer disease.
- Acute pancreatitis.
- Biliary colic.

In contrast, lower abdominal pain is suggestive of:

- Gynaecological problems, e.g. acute salpingitis.
- Acute appendicitis.
- Acute diverticulitis.
- Acute urinary retention.

Particular sites of pain are generally associated with particular conditions, for example:

- Pain in the right iliac fossa due to appendicitis.
- Pain in the right upper quadrant due to acute cholecystitis.
- Pain in the left iliac fossa due to acute diverticulitis.
- Pain in the loin due to renal colic.

Generalized pain is more likely to be due to a metabolic cause or peritonitis from perforation or infarction.

Radiation of pain

Pain due to certain conditions characteristically radiates to particular sites. For example:

- Pancreatic pain radiates 'through' to the middle of the back.
- Gall bladder pain commonly radiates around the right side to back.
- Myocardial pain, when caused by ischaemia in the diaphragmatic surface, radiates to the epigastrium.
- Renal pain starts in the loin but radiates to the groin.

Character of the pain

The character may be difficult to ascertain and is not always reliable, but the following may be useful:

- 'Colicky' describes pain that builds to a peak and wanes. It is characteristic of hollow organ pain, e.g. distension of the bowel, bile duct, or ureter wall in obstruction.
- A sharp stabbing pain worsened by movement or respiration suggests pleural or peritoneal irritation, e.g. peritonitis from acute appendicitis or cholecystitis.

Generalized peritonitis has a similar characteristic, but is less well localized and is seen with perforation or ruptured aortic aneurysm.

Relieving and exacerbating factors

These are not often helpful in the acute situation. With any painful condition, the patient will usually adopt the most comfortable posture:

- There may be a history of peptic ulcer disease or pain exacerbated or relieved by food.
- Acute pancreatitis is often relieved by sitting forward while holding the abdomen.
- Vomiting may relieve the pain of bowel obstruction.

Past medical history

Past history and risk factors are important, for example:

- In an elderly patient with known abdominal aortic aneurysm, a sudden onset of abdominal pain may be due to rupture.
- A patient with a history of constipation may present with acute obstruction.

Risk factors for acute pancreatitis include:

- Gallstones.
- Alcohol.
- Recent endoscopic retrograde cholangiopancreatography (ERCP).

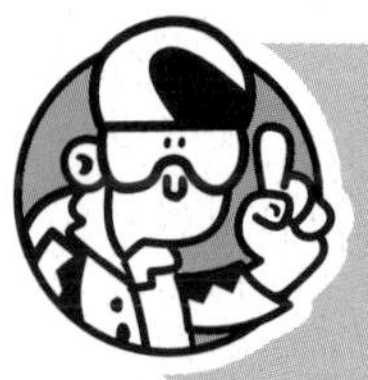

A menstrual history is essential to exclude the possibility of a ruptured ectopic pregnancy.

Family history

This may be relevant, for example porphyria is a hereditary condition that commonly presents with acute abdominal pain.

EXAMINING THE PATIENT WITH ACUTE ABDOMINAL PAIN

A general inspection can reveal a lot about your patient while you are taking the history and instigating management. Decide whether the patient looks 'ill'. This is a good indicator of serious underlying pathology. Other pointers are:

- Is the patient lying still with shallow breathing (generalized peritonitis)?
- Is the patient agitated and restless (colicky pain) or holding a particular part of the abdomen (localized peritonitis)?
- Is the patient hypotensive or in shock (ruptured abdominal aneurysm, ectopic pregnancy)?
- Is there any external bruising (acute pancreatitis)?

Guarding and rebound tenderness

If the patient tends to hold the abdominal muscle rigid (guarding), this may suggest peritonitis is present. The abdomen will be tender but the patient will allow gradual gentle pressure. Sudden removal of the palpating hand produces rebound tenderness—this is an important sign of peritonitis which can also be elicited by the patient being reluctant to 'blow out' the abdomen to touch your hand positioned at about 5 cm above the resting abdomen.

Site of tenderness

If tenderness is more localized, think of the underlying structure, for example:

- Appendix in the right iliac fossa.
- Descending colon in the left iliac fossa.
- Ovaries in lower abdomen.
- Stomach or pancreas in the upper abdomen.

Pulsation

A pulsating or expansile mass may suggest an aortic aneurysm, but in some cases of rupture, the pulsation may be absent. Peripheral pulses should be palpated.

Distension

In the presence of chronic liver disease, ascites may be present and can become infected (spontaneous bacterial peritonitis, SBP). Acute onset of painful ascites is sometimes seen in hepatic vein thrombosis (Budd–Chiari syndrome).

Internal examination

Rectal examination is essential to exclude melaena from acute upper gastrointestinal ulceration. Constipation may give a clue about obstruction or a tender rectal examination may be due to a locally inflamed appendix.

Vaginal examination may be indicated in certain circumstances, e.g. a tender fornix may suggest torsion or rupture of an ovarian cyst.

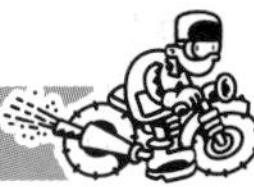

INVESTIGATING ACUTE ABDOMINAL PAIN

Investigations are usually important to confirm your diagnosis or to determine the severity of the illness.

Full blood count

A full blood count may aid diagnosis:

- A raised white cell count may support a diagnosis of underlying sepsis or peritonitis, but most sick patients will have a raised white cell count. There may be haemoconcentration due to dehydration or vomiting.
- Platelets will be high in inflammatory disease.
- A low haemoglobin should raise suspicion of bleeding in association with the acute abdominal pain.

Biochemistry

Specific biochemical tests and their correct interpretation in the context of acute abdominal pain can be very helpful:

- A raised amylase is important to support a diagnosis of acute pancreatitis, but it can be slightly raised in cholecystitis and biliary colic.
- Urea and electrolytes may be disturbed if the patient is ill or dehydrated. The combination of hyperkalaemia with hyponatraemia should suggest the possibility of Addison's disease.
- A high sugar with acidosis in a patient with acute abdominal pain may be due to diabetic ketoacidosis.
- Raised liver enzymes may point to a diagnosis of obstructive jaundice due to gallstones or acute cholestasis associated with Budd–Chiari syndrome.
- Urine analysis may reveal haematuria suggestive of renal colic.
- Urinary porphyrin estimation has been superseded by measurement of specific enzyme activity in the blood.
- A pregnancy test is mandatory in women of a child-bearing age.

Radiology

A chest X-ray is essential to exclude air under the diaphragm, indicative of perforation of a viscus (Fig. 3.1).

A plain abdominal X-ray may reveal:

- Dilated bowel loops indicative of obstruction (Fig. 3.2).
- Faecal loading associated with constipation or obstruction.
- Calcification in gallstones, ureteric stones, or aortic aneurysm.

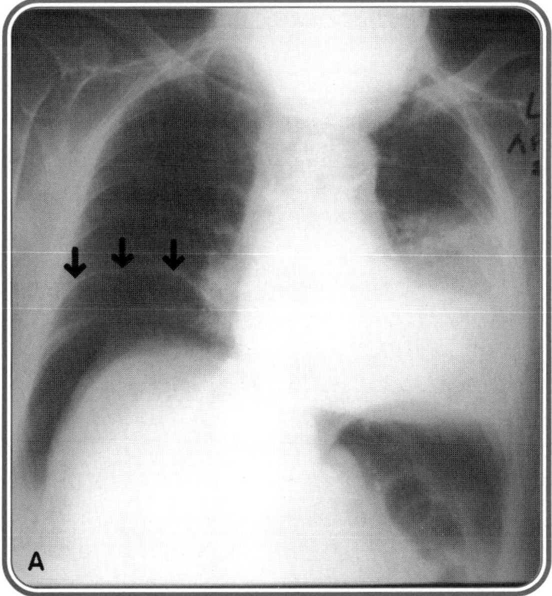

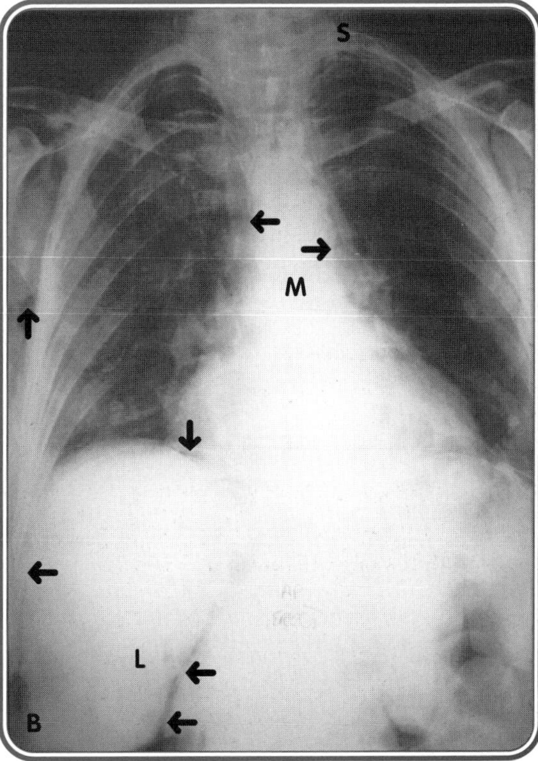

Fig. 3.1 Chest X-rays. (A) A patient with acute abdominal pain due to visceral perforation. Air under the diaphragm is more obvious on the right side above the liver (arrows). (B) A patient with retroperitoneal perforation: arrows show where air tracks up around the liver (L), into the mediastinum (M), and subcutaneously (S) (felt as crackling under the skin.

Ultrasound is not routinely performed as an emergency, but may be helpful in confirming:

- Dilated bile ducts due to stones.
- Stones in gallbladder.
- Congested liver (Budd–Chiari).
- Ovarian cysts.

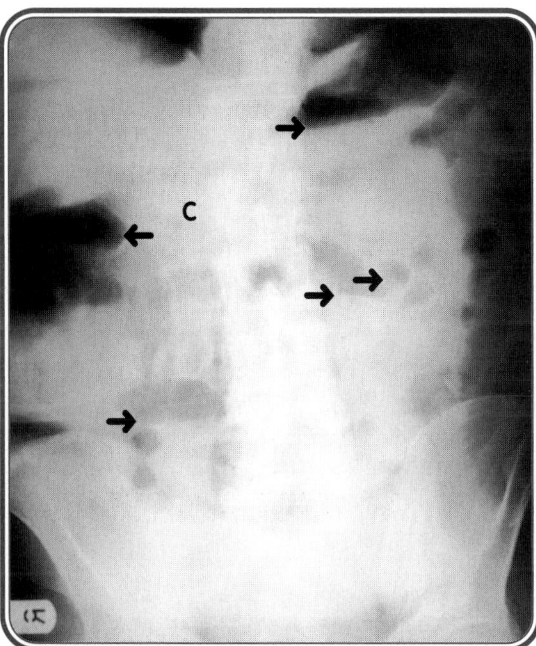

Fig. 3.2 Abdominal X-ray from a patient with intestinal obstruction, showing fluid levels in the bowel (arrows), a grossly distended caecum (C), and a collapsed colon.

A computed tomography scan similarly is rarely needed in the emergency situation, but can be useful when the diagnosis is not apparent, e.g. ruptured liver or renal cysts.

Electrocardiography

All patients who present with chest or abdominal pain should have an electrocardiogram to exclude myocardial infarction (Fig. 3.3). Some T-wave changes are non-specific and can be seen in many causes of acute abdominal pain.

Endoscopy

Gastroscopy may be indicated if peptic ulcer disease is suspected but would be contraindicated in many causes of acute abdominal pain, e.g. perforation.

Urgent ERCP may be indicated for suspected gallstone pancreatitis or acute cholangitis.

In both conditions, emergency sphincterotomy has been shown to be effective.

Surgery

Many of the causes of acute abdominal pain are surgical emergencies. Occasionally no cause is apparent and diagnostic laparotomy or laparoscopy can be useful in these situations, e.g peritonitis of uncertain cause.

Summary

An algorithm summarizing the investigation of acute abdominal pain is shown in Fig. 3.4.

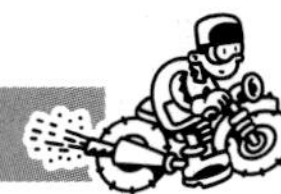

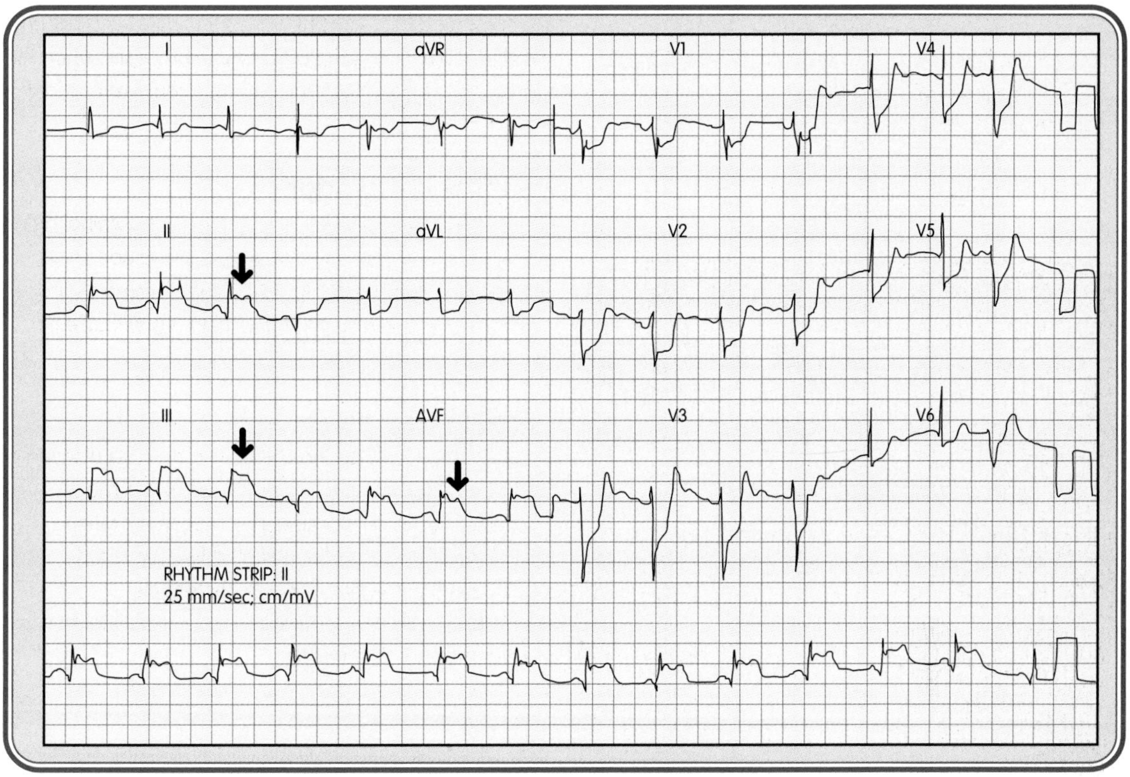

Fig. 3.3 ECG from a patient presenting with acute abdominal pain. ST segment elevation in leads II, III, and AVF (arrows) support a diagnosis of inferior myocardial infarction.

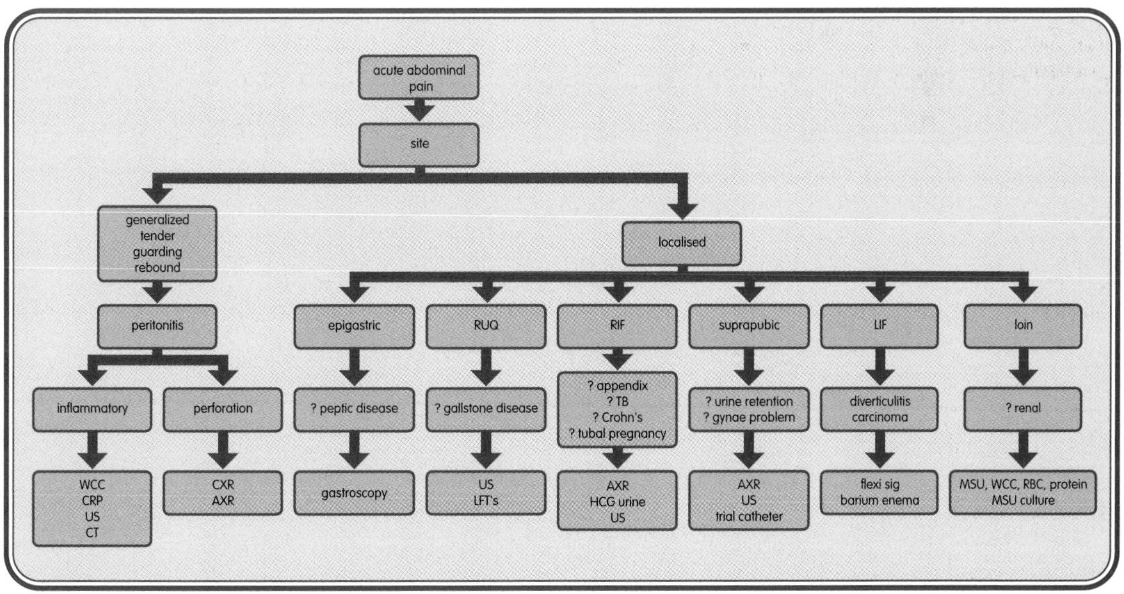

Fig. 3.4 Algorithm for the investigation of acute abdominal pain. (WCC, white cell count; CRP, C-reactive protein; US, ultrasound; CT, computed tomography; CXR, chest X-ray; AXR, abdominal X-ray; LFTs, liver function tests; HCG, human chorionic gonadotrophin (pregnancy test); RUQ, right upper quadrant; LIF, left iliac fossa; RIF, right iliac fossa; MSU, midstream urine; RBC, red blood cells.)

4. Chronic Abdominal Pain

Chronic abdominal pain is a common complaint that accounts for about 40% of referral to gastroenterology outpatient clinics. The symptoms are often of an intermittent nature, with pain-free periods in between. The list of differential diagnoses is vast, and only those commonly seen in clinical practice are discussed here. There is considerable overlap between some of these symptoms and 'indigestion' discussed in Chapter 1, but pain is not really a prominent symptom in dyspepsia and is discussed in more detail here.

The common differential diagnoses for chronic abdominal pain include:

- Peptic ulcer disease.
- Chronic pancreatitis.
- Chronic cholecystitis.
- Chronic appendicitis.
- Irritable bowel syndrome.
- Constipation.
- Subacute bowel obstruction.
- Crohn's disease.
- Intestinal malignancy.
- Mesenteric ischaemia.
- Gynaecological causes, e.g. endometriosis, pelvic inflammatory disease.

HISTORY OF THE PATIENT WITH CHRONIC ABDOMINAL PAIN

As with acute abdominal pain, a detailed history is essential to focus the differential diagnois. Several important features need to be discovered, and these are discussed below.

Site and radiation of the pain

The most obvious clue to the aetiology is the site of the pain and its radiation.

Chronic pain in the upper abdomen is suggestive of:

- Peptic ulcer disease.
- Chronic cholecystitis.
- Chronic pancreatitis.

Pain at particular sites may be even more specific:

- Pain in the right upper quadrant is commonly of liver or biliary origin.
- Pain in the right iliac fossa may suggest Crohn's disease.
- Pain in the loin may be due to chronic pyelonephritis.
- Pain in the lower abdomen is usually due to colonic or gynaecological problems.

Character

The character of chronic pain is often vague, but certain features are helpful:

- Most chronic abdominal pain is described as a dull ache which is suggestive of visceral peritoneal involvement, e.g. chronic pancreatitis, intestinal malignancy, gynaecological causes.
- Sharp, stabbing, or colicky pain may be associated with distension of a viscus, e.g. biliary colic, constipation, or irritable bowel syndrome.

Exacerbating and relieving factors

These are sometimes helpful. The patient may have had the pain for some time and may have experimented with ways to relieve or exacerbate the pain, such as with food or alcohol.

Food can have the following effects:

- It may aggravate biliary causes, characteristically occurring 20–30 minutes after a meal, and there may be fat intolerance, although this is not specific for any diagnosis.
- Patients may notice that pain occurs 1–2 hours after food in mesenteric ischaemia ('abdominal angina') and this results in them being afraid to eat.
- It can relieve the pain of a duodenal ulcer, in particular, when the patient drinks milk at bedtime.

Alcohol:

- Worsens chronic pancreatitis and gastritis, but the patient does not always modify his or her behaviour.

Defaecation or passage of flatus:

- Relieves lower abdominal pain of constipation or irritable bowel.
- May exacerbate pain due to local inflammatory conditions of the anus or rectum, or in obstruction.

Menstruation:
- Painful periods should be obvious but ectopic areas of endometriosis may also induce pain at time of menstruation.
- Pain in mid-cycle can occur with ovulation ('mittelschmerz') or occasionally with ovarian cysts.

Associated features

Patients may not notice other problems or their significance in relation to the pain may not be obvious to them. It is important to ask specifically about:
- Distension or bloating—if intermittent, this is suggestive of irritable bowel syndrome or subacute obstruction; if progressive, it may indicate development of a mass or ascites.
- Weight loss—think of underlying malignancy, i.e. pancreatic or intestinal, especially in elderly patients. In younger patients, think of Crohn's disease or lymphoma. Weight loss may also result from avoidance of food.
- Change in bowel habit—alternating constipation or diarrhoea may be due to a change in diet but intestinal malignancy must be excluded in patients over 45 years old.
- Vaginal discharge—pelvic inflammatory disease is something the patient may be embarrassed to volunteer information about.

EXAMINING THE PATIENT WITH CHRONIC ABDOMINAL PAIN

On general inspection, important features to note include:
- Obvious signs of weight loss.
- Pigmentation, pallor or jaundice.
- Signs of dehydration.

In the neck, look for:
- Lymphadenopathy.
- Goitre.
- Weight loss and skin turgor.

Abdominal inspection and palpation may reveal:
- Scars from previous surgery—patients occasionally omit information about previous operations.
- Distension—is it uniform due to ascites or asymmetrical due to a mass?
- Peristalsis can be obvious in thin people with intestinal obstruction.
- A mass may be present, and its anatomical location usually indicates the aetiology, e.g. epigastric in gastric malignancy, right iliac fossa in Crohn's disease, or an appendix mass.
- Stigmata of chronic alcohol misuse may be present (spider naevi, umbilical varices).

Other features to note are:
- Signs of peripheral vascular disease which may accompany mesenteric ischaemia.
- Tenderness in the fornix or vaginal discharge, suggesting pelvic inflammatory disease.
- Rectal examination should always be performed for patients with lower abdominal pain.

INVESTIGATING CHRONIC ABDOMINAL PAIN

Full blood count

Anaemia may be due to blood loss, and a microcytic picture is usually present. In malignant disease, a normocytic anaemia may also occur. Raised white cell count is indicative of underlying infection. Platelets can be raised in chronic inflammatory disease.

Biochemistry

Often a range of biochemistry tests is undertaken as a routine, but correct interpretation is essential. The following may be helpful:
- Electrolytes can be disturbed if diarrhoea or vomiting have occurred.
- Calcium is raised in malignant disease, but hypercalcaemia for other reasons, e.g. hyperparathyroidism, may also cause chronic abdominal pain.
- Amylase can be raised slightly and non-specifically with many causes of abdominal pain. It is usually normal in chronic pancreatitis, in contradistinction to acute pancreatitis
- Liver enzyme abnormalities are common with cholangitis or gallstone problems.
- Urea may be raised if dehydration is present, or low if the patient has been anorectic or has malabsorption.
- A thyroid function test should be performed because hypothyroidism is an occasional cause of abdominal pain.
- Tumour markers such as CEA or CA19.9 may be useful, but need to be interpreted in context.

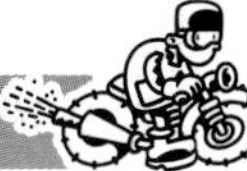

Radiology

Plain abdominal X-ray may reveal:

- Calcification indicative of chronic pancreatitis, gallstones, or aortic aneurysm (Fig. 4.1).
- Faecal loading suggestive of chronic constipation.
- Dilated bowel indicative of subacute obstruction.

Abdominal ultrasound is useful to identify:

- Gallstones causing chronic cholecystitis or bile duct obstruction.
- Liver metastases which usually arise from colon or breast (Fig. 4.2).
- Chronic pancreatitis or carcinoma of the body of pancreas.

Barium enemas may be used:

- Small bowel barium enema can be used to identify stricture in the terminal ileum due to Crohn's disease.
- Large bowel barium enema is used to confirm diverticular disease or exclude colonic carcinoma.

Computed tomography of the abdomen may be required to visualize chronic pancreatitis or pancreatic carcinoma and to search for lymphoma.

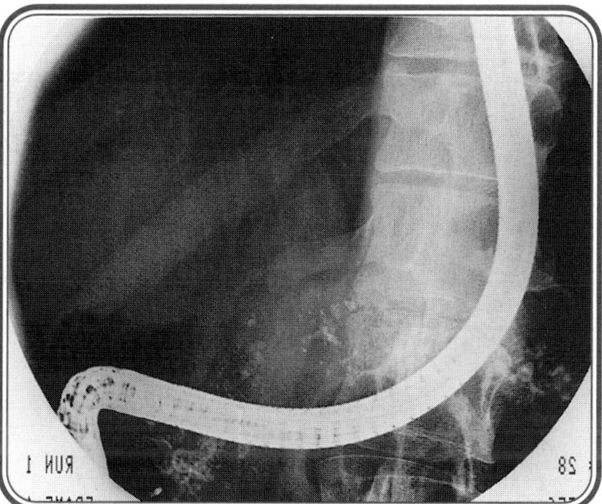

Fig. 4.1 Abdominal calcification is seen across the pancreatic area in a pre-injection endoscopic retrograde cholangiopancreatogram.

Endoscopy

Gastroscopy is useful to find causes of dyspepsia and to exclude gastric carcinoma. Colonoscopy may be required to confirm diverticular disease or to exclude colonic carcinoma.

Surgery

Despite extensive (and sometimes expensive!) investigation, no cause for chronic abdominal pain may be found. In this situation, after careful consideration, a diagnostic laparoscopy can be useful, e.g. to identify endometriosis

Summary

An algorithm summarizing the investigation of chronic abdominal pain is shown in Fig. 4.3.

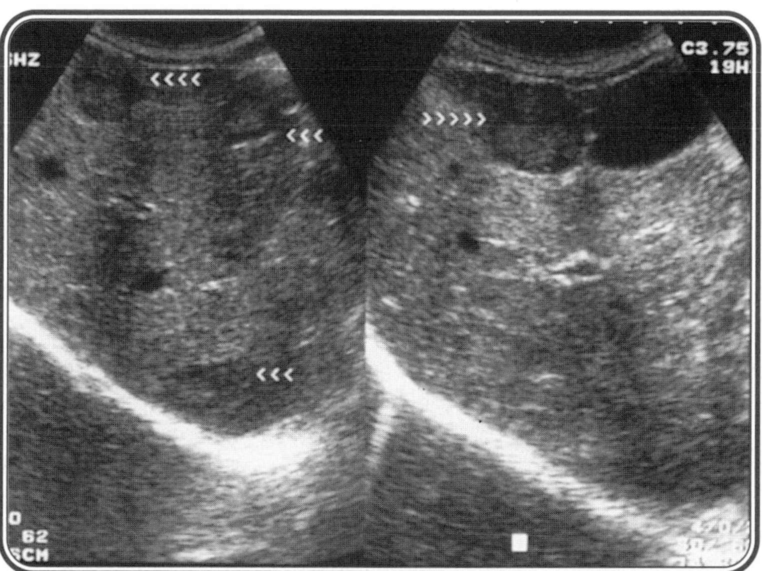

Fig. 4.2 Ultrasound scan showing multiple areas of different echogenicity and size in the liver suggestive of metastases.

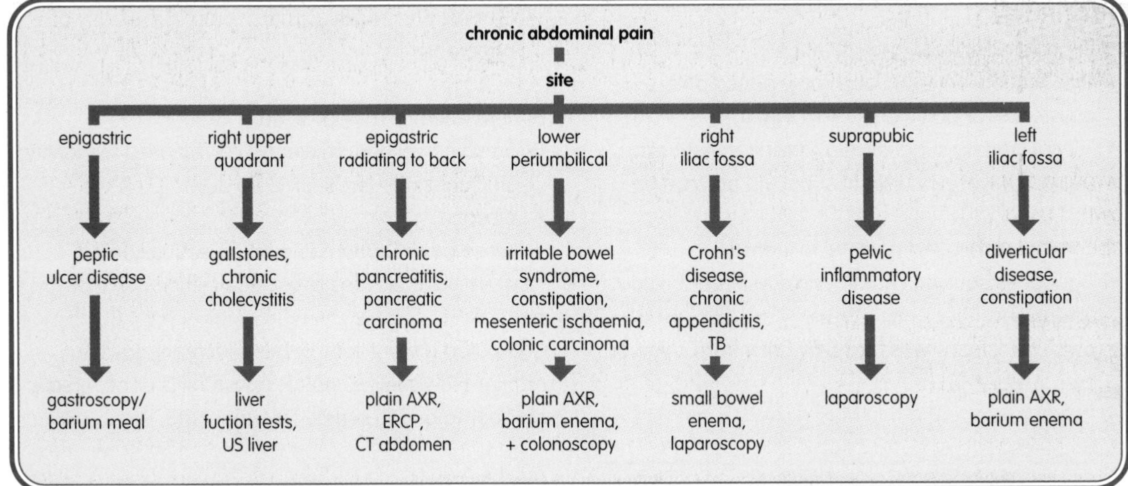

Fig. 4.3 Algorithm for the investigation of chronic abdominal pain. (AXR, abdominal X-ray; CT, computed tomography; ERCP, endoscopic retrograde cholangiopancreatogram; US, ultrasound.)

5. Abdominal Distension

Swelling of the abdomen only rarely presents on its own: it usually accompanies other symptoms such as abdominal pain or diarrhoea.

HISTORY OF THE PATIENT WITH ABDOMINAL DISTENSION

Patients may complain that their abdomen is abnormally distended. They may have noticed that their clothes are fitting too tightly. Others may have commented that they have put on weight or look pregnant.

Occasionally, patients do not realize they have abdominal distension until you or someone else finds it on examination. Several specific features in the history can give important clues to the aetiology or pathogenesis.

Traditionally, all medical students are taught abdominal distension is caused by Fat, Faeces, Flatus, Fluid, or Fetus (the 5 F's) and, although this is not strictly accurate, it is worth remembering, especially when one comes across a difficult examiner!

Onset of symptoms

The onset may give a clue about its cause:

- Distension caused by ascites often takes several days or weeks to develop and gradually worsens with time.
- Acute abdominal distension accompanied by pain suggests the diagnosis of Budd–Chiari syndrome, i.e. hepatic vein thrombosis.
- Distension due to acute bowel obstruction may only have a relatively short period of onset, i.e. 12–24 hours, and will have associated features such as vomiting and abdominal pain.
- Menstrual history is important in women of child-bearing age: unexpected pregnancies occur and have occasionally gone unnoticed or been denied, even up to full term.
- Intermittent distension is suggestive of subacute obstruction or, more commonly, irritable bowel syndrome, in which patients obtain relief from opening their bowels.

Bowel habit

Abdominal distension due to gastrointestinal disease will usually be associated with disturbed GI function.

A long history of constipation may suggest that the distension is due to faeces. In severe cases, subacute or acute obstruction occurs and the distension is further aggravated by flatus. Abdominal pain and vomiting may also be a prominent feature.

Alternating diarrhoea and constipation associated with intermittent distension and borborygmi are highly suggestive of irritable bowel syndrome.

Past history

As always, the patient's past medical history can give helpful clues:

- A history of liver disease may suggest ascites.
- Pericardial disease due to rheumatic fever in the past, or even tuberculosis, can produce constrictive pericarditis, and is often forgotten as a cause of ascites.
- Cardiac failure can also cause ascites.
- Nephrotic syndrome can result in hypoproteinaemic ascites.

A family history may be important, e.g. polycystic kidney or polycystic liver disease, which can produce distension if cysts are large. The condition is autosomal dominant.

EXAMINING THE PATIENT WITH ABDOMINAL DISTENSION

On general examination, several features can be helpful:

- Presence of jaundice, parotitis, or encephalopathy suggests the possibility of liver-related ascites.

- The patient may not be able to lie down flat for the examination due to congestive cardiac failure.
- Truncal obesity together with abdominal striae may alert one to the diagnosis of Cushing's disease.
- Paradoxical jugular venous pulsation in the neck may suggest constrictive pericarditis, and the heart sounds may be diminished.

On examination of the abdomen:

- Look for any asymmetry present—is the lower abdomen more distended? This may be the case in pregnancy; ovarian tumour or fibroids protruding from the pelvic cavity (Fig. 5.1).
- Look for scars that may be present—has the patient had previous surgery for malignancy or obstruction?
- Faecal loading is often palpable over the descending colon and can be indented, unlike a malignant mass.
- Hepatosplenomegaly may be evident if underlying cirrhosis or right ventricular failure is present.
- A rectal examination is mandatory for masses arising from the pelvis.
- Supplemental vaginal examination may be required if an ovarian or uterine origin is suspected.

Percussion of the abdomen is most helpful in differentiating flatulent distension:

- A tympanitic note is produced by flatulence.
- A dull note is produced by a solid mass.
- If the dull note can be made to move by rolling the patient to one side, a moveable fluid collection such as ascites is likely, i.e. shifting dullness.

Auscultation can be useful in complete obstruction, when bowel sounds may be hyperactive or absent.

INVESTIGATING ABDOMINAL DISTENSION

The investigation largely depends on the clinical scenario, but radiology is the most important means of sorting out causes of abdominal distension.

Radiology

Different imaging modalities may be used for diagnosis:

- Chest X-ray is useful to demonstrate an enlarged

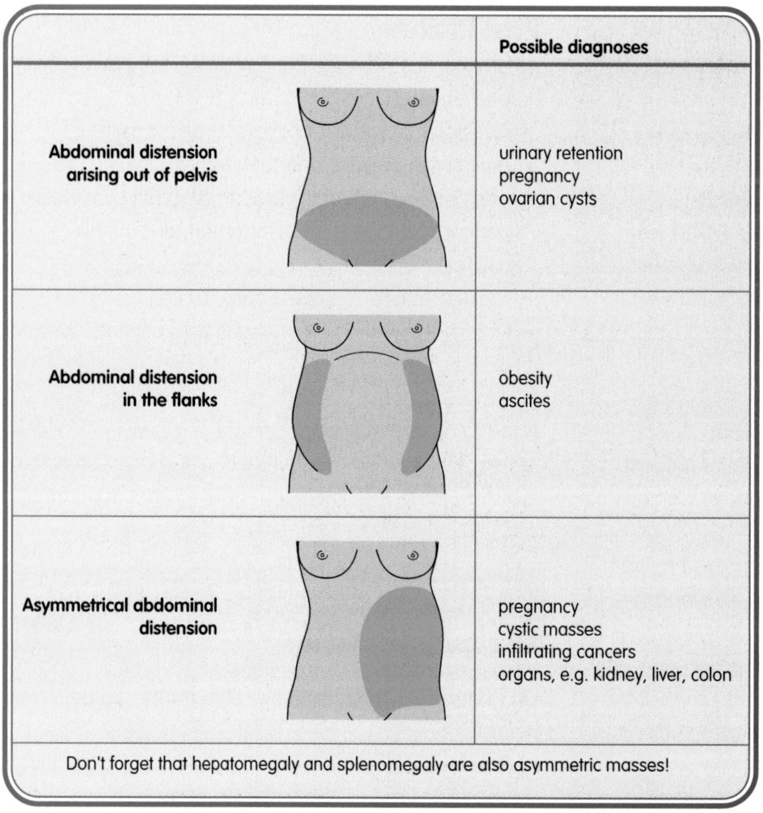

	Possible diagnoses
Abdominal distension arising out of pelvis	urinary retention pregnancy ovarian cysts
Abdominal distension in the flanks	obesity ascites
Asymmetrical abdominal distension	pregnancy cystic masses infiltrating cancers organs, e.g. kidney, liver, colon

Don't forget that hepatomegaly and splenomegaly are also asymmetric masses!

Fig. 5.1 Illustration of patterns of abdominal distension.

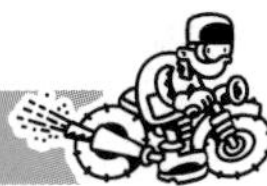

heart or signs of cardiac failure. The heart size may be normal in constrictive pericarditis.

- Plain abdominal X-ray is indicated if the patient is suspected clinically of having bowel obstruction, when fluid levels in the bowel will be obvious. Occasionally, a calcified mass may be seen in the pelvis due to fibroids or dermoid cysts of the ovaries. Faecal loading may also be shown in the colon.
- Abdominal ultrasound is the diagnostic modality of choice to identify ascites. It is also helpful to differentiate pelvic from intra-abdominal masses.
- A computed tomography or magnetic resonance imaging scan of the abdomen may be indicated for some patients when ultrasound is equivocal (Fig. 5.2) or for a diagnosis of underlying malignancy.

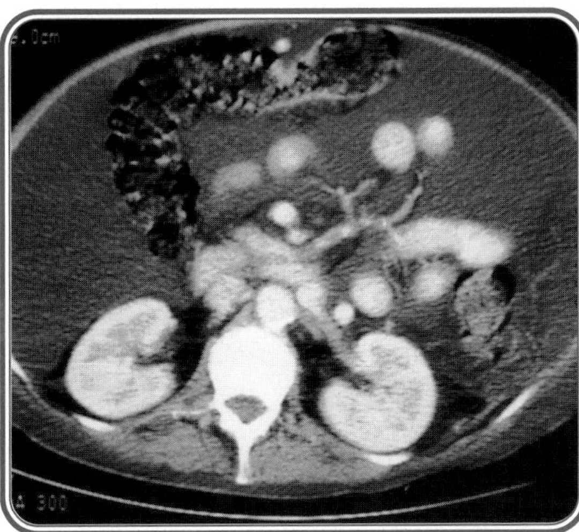

Fig. 5.2 Distension caused by ascites (ground glass appearance). Small bowel is floating in the fluid.

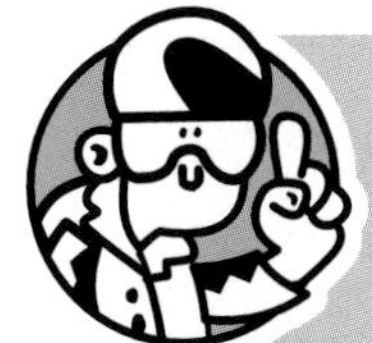

A pregnancy test is essential if the cause of abdominal distension is not obvious for other reasons in women of child-bearing age. This is achieved by measuring the level of human chorionic gonadotrophin in the urine. Protein in the urine should alert one to the possibility of nephrotic syndrome.

Cardiac investigation

Further tests may be necessary if cardiac failure or constrictive pericarditis is considered likely. Electrocardiogram (ECG) may show:

- Elevated ST segment.
- T wave changes.
- Low voltage (if a pericardial effusion is present).

Echocardiography is useful to demonstrate:

- Valvular stenosis or regurgitation.
- Pericardial effusion.
- Pericardial thickening.
- Poor ventricular myocardial function.

Summary

An algorithm summarizing the investigation of abdominal distension is shown in Fig. 5.3.

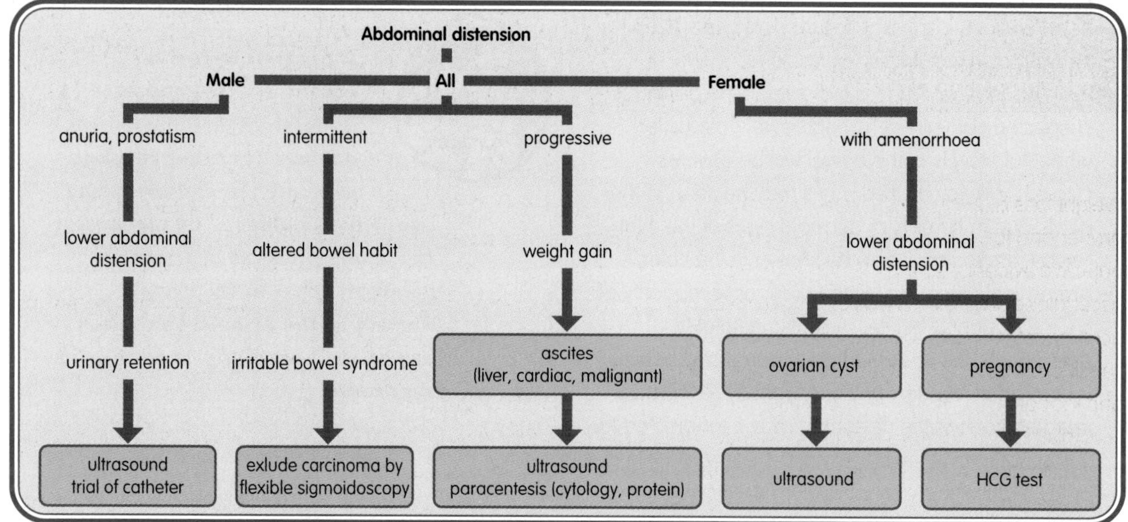

Fig. 5.3 Algorithm for the investigation of abdominal distension. (HCG, human chorionic gonadotrophin.)

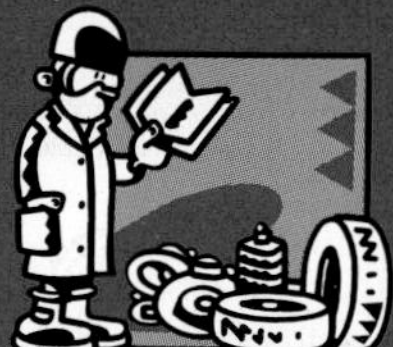

6. Weight Loss and Anorexia

Weight loss is a very subjective symptom, and for a proper and full investigation, it is important to try to obtain objective evidence so that the rate of weight loss can be ascertained. Anorexia is loss of appetite which commonly accompanies weight loss, and it is appropriate to consider these entities together. The causes are myriad and include:

- Malignancy of any variety due to hypermetabolic effects; gastrointestinal malignancy clearly can also cause weight loss by interfering with the digestive process.
- Endocrine causes, e.g. diabetes mellitus, hyperthyroidism, adrenal insufficiency.
- Malabsorption, e.g. coeliac disease, Crohn's disease, bacterial overgrowth, intestinal parasitosis.
- Infection, e.g. underlying abscess, tuberculosis.
- Psychiatric cause, e.g. anorexia nervosa or bulimia, depression.
- Neurological cause, e.g. bulbar palsy, myasthenia causing difficulty in swallowing.

Documentation of weight over a period of time is often extremely useful, e.g. clinic notes, GP records. For reasons of posterity, it is important to document weight at every opportunity when you clerk a patient.

HISTORY OF THE PATIENT WITH WEIGHT LOSS

A careful history is required in order to assess weight loss objectively. Important aspects to enquire about include:

- How much weight loss and over how long? Weight loss of 10 kg over 2 months is much more significant than over 1 year.
- Do their clothes fit them more loosely? How much tighter do belts have to be?
- Do they have any recent photographs to compare weight over a period of time?
- Has there been excessive thirst (polydipsia) or excessive passage of urine (polyuria) suggestive of diabetes mellitus?

Anorexia

It is very important to assess appetite when considering weight loss. The following should be considered:

- Are there any features of psychiatric illness such as distorted body image, early wakening, depression, behavioural changes?
- Is appetite out of step with weight loss? Hyperthyroidism causes increased appetite with weight loss. Brain tumours occasionally present with 'omniphagia'.

Associated features

These may give a clue to underlying disease, especially those resulting in malabsorption. Look for any gastrointestinal symptoms such as:

- Diarrhoea (malabsorption, hyperthyroidism).
- Vomiting.
- Change in bowel habit (possible malignancy).
- Increased activity due to change of lifestyle.

Has there been fever or heat intolerance, suggesting underlying infection or malignancy?

Past medical history

A history of previous gastrointestinal surgery, particularly partial gastrectomy or small bowel resection, is important, because this may interfere with normal digestion. Patients who have had a stroke or neuromuscular problem such as myasthenia may find eating difficult.

EXAMINING THE PATIENT WITH WEIGHT LOSS

There may be obvious cachexia or weight loss when looking at the patient. Look out for additional signs such as:

- Pallor indicative of anaemia, which may accompany

malabsorption or malignancy.

- Lymphadenopathy, suggestive of malignancy or lymphoma.
- Tremor with exophthalmos and a goitre, suggestive of thyrotoxicosis.
- Pigmentation of the skin and buccal membrane with postural hypotension, suggesting adrenal insufficiency.
- Hepatomegaly, ascites, or jaundice, suggesting possible malignancy or liver abscess.
- Lack of eye contact, withdrawn demeanour, or unkempt appearance, suggestive of depression or self-neglect.

Abdominal and particularly rectal examination must not be omitted when considering weight loss.

In a young female who is very thin, the following features ought to arouse suspicion of anorexia nervosa or bulimia:

- A history of excessive dieting or of binge eating.
- Delayed sexual maturation or amenorrhoea.
- Tooth erosion (due to acidic vomiting).
- Wearing loose clothes to disguise a perceived distorted body image.
- Lanugo hair on the arms and trunk.
- Callosities on dorsum of fingers from repeated self-induction of gag-reflex vomiting.

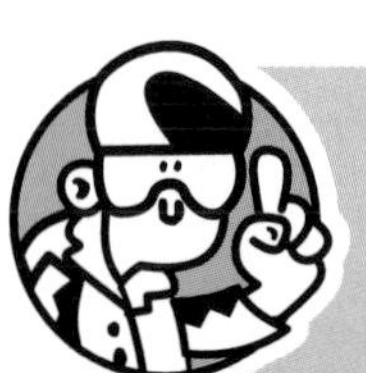

Although amenorrhoea is characteristic of anorexia nervosa, it will occur with any condition causing profound weight loss. It should also be differentiated from primary amenorrhoea or pituitary failure.

INVESTIGATING WEIGHT LOSS

Wide-ranging investigation may be necessary to find the cause of weight loss. Here, investigations are confined to weight loss of GI causes and that which may present to a gastroenterologist.

Blood tests

The following blood tests may aid diagnosis:

- A full blood count is important to look for anaemia. A pancytopaenia may be indicative of marrow failure or malabsorption of vitamin B_{12}.
- Erythrocyte sedimentation rate is a useful test in this context because it is almost always raised if significant malignant or infectious pathology is present. C-reactive protein is a better marker of inflammatory disease.
- A coagulopathy and low blood urea is indicative of profound malabsorption or malnutrition.
- Measurement of blood sugar is essential to exclude diabetes mellitus.
- Hyperkalaemia with hyponatraemia should arouse suspicion of adrenal insufficiency. A Synacthen test may be indicated.
- Raised liver enzymes in the absence of discernible liver problems should arouse suspicion of malignant disease.
- Thyroid function tests are essential to exclude hyperthyroidism.
- Gonadal function tests may be useful to differentiate primary and secondary causes of amenorrhoea.
- Tumour markers can be helpful if no cause is found on other investigation, but need to be used with caution.

Radiology

The tests that will be most helpful depend on the clinical context:

- Chest X-ray is important to exclude occult lung tumour, lymphadenopathy (lymphoma), or tuberculosis.
- Ultrasound of the abdomen and pelvis is useful to look for underlying malignancy.
- Barium enema should be undertaken by elderly patients to exclude colonic malignancy. In younger patients, a small bowel enema may be necessary to exclude Crohn's disease.
- Computed tomography of the abdomen is the best modality to look for occult malignancy such as pancreatic tumours and intra-abdominal lymphadenopathy.

Endoscopy

Gastroscopy:

- May be important to exclude occult gastric carcinoma in elderly patients.

- Is a useful investigation in younger patients allowing a small bowel biopsy to be taken to exclude coeliac disease.

Colonoscopy may be necessary to evaluate further any lesion in the colon found on barium enema.

Summary

An algorithm summarizing the investigation of weight loss is shown in Fig. 6.1.

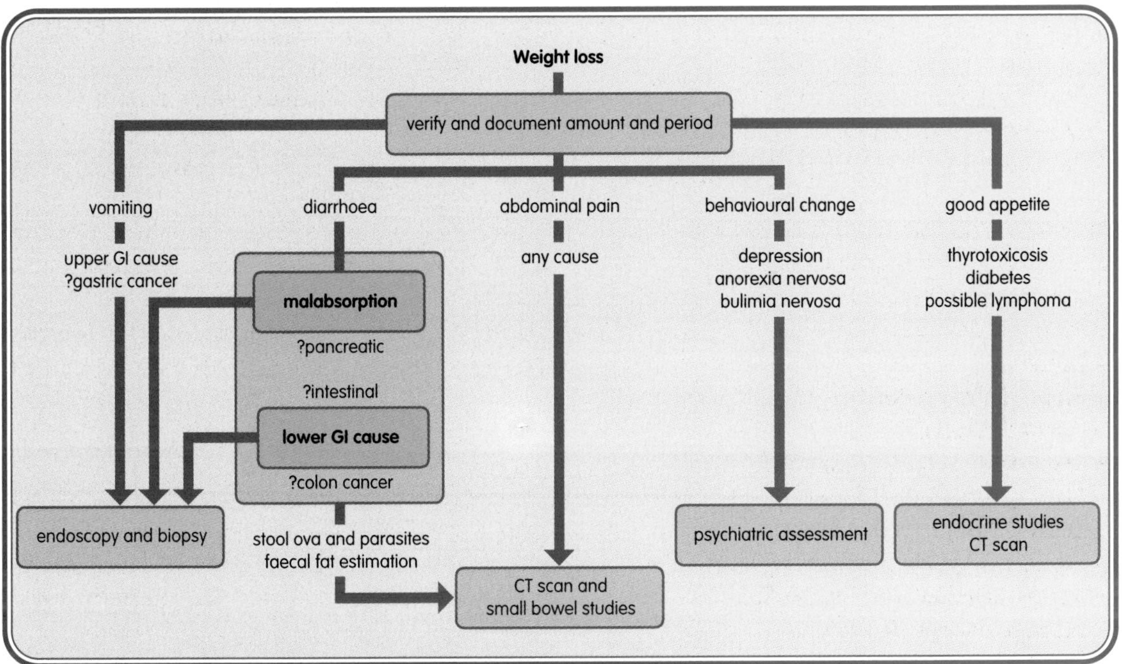

Fig. 6.1 Algorithm for the investigation of weight loss. (CT, computed tomography.)

7. Vomiting

Vomiting is the forceful evacuation of gastric contents. It is most often mediated through a vagal reflex involving chemoreceptor trigger zones in the medulla of the brain. It can be differentiated from regurgitation of oesophageal contents due to obstruction or pouch because of its greater force and volume. It is frequently preceded by nausea or abdominal pain. Vomiting can also occur because of intracranial phenomena or direct toxic effects on the trigger zone by drugs.

The common causes of vomiting include:

- Raised intracranial pressure or inflammation of the brain lining: meningitis or encephalitis.
- Migraine.
- Vestibular disturbances.
- Gastric causes such as gastritis due to for example alcohol, noxious substances, viral infection, bile, non-steroidal anti-inflammatory drugs [NSAIDs].
- Gastrointestinal obstruction due to malignancy or pyloric stenosis.
- Liver disease such as acute hepatitis or hepatic failure.
- Gastroparesis secondary to diabetes.
- Metabolic cause, e.g. adrenal insufficiency, uraemia, hypercalcaemia, porphyria, diabetic ketoacidosis.
- Drug toxicity, e.g. digoxin, cytotoxics, opiates.
- Pregnancy.
- Psychogenic vomiting.

HISTORY AND DIFFERENTIAL DIAGNOSIS OF VOMITING

A detailed history is important to differentiate gastrointestinal (GI) from central nervous systems (CNS) causes. Psychogenic or metabolic causes can be very difficult to discern, but are often more chronic or recurrent than is the case with GI causes. Features to consider are discussed below.

Onset and duration

Onset is an important feature: a short history is more likely to be due to an acute cause similar to those seen in acute abdominal pain, e.g. infection or acute obstruction.

Drugs and alcohol

A drug history is essential: probably the most common cause of nausea and vomiting.

The list of drugs causing nausea or vomiting is very long but particular ones to note are:

- Opiates.
- Cytotoxic drugs.
- Antibiotics.
- Digoxin.

Alcohol excess results in gastritis, and vomiting commonly occurs the morning after excessive alcohol intake.

Infections and toxins

Recent contact with people with similar symptoms should alert you to viral gastritis or food poisoning. Food poisoning is caused by ingestion of bacteria or their toxins in contaminated food. The time course of symptoms in relation to a meal is important:

- Symptoms occuring 1–4 hours after a meal is indicative of toxin such as heat-stable enterotoxin from *Staphylococcus aureus*.
- Symptoms occurring 12–48 hours after a meal are more often due to direct bacterial effects, although with some (e.g. *Shigella*), toxins also play a role. Most will also cause diarrhoea. *Salmonella spp.* is possibly the most common bacterial contaminant causing vomiting.

Past history

In addition to the fact that the patient may have a condition for which he or she is taking medication that could cause vomiting, the following may be relevant:

- Previous gastric surgery may give rise to biliary gastritis causing vomiting.
- Chronic duodenal ulceration can cause pyloric stenosis with gastric outlet obstruction.
- Chronic liver disease progressing to hepatic failure can also cause vomiting.
- Long-standing diabetes can result in gastroparesis and obstruction due to autonomic neuropathy.

Associated features

These can often give a clue to the underlying abnormality:

- Diarrhoea is common with vomiting induced by food poisoning.
- Weight loss may be prominent if underlying malignancy is present.
- Postural hypotension may be apparent if adrenal insufficiency is the cause.
- Headache is usually prominent with any CNS cause.
- Psychological factors, particularly in young females, may have a role in recurrent vomiting without anorexia nervosa.

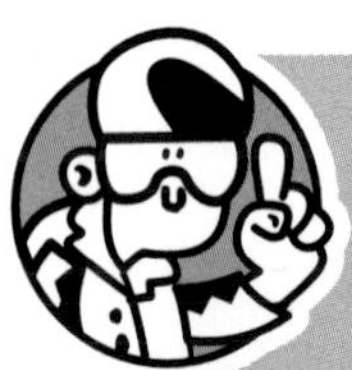

Pregnancy is a very common cause of early morning sickness and vomiting in young women. Don't forget to take a menstrual history, but you cannot always rely on it—if in doubt do a pregnancy test!

EXAMINING THE PATIENT WITH VOMITING PROBLEMS

General examination is important to ascertain whether a systemic condition is responsible for the vomiting. Important points to consider are:

- Photophobia due to meningitis or migraine.
- Neck stiffness or purpuric rash indicative of bacterial meningitis.
- Cachexia may suggest underlying malignancy.
- Pallor or pigmentation indicating anaemia, hypoadrenalism, or renal failure.
- Dehydration may indicate that vomiting has been severe and prolonged.
- Pyrexia or tachycardia possibly indicative of sepsis.

Abdominal examination is important to identify any masses that may cause obstruction.

A succussion splash may be present with gastric outlet obstruction.

INVESTIGATING VOMITING PROBLEMS

Investigation may be necessary both to identify the cause of vomiting and to monitor its metabolic effects.

Blood tests

Consider the following blood tests:

- Full blood count may confirm dehydration if haematocrit is high. Raised white cell count can indicate infection.
- Blood urea is mildly raised in dehydration, but higher levels may be indicative of renal failure or obstructive uropathy which can both cause vomiting.
- Blood glucose is high in diabetic ketoacidosis.
- Hyperkalaemia with hyponatraemia may suggest adrenal insufficiency. Persistent vomiting will also cause hypokalaemia.
- Hypercalcaemia from any cause can produce vomiting due to metabolic alkalosis.
- Liver enzymes may reveal a pattern of acute hepatitis which sometimes presents with vomiting.

Microbiological tests

Blood cultures and cerebrospinal fluid tap may be indicated if the patient is very ill or if meningitis is suspected.

Radiology

Plain abdominal X-ray is useful to exclude obstruction, e.g. due to pyloric stenosis.

A CT scan of the head may be indicated by the clinical picture.

Summary

An algorithm summarizing the investigation of vomiting is shown in Fig. 7.1.

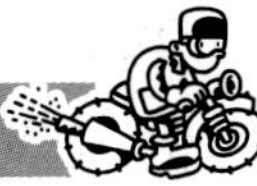

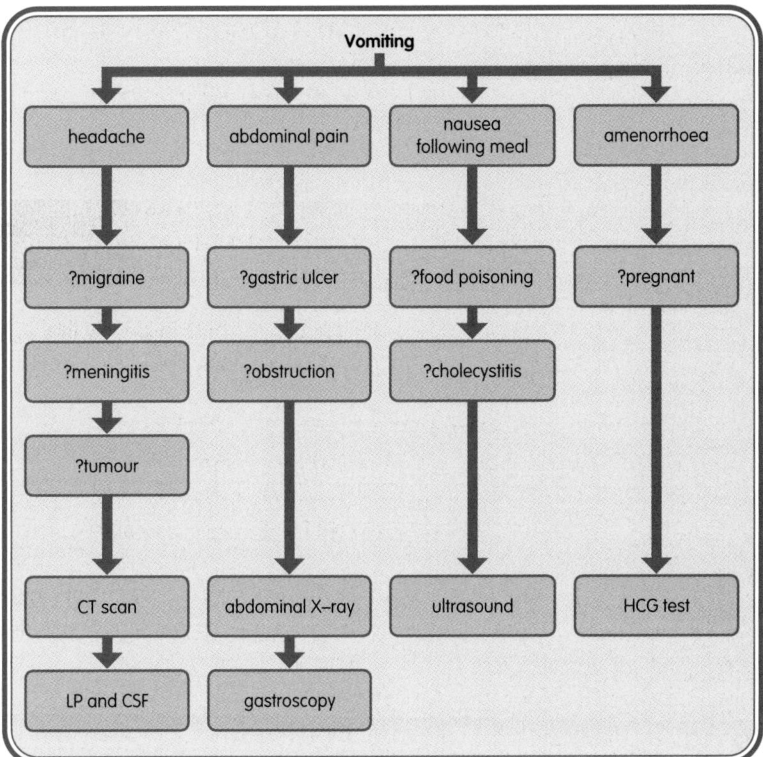

Fig. 7.1 Algorithm for the investigation of vomiting. (LP, lumbar puncture; CSF, cerebrospinal fluid; CT, computed tomography; HCG, human chorionic gonadotrophin or pregnancy test.)

8. Haematemesis and Melaena

Haematemesis refers to the vomiting of blood. Melaena is the passage of black tarry and foul-smelling stools, resulting from the effect of the digestive process on fresh blood. Haematemesis and malaena are usually caused by upper gastrointestinal (GI) bleeding.

Common causes include:

- Reflux oesophagitis.
- Mallory–Weiss tear.
- Oesophageal varices.
- Gastric ulcers or erosions.
- Gastric carcinoma.
- Duodenal ulcer disease.
- Hereditary telangiectasia.

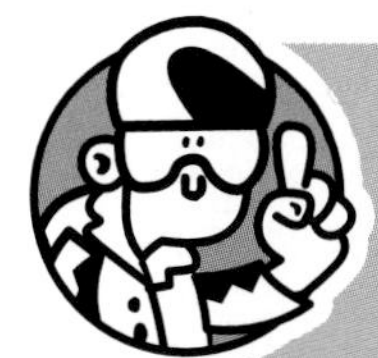

Iron tablets can be confused with melaena, as they produce dark or black stool. However, iron stools have a sticky or grainy consistency unlike the tarry, runny nature of melaena. Melaena also has a characteristic odour!

HISTORY OF THE PATIENT WITH HAEMATEMSIS

The first fact that needs to be established is whether it is a true haematemesis.

- Haemoptysis is coughing of blood and can sometimes be confused with haematemesis.
- Epistaxis (nose bleed), especially if it is severe where the blood is often swallowed, can be difficult to differentiate from true haematemesis.
- Melaena should always follow a true haematemesis, but must not be confused with bleeding from the colon or rectum, which produces dark or bright red blood, respectively.

There are a few clues to help to decide the cause of bleeding. These are discussed below.

Volume of blood loss

Try to estimate this in terms that the patient can understand, i.e. 1/2 cupful, 2 cupfuls etc. Beware that the amount of blood is often overestimated.

- The larger the amount, the more significant the GI bleed and the more likely it is due to oesophageal varices or an arterial bleed from a peptic ulcer.
- A small bleed may manifest itself as altered blood if it has been present in the stomach for some time. The patient may complain of vomiting 'coffee grounds'.

Past medical history

Find out whether the patient suffers from chronic liver disease. This results in portal hypertension. Oesphageal variceal haemorrhage is more likely, although these patients also get peptic ulcers.

Patients themselves or other family members may give a history of recurrent GI bleeds due to hereditary haemorrhagic telangiectasia.

Drug history

Pay particular attention to non-steroidal anti-inflammatory drugs (NSAIDs) that may predispose to reflux oesophagitis, gastritis, and gastric erosions, especially in elderly people, they cause both occult or manifest haemorrhage.

Patients on warfarin for previous cardiovascular accident or atrial fibrillation may have large haemorrhages from very minor gastric erosions.

Associated features

Vigorous vomiting or retching preceding the haematemesis is suggestive of a Mallory–Weiss tear of the mucosa across the gastro-oesophageal junction. This can result in significant haemorrhage, although it is usually self-limiting.

A history of preceding abdominal pain is suggestive of peptic ulcer disease or gastritis.

Heartburn may be due to acid reflux causing reflux oesophagitis.

The priority in managing haematemesis is to make sure you have adequate intravenous access to resuscitate the patient, even before you take a full history. The airway should also be protected.

EXAMINING THE PATIENT WITH HAEMATEMESIS

If the haemorrhage has been severe, it will be necessary to examine and resuscitate the patient while trying to ascertain the cause. Important features to look for are:

- Hypotension—systolic blood pressure <100 mmHg.
- Tachycardic—heart rate >100 bpm.
- Pallor.
- Cold, clammy peripheries.

Features of liver disease suggesting the presence of oesophageal varices may be obvious such as:

- Parotitis.
- Spider naevi.
- Palmar erythema.
- Hepatosplenomegaly.
- Ascites.

Peri-oral telangiectasia may suggest hereditary haemorrhagic telangiectasia.

Rectal examination is important to establish the presence of melaena.

INVESTIGATING HAEMATEMESIS

Endoscopy is the definitive test for all GI bleeding. If haematemesis and melaena are obvious or significant, then urgent endoscopy is indicated to establish the cause and stop the bleeding. However, the patient should always be resuscitated first.

Blood tests

Certain blood tests may give clues to the cause:

- Full blood count can be surprisingly normal due to haemoconcentration, but should be rechecked once the patient is rehydrated.
- Low platelets should alert one to the possibility of hypersplenism, due to portal hypertension, associated with bleeding oesophageal varices.
- Biochemistry may reveal an elevated urea disproportionate to serum creatinine. This is due to the 'high protein meal' provided by blood in the GI tract and is characteristic of upper gastrointestinal bleeding.
- Liver enzymes may be abnormal, but can be normal even in the presence of cirrhosis. In chronic liver disease with oesophageal varices, hepatic synthetic function may be impaired and is reflected in a low serum albumin and a coagulopathy.

Summary

An algorithm summarizing the investigation of upper GI bleeding is shown in Fig 8.1.

haematemesis and/or melaena
establish 'true' nature of symptoms
manage in parallel
drug history
preceding history of pain
vomiting first
liver disease
assess shock
walfarin/NSAIDs
good IV access
peptic ulcers
oesophageal varices
gastric erosions
Mallory–Weiss tear
colloid
group and cross-match
transfuse if anaemic
gastroscopy after resuscitation

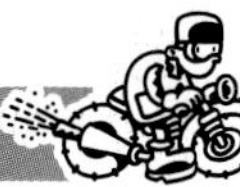

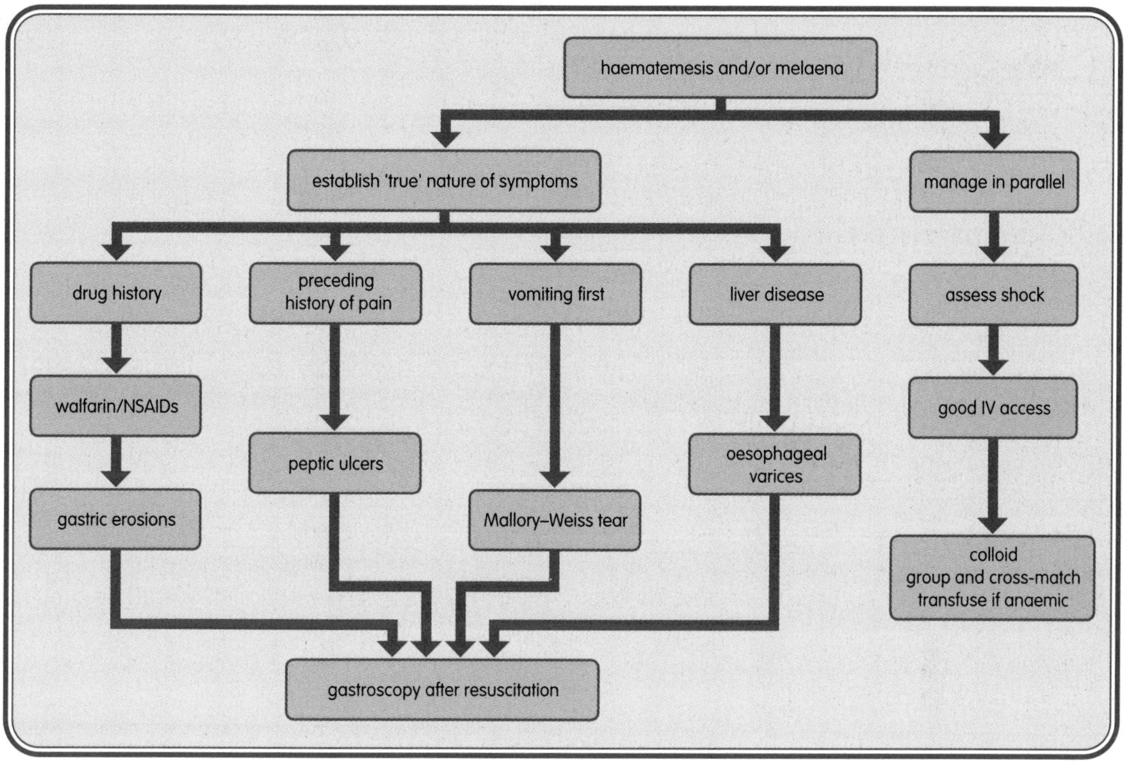

Fig. 8.1 Algorithm for investigation of upper GI bleeding. (NSAIDs, non-steroidal anti-inflammatory drugs.)

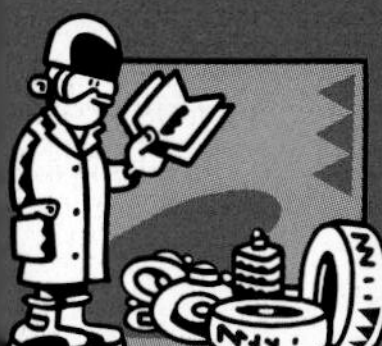

9. Diarrhoea

Diarrhoea is broadly defined as an increased frequency or volume of bowel excretion. A more precise definition is the passage of 300 ml of motion of altered consistency in 24 hours. It is a common condition which affects most people at some point in their lives. Most cases are due to an underlying infective cause, which is usually self-limiting and requires no treatment. However, more prolonged cases need further investigation to exclude a more serious pathology.

The possibilities include:

- Infection, i.e. viral, bacteria, protozoal, or parasitic.
- Malabsorption due to small bowel or pancreatic disease.
- Colonic carcinoma or polyps.
- Endocrine causes such as thyrotoxicosis, adrenal insufficiency, or endocrine tumours of the bowel.
- Neuropathic causes such as vagotomy or diabetic autonomic neuropathy.
- Drug-related, e.g. antibiotics (especially pseudomembranous colitis), purgative abuse.
- Radiation enteritis.
- Postsurgical, e.g. postvagotomy, terminal ileal resection (including bile salt diarrhoea).
- Overflow diarrhoea (secondary to constipation).

HISTORY OF THE PATIENT WITH DIARRHOEA

It is essential to establish whether the patient's meaning of diarrhoea is the same as yours. Often a patient presents to a gastroenterology clinic complaining of 'diarrhoea' when in reality the problem is that the frequency or consistency of stool, although within the normal range, has changed for that patient.

Features to consider are discussed below.

Onset

Acute onset of diarrhoea is usually of an infective cause, and in the majority of cases an underlying precipitating factor can be found, for example:

- Ingestion of suspicious food.
- Foreign travel.
- Contact with another person with similar symptoms.

Diet

Has the patient's diet changed in any way recently:

- Increased ingestion of dairy produce.
- High-fibre cereals.
- Stimulants such as coffee.

It is surprising how often many patients fail to link intake to output!

Drug history

Diarrhoea commonly occurs with certain drugs:

- Colchicine
- Digoxin.
- Purgatives.

Broad-spectrum antibiotics such as erythromycin and penicillins commonly cause diarrhoea due to alteration in gut flora and, in severe cases, pseudomembranous colitis occurs as a result of *Clostridium difficile* overgrowth.

Past medical and surgical history

Find out about:

- Gastric or intestinal surgical resection are relevant because they interfere with motility and absorption.
- Previous radiation treatment for non-gastrointestinal cancer may affect the bowel years later.
- Systemic conditions such as diabetes or collagen-vascular disease may also cause diarrhoea.
- HIV predisposes to atypical infections causing diarrhoea.

Type of diarrhoea and associated features

Bloody diarrhoea with mucus is suggestive of mucosal inflammation, as seen in ulcerative colitis, radiation colitis, and pseudomembranous colitis. Colonic carcinoma can also give rise to blood-stained diarrhoea.

Pale, greasy diarrhoea due to a high fat content (steatorrhoea) is highly indicative of malabsorption, either due to small bowel disease or pancreatic insufficiency.

Ask the patient whether:

- There is a history of coeliac disease in the family.
- He or she has abused alcohol in the past.

There may be associated features that give some clue to the underlying diagnosis, such as:

- Joint pains, mouth ulcers, or uveitis in inflammatory bowel disease.
- Diabetes mellitus with peripheral neuropathy in autonomic bowel neuropathy.
- Scleroderma causing hypomotility with malabsorption.
- Jaundice with steatorrhoea due to pancreatitis or pancreatic carcinoma.

EXAMINING THE PATIENT WITH DIARRHOEA

General features to look for include:

- Dehydration is common in acute onset diarrhoea because gastroenteritis is usually associated with vomiting and hence a substantial fluid loss. Large amounts of fluid can also be lost in severe diarrhoea seen in inflammatory bowel disease and VIPomas (tumours that secrete vasoactive intestinal peptide).
- Pallor due to anaemia may be seen in inflammatory bowel disease and colonic malignancy due to chronic blood loss. Malabsorption will also cause anaemia due to deficiency of iron and vitamin B_{12}/folate.
- Weight loss associated with chronic diarrhoea is a common feature of malabsorption from all causes. Underlying malignancy should also be excluded.
- Associated features of inflammatory bowel disease may be apparent, such as aphthous ulcers, pyoderma gangrenosum, and uveitis.
- Associated features of endocrine disease include skin pigmentation in adrenal insufficiency, proptosis in thyrotoxicosis, and peripheral neuropathy in diabetes.
- Clinical features of alcoholic liver disease or of cystic fibrosis may suggest pancreatic insufficiency.

Check for abdominal scars from previous surgery, suggesting postvagotomy diarrhoea, or terminal ileal resection for Crohn's disease which pre-disposes to bile salt diarrhoea. Previous surgery for intra-abdominal malignancy, e.g. ovarian, may be followed by radiotherapy causing radiation enteritis (skin burns may be present) (Fig. 15.10).

Palpate for abdominal masses or tenderness. Most gastroenteritis will have associated abdominal discomfort. A mass in the right iliac fossa may be present in Crohn's disease as well as caecal carcinoma. Rectal examination must be carried out in all patients presenting with diarrhoea, especially in elderly people, because overflow diarrhoea is a common cause. Faecal impaction or a rectal mass due to rectal carcinoma may be palpated.

INVESTIGATING DIARRHOEA

The extent of investigation is guided by the severity of diarrhoea and by the information found out from the history and examination. As always, interpretation of results is most important.

Haematology

Haematology tests may aid diagnosis:

- Full blood count may indicate microcytic or macrocytic anaemia due to iron and vitamin B_{12} or folate deficiency, respectively.
- Microcytic anaemia with rectal bleeding and mucus associated with the diarrhoea favours a diagnosis of inflammatory bowel disease.
- Steatorrhoea with iron deficiency may suggest coeliac disease.

Biochemistry

Consider the following tests:

- Electroytes may be disrupted if diarrhoea has been severe and prolonged or is caused by adrenal insufficiency.
- Urea is low if malabsorption or malnutrition is present. It is mildly raised in dehydration or in the presence of melaena.
- Iron, ferritin, vitamin B_{12}, and folate levels may help to interpret associated anaemia (for anaemia see Chapter 11).
- Thyroid function tests should be performed for any patients who do not appear to have an obvious cause for the diarrhoea.
- Urinary 5-hydroxy-indole acetic acid (5HIAA) is a metabolite of serotonin, which is elevated in carcinoid syndrome (see p. 129).
- Liver enzyme elevation in serum may be associated with pancreatic insufficiency secondary to chronic alcohol abuse.

Microbiology

Stool culture is necessary to exclude an underlying infective cause. However, most infective causes are viral and self-limiting, hence viral cultures are rarely done. Stool microscopy looking for ova and cysts seen in parasitic infections such as *Giardia*.

Clostridium difficile **toxins can be detected by a specific assay, and should be requested in severe postantibiotic diarrhoea to exclude pseudomembranous colitis.**

Radiology

Plain abdominal X-ray can be done:

- To confirm faecal impaction.
- More commonly, to see whether there is a megacolon associated with inflammatory ulcerative colitis, especially if the patient is clinically unwell.

Calcification of the pancreas is suggestive of pancreatic insufficiency in patients with steatorrhoea secondary to chronic pancreatitis.

Further investigation at this point is usually guided by the clinical presentation and results of the above enquiry. Investigations to consider include:

- Rigid sigmoidoscopy, where inflammation of the mucosa can be directly visualized and biopsies can be taken. Rectosigmoid carcinoma or polyps can also be seen and appropriate biopsies taken. Extensive melanosis coli can sometimes be seen in chronic purgative abuse.
- Small bowel barium study, barium enema, or colonoscopy is indicated for patients with bloody diarrhoea and iron deficiency anaemia to look for inflammatory bowel disease. This investigation will also detect underlying colonic malignancy, but bloody diarrhoea is rare.
- Duodenal biopsy is carried out to exclude coeliac disease, which usually presents with steatorrhoea associated with folate deficiency and anaemia.
- Breath tests using ^{14}C-glycholate or lactulose are used to exclude bacterial overgrowth in patients with steatorrhoea and vitamin B_{12} deficiency.
- Pancreatic function tests, e.g. Lundh meal or para-aminobenzoic acid (PABA) test, can be used to assess malabsorption due to pancreatic insufficiency causing steatorrhoea.

Summary

An algorithm summarizing the investigation of diarrhoea is given in Fig. 9.1.

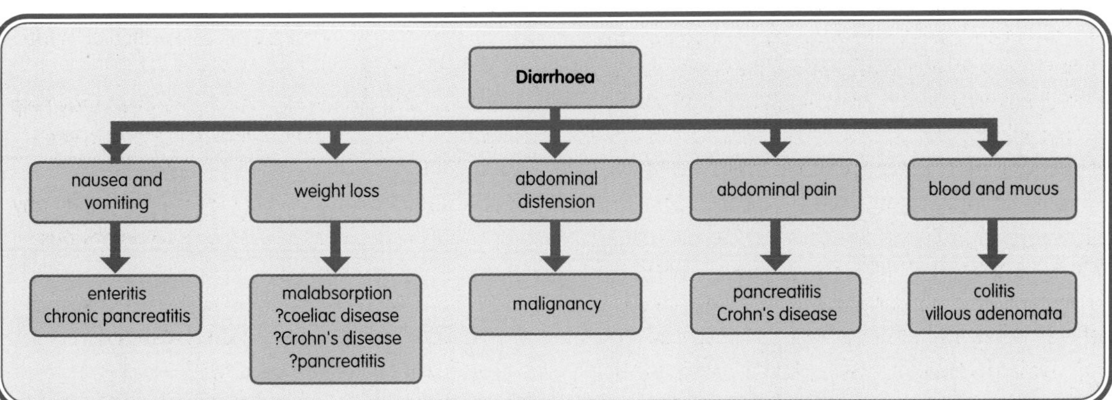

Fig. 9.1 Algorithm for the investigation of diarrhoea.

10. Rectal Bleeding

Rectal bleeding usually refers to bright red bleeding, and is usually due to anorectal pathology. A clear precise history will determine the site and the underlying cause in most cases.

Any rectal bleeding other than bright red blood indicates that the blood has been altered by bacterial or enzymatic digestion higher up in the colon or small bowel. The importance of distinguishing altered blood from just rectal bleeding cannot be overemphasized.

Causes of bright red rectal bleeding include:

- Haemorrhoids.
- Anal fissure.
- Anorectal carcinoma or polyps.
- Angiodysplasia.
- Diverticular disease.
- Inflammatory bowel disease.

HISTORY OF THE PATIENT WITH RECTAL BLEEDING

Establish the relationship between the onset of rectal bleeding and passage of stool, as this will give important clues about the aetiology:

- 'Spotting' of bright red blood appearing on toilet paper only after the passage of stool is highly suggestive of haemorrhoids or anal fissure if there is associated pain on defaecation.
- Presence of blood that is separate from faeces (often noticed as bright red fresh blood in the toilet pan) is associated with low rectal lesions such as haemorrhoids and anorectal carcinoma, where passage of mucus is also common. Pain is not usually a feature, except where anal fissure is also present with the haemorrhoids.
- Passage of dark red blood mixed in with the stool is suggestive of a high rectal lesion such as carcinoma, angiodysplasia, or an inflamed diverticula.

Associated features such as weight loss, diarrhoea, or abdominal pain suggest serious pathology rather than simple anorectal conditions.

EXAMINING THE PATIENT WITH RECTAL BLEEDING

A general examination looking for anaemia and cachexia should be followed by an abdominal examination. Faecal masses may be palpable due to underlying constipation, which predisposes to haemorrhoids and anal fissure. Tenderness with or without guarding and rebound over the left iliac fossa may suggest underlying inflamed diverticula.

- Rectal examination is mandatory in this situation; take particular note of the external area on parting of the anal cleft. Anal tags are suggestive of previous thrombosed haemorrhoids.
- Mucus discharge may be seen in inflammatory bowel disease and anorectal carcinoma.
- Increased anal tone and pain on rectal examination is highly indicative of anal fissure.
- Hard faeces in the rectum may suggest chronic constipation or anal fissure.
- Masses due to rectal carcinoma or polyp can also be palpated on rectal examination.

Proctoscopy enables examination of the position of haemorrhoids, which may be treated with sclerotherapy. Anal fissures can also be seen, although it is unlikely that the patient with this painful condition will tolerate the passage of a proctoscope.

Rigid sigmoidoscopy can visualize up to 15–20 cm from the anal margin, and biopsies can be taken of any suspicious lesion to exclude carcinoma.

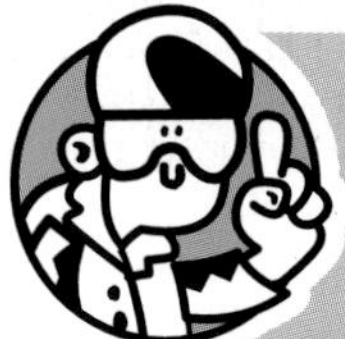

Blood loss from haemorrhoids is usually not severe enough to cause anaemia. Rectal bleeding with anaemia is more likely to be due to carcinoma or angiodysplasia.

INVESTIGATING RECTAL BLEEDING

The majority of conditions can be diagnosed on history and examination with proctoscopy and sigmoidoscopy. However, further investigation may be required if the diagnosis is equivocal:

- Full blood count to establish whether anaemia is present is essential.
- Colonoscopy or flexible sigmoidscopy allow higher sigmoid lesions, and many vascular lesions such as angiodysplasia to be seen. More than two-thirds of all colonic polyps and tumours occur within 60 cm of the anal margin.
- Angiography is only performed if there is a high index of suspicion and the patient is actively bleeding at the time to locate the lesion of angiodysplasia.

Summary

An algorithm summarizing the investigation of rectal bleeding is shown in Fig. 10.1.

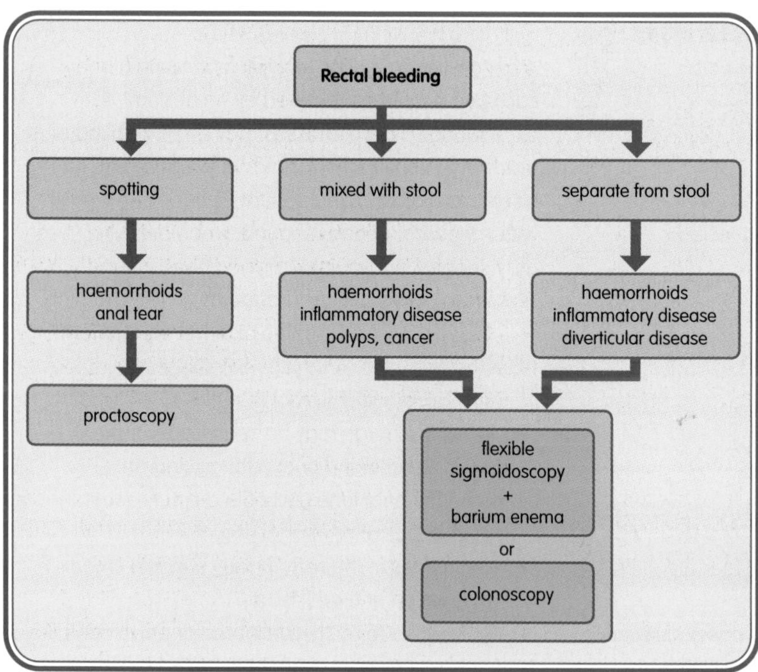

Fig. 10.1 Investigation of rectal bleeding.

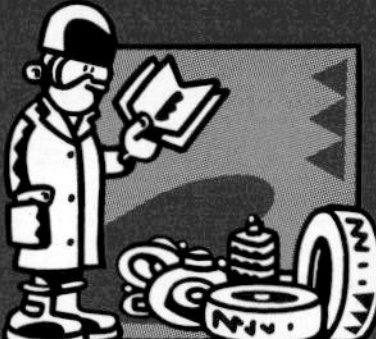

11. Anaemia

Anaemia is a reduction of the haemoglobin concentration in plasma. It is commonly caused by reduced numbers of red blood cells or of their iron content. The symptoms of anaemia are caused by the reduced oxygen-carrying capacity of blood and therefore the reduced delivery of oxygen to tissues. Gastrointestinal causes of anaemia include:

- Reduced intake, e.g. dietary deficiencies of iron, folate, and vitamin B_{12}.
- Reduced absorption, e.g. pernicious anaemia, small bowel disease such as Crohn's, coeliac disease, or bacterial overgrowth, achlorhydria following gastrectomy.
- GI blood loss, e.g. from peptic ulcer disease, oesophagitis, occult carcinoma, or angiodysplasia.

HISTORY OF THE PATIENT WITH ANAEMIA

Depending on the severity of anaemia and coincidence of other pathology, the patient can present with symptoms of anaemia such as:

- Fatigue.
- Palpitation.
- Shortness of breath.
- Angina pectoris.

Often, anaemia is an incidental finding on a routine blood test when the patient presents with unrelated symptoms.

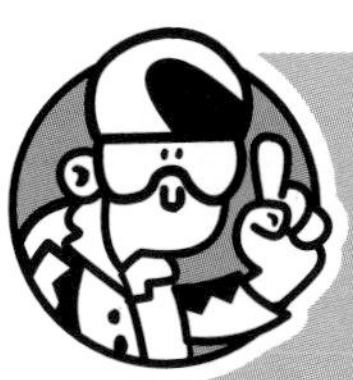

Symptoms of anaemia such as fatigue are thought to require a reduction in haemoglobin concentration of about 25%. For practical purposes this means that symptoms are uncommon unless haemoglobin is <8 g/dl (females) or <10 g/dl (males).

The following aspects of history should be considered in detail.

Diet

Check whether the patient has a well-balanced diet:

- Meat contains haem iron, which is more readily bioavailable than non-haem iron.
- Strict vegans are particularly at risk of iron deficiency.
- Fresh vegetables and fruit are important sources of the reductants necessary to make iron bioavailable.

Past medical and surgical history

Clearly important is previous surgery such as:

- Partial gastrectomy resulting in achlorhydria and thus preventing reduction of iron.
- Terminal ileal resection, resulting in vitamin B_{12} malabsorption.

Previous medical history is important for similar reasons:

- Long-term antisecretory medication could theoretically precipitate anaemia if iron stores were already low.
- Crohn's disease could affect terminal ileal absorption.
- Use of non-steroidal anti-inflammatory agents is associated with chronic occult blood loss.

Associated features

Consider the following associated features:

- Diarrhoea with anaemia is a common manifestation of malabsorption. Chronic diarrhoea due to giardiasis or hookworm infestation is a common cause of anaemia worldwide. Coeliac disease is possibly the most common cause of malabsorption presenting with anaemia in the Western world.
- Abdominal pain or dyspepsia may be present, suggesting acid reflux or peptic ulcer disease causing chronic gastrointestinal blood loss, although these are not common causes of anaemia. Pain may also be present if a luminal tumour is the cause.
- Haematemesis is not usually ignored by patients but melaena occasionally is. This may be caused by gastric ulcer or erosion, angiodysplasia of the stomach, or a right-sided colonic tumour.

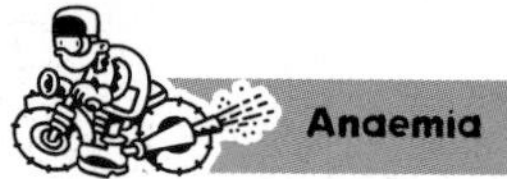

EXAMINING THE PATIENT WITH ANAEMIA

Look for features of anaemia such as:

- Pallor.
- Koilonychia.
- Atrophic glossitis.
- Tachycardia.

Check whether there are any abdominal scars from surgery (see Fig. 15.10). The patient may have forgotten about operations, so consider particularly:

- Midline scar of gastric surgery.
- Right lower abdominal or midline scar from a ileal resection.

Is there any abdominal tenderness and does its position suggest underlying peptic ulcer disease or a caecal carcinoma (see Fig. 14.1)?

Are there features of chronic liver disease such as spider naevi, parotitis, gynaecomastia which may alert you to underlying oesophageal varices or portal hypertensive gastropathy?

A rectal examination is mandatory in any patient presenting with iron deficiency anaemia to exclude anorectal carcinoma.

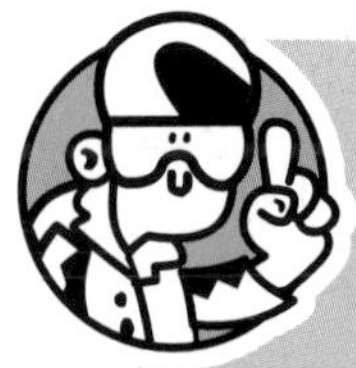

Pale conjunctivae correlate very poorly with haemoglobin concentration and cannot be relied on as a sign.

INVESTIGATING ANAEMIA

The most important key to exploring anaemia is the full blood count. The extent or severity of the anaemia may be determined by haemoglobin and haematocrit. Important clues to the aetiology are often given by the red blood cell size and haemoglobin content. Thus:

- Microcytic hypochromic picture is due to iron deficiency. This can result from dietary deficiency, failure of absorption, or blood loss.
- Normocytic normochromic picture is commonly associated with chronic inflammatory disease, in which iron stores are adequate but not available for use.
- Macrocytic picture, which can be due to folate or vitamin B_{12} deficiency, alcohol, or certain drugs.

Further studies therefore depend on the full blood count.

As full blood counts are automated, macrocytosis can be spurious if there are increased numbers of larger cells, such as reticulocytes, or very large numbers of white cells (as found in certain leukaemias) present. If in doubt, ask for a reticulocyte count or a blood film examination.

Biochemistry

Biochemistry tests may aid diagnosis:

- Serum iron is used to confirm iron deficiency.
- Serum ferritin is low in iron deficiency but is often high in the presence of anaemia due to chronic inflammatory disease.
- Serum folate should be measured in any patient with macrocytosis. Deficiency is usually due to malabsorption (most commonly coeliac disease), poor dietary intake, excessive use as in pregnancy, or increased cell turnover in malignancy. Antifolate drugs such as methotrexate and anticonvulsants also cause folate deficiency.
- Vitamin B_{12} must also be measured in patients with macrocytosis. If deficient, a Schilling test (see Chapter 17) may be helpful in deciding the cause.
- Urea in blood is a useful, although not completely reliable, indicator of nutrition—low levels occur in malabsorption.
- Faeces can be tested for occult blood loss.

Endoscopy

Gastroscopy should be undertaken in all cases of iron deficiency anaemia, unless another cause is obvious, to exclude oesophagitis, gastric ulcer or erosions, and carcinoma.

If macrocytic anaemia is due to vitamin B_{12} deficiency because of bacterial overgrowth, serum folate will be elevated. Otherwise, folate is usually also deficient.

The presence of a duodenal ulcer is an insufficient explanation for iron deficiency anaemia. A small bowel biopsy can be taken at the same time, to exclude coeliac disease.

Colonoscopy is the preferred large bowel investigation, as it should identify all lesions resulting in blood loss, including angiodysplasia. When it is not practical, barium examination should be undertaken.

Radiology

A barium meal is indicated if there is suspicion of gastric carcinoma and gastroscopy is not possible. Similarly, a barium enema will demonstrate the presence of diverticular disease, polyps, and carcinoma, but endoscopy is preferable in order to ascribe the cause of bleeding to a particular lesion or to identify angiodysplasia.

Angiography is helpful in the presence of active bleeding, but is not generally rewarding in the investigation of chronic anaemia

Other tests for anaemia

Other tests may be useful:

- A Schilling test may help differentiate the different causes of vitamin B_{12} deficiency (see Chapter 17).
- A ^{14}C-glycocholic acid breath test or a lactulose hydrogen breath test may be used to investigate bacterial overgrowth (see Chapter 17).
- A ^{99}Tc radioisotope scan is helpful if a Meckel's diverticulum is suspected of causing chronic anaemia in a young patient.
- A ^{51}Cr-labelled red cell scan may give a clue to the general location of occult blood loss, but is not helpful to identify the nature of the lesion or the precise anatomical location.

Summary

An algorithm summarizing the investigation of anaemia is given in Fig. 11.1.

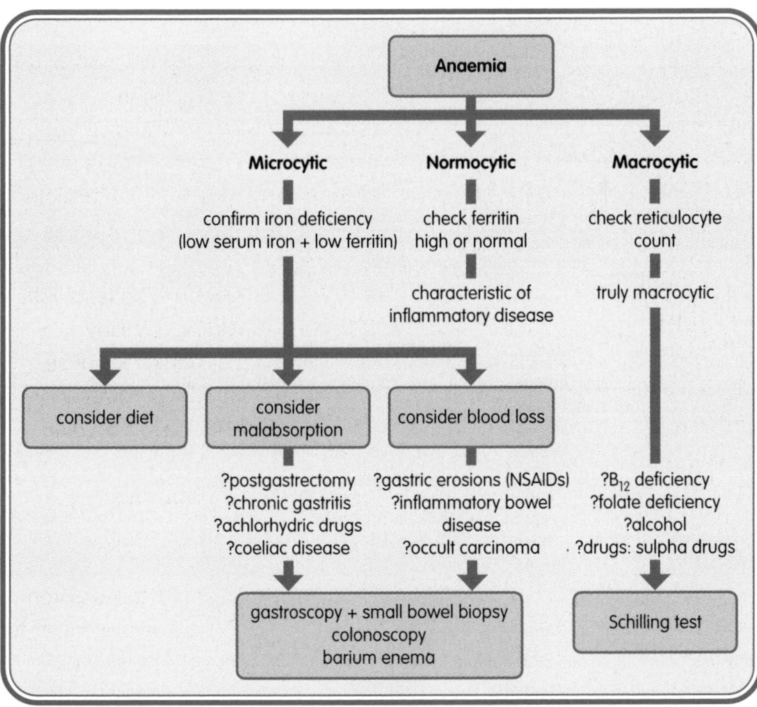

Fig. 11.1 Algorithm for the gastrointestinal investigation of anaemia. (NSAIDs, non-steroidal anti-inflammatory drugs.)

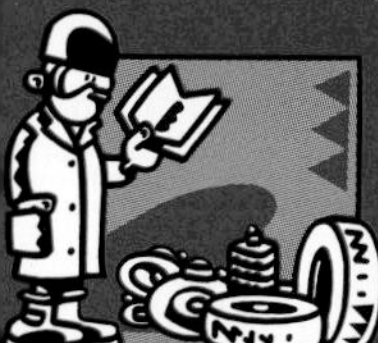

12. Jaundice

Jaundice is a yellow colouring of the skin and sclerae due to elevated levels of bilirubin in plasma. Jaundice is detectable clinically if serum bilirubin exceeds 40 mmol/L (about twice the normal upper limit). There are numerous causes of jaundice, and a careful history and examination is vital so that unnecessary invasive investigations can be avoided.

The more common causes include:

- Haemolytic anaemias such as sickle cell anaemia or thalassaemia.
- Congenital hyperbilirubinaemia due to enzyme defects, most commonly Gilbert's syndrome.
- Extrahepatic bile duct obstruction due to gallstones, pancreatitis, or pancreatic cancer.
- Sclerosing cholangitis.
- Intrahepatic cholestasis due to drugs, alcohol, hepatitis, or chronic liver disease.

HISTORY OF THE PATIENT WITH JAUNDICE

All aspects of the history should be taken with care as there are times when certain facts can appear to be trivial, yet may later become vital in the diagnosis. The following features help to differentiate causes of jaundice

Age

Younger patients are more likely to have congenital hyperbilirubinaemia or viral hepatitis than carcinoma of the pancreas, which is a disease of advancing years.

Onset of symptoms

The onset of symptoms may give clues to the diagnosis:

- An acute onset is more likely to be an infective cause.
- A slow insidious onset is more likely to be due to chronic active hepatitis, e.g. caused by autoimmune disease or alcohol.

Infectious contact and risk behaviour

It is important to establish whether the patient has any risk factors for developing jaundice:

- Find out whether there has been contact with other people with jaundice, such as occurs in epidemics of hepatitis A and E or infectious mononucleosis.
- Has there been high-risk behaviour for contact with hepatitis B (promiscuous sexual activity or shared needles)?
- A history of recent travel abroad is usually sought for the same reasons: ingestion of seafood abroad is a common source of infectious hepatitis. Don't forget exotic causes such as yellow fever from Africa!
- Occupational or recreational history may be relevant: sewage and farm workers are at risk of leptospirosis, as well as windsurfers and people who go pot-holing.
- A history of habitual alcohol intake must be excluded, if necessary by interviewing relatives.

The most common mode for transmission of hepatitis B worldwide is not sexual or intravenous drugs but 'vertical' transmission from mother to baby. This takes place in the birth canal and presents the best opportunity to prevent transmission of hepatitis B virus by immunizing the neonate.

Past medical history

This may immediately suggest a diagnosis. For example:

- Previous cholecystectomy could suggest a bile duct stone or stricture.
- Ulcerative colitis can predispose to sclerosing cholangitis.
- Recent anaesthetic with halothane can precipitate jaundice.
- Patients often forget that they have had antibiotics recently.

Drugs

Many drugs are metabolized in the liver, and some cause idiosyncratic reactions, resulting in jaundice. Others have a dose-related effect, resulting in liver damage and jaundice. Important drugs to consider include:

- Antibiotics such as co-amoxiclav or flucloxacillin.
- Antituberculous drugs such as isoniazid or rifampicin.
- Anti-neuroleptics such as chlorpromazine.
- Paracetamol in excess of therapeutic dose.
- Anabolic steroids—these are occasionally illegally used by bodybuilders and cause jaundice.

Family history

A history of intermittent jaundice in the family suggests congenital hyperbilirubinaemia. Also enquire about Wilson's disease and alpha-1-antitrypsin deficiency.

Associated features

A number of features may suggest underlying pathology, such as:

- Presence of abdominal pain, especially located to right upper quadrant, suggests bile duct stones.
- Acute onset abdominal distension with jaundice may indicate acute hepatitis or hepatic vein thrombosis.
- Absence of pain with weight loss in older patients is suggestive of carcinoma of the pancreas.
- Dypsnoea and peripheral oedema due to cardiac failure may indicate a congested liver with jaundice.

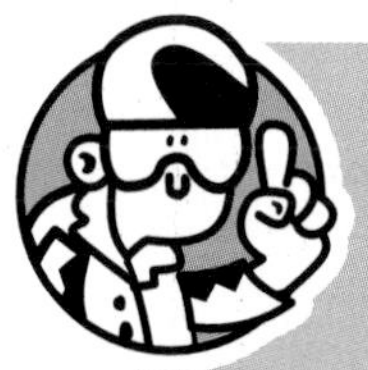

Acholuric jaundice is the term given to jaundice without dark urine and pale stool. The presence of these features indicates that the jaundice is cholestatic in nature. Obstructive jaundice is only one cause of cholestatic jaundice.

EXAMINING THE PATIENT WITH JAUNDICE

Assess the severity of the jaundice clinically:

- Acute jaundice has a bright yellow hue.
- Chronic jaundice has a dusky appearance and if severe, the patient looks green.

Look for anaemia, which may indicate underlying haemolysis.

Generalized lymphadenopathy may be due to EpsteinBarr, cytomegalovirus (CMV), or toxoplasmosis.

Are there features of chronic liver disease or cirrhosis (see Chapter 22) such as:

- Parotitis.
- Spider naevi.
- Gynaecomastia.
- Loss of secondary sexual hair.
- Palmar erythema.
- Hepatomegaly.
- Ascites (may be acute in Budd–Chiari syndrome).

The gall bladder may be palpated in a patient with progressive painless jaundice due to obstruction. In elderly patients, painless jaundice with distension of the gall bladder is commonly due to carcinoma of the head of the pancreas (Courvoisier's law).

Associated systemic signs may suggest particular syndromes with liver involvement:

- Chronic respiratory disease with jaundice may occur with cystic fibrosis or alpha-1-antitrypsin deficiency.
- Neurological signs with jaundice may suggest hepatolenticular degeneration (Wilson's disease).

Kayser–Fleischer rings are present in 70% of patients with Wilson's disease. They are seen as a brown ring around in the periphery of the cornea, most often at the top. Slit lamp examination may be necessary.

INVESTIGATING JAUNDICE

Abdominal ultrasound is the key investigation in a patient with jaundice as it will differentiate obstructive jaundice from other causes, and the subsequent approaches to management are different. If the bile ducts are not dilated, then blood tests become useful to differentiate causes of jaundice:

- Liver biochemistry is helpful to confirm jaundice and to confirm unconjugated hyperbilirubinaemia in cases of congenital or haemolytic jaundice. A high alkaline phosphatase is indicative of cholestasis, whereas high levels of transaminases are suggestive of a hepatitic cause. However, a mixed picture is often the case, hence too much emphasis should not be given to blood results alone.
- Prothrombin time is the most easily available test that gives some indication of hepatic synthetic function because all of the clotting factors are made in the liver. It correlates well with outcome in acute liver failure.

Prothrombin time is influenced by vitamin K, as this is a required co-factor for coagulation factors II, VII, IX, and X. The absorption of vitamin K, a fat-soluble vitamin, is reduced in cholestatic or obstructive bile duct disease in which sufficient bile does not reach the small intestine. In this situation, a single dose of intravenous vitamin K may correct the prothrombin time; it will have no effect if the coagulopathy is due to deficient synthesis of coagulation factors, as in parenchymal liver diseases.

- Albumin, also made in the liver is reduced in any 'sick' state and correlates less well with liver pathology. Similarly, blood urea is usually low but not very informative.
- Serum bilirubin does not necessarily reflect the degree of liver damage particularly in the acute situation. In chronic liver disease, it gives a reasonable indication of the stage of progression.
- Full blood count may reveal anaemia. This may be spuriosly macrocytic if accompanied by a significant reticulocytosis, as in haemolytic disease. Reticulocyte count should be checked. Macrocytosis with low platelets is suggestive of hypersplenism associated with the portal hypertension of chronic liver disease. Increased monocytes may be due to Epstein Barr infection. A blood film may be appropriate to look for signs of haemolysis or sickle cells.
- Serology should be reserved to look for viral markers of acute hepatitis A to E, and for Epstein Barr, cytomegalovirus, and toxoplasmosis. A monospot test can give a rapid diagnosis of infectious mononucleosis. Markers for leptospirosis should also be done if clinically indicated.
- Autoantibodies to nuclear proteins and smooth muscle indicate an acute autoimmune hepatitis. They will usually be accompanied by elevated IgG levels. IgA is commonly elevated in alcoholic hepatitis.
- Elevated urinary copper and low serum caeruloplasmin levels indicate the possibility of Wilson's disease which is fatal if undetected and untreated.
- Percutaneous liver biopsy gives valuable information about the cause of parenchymal liver damage and its extent. It can be performed with or without ultrasound guidance. Special staining for copper and alpha-1-antitrypsin can be done on histological sections.
- A computed tomography scan of the abdomen is mainly used to assess pancreatic masses and nodes at the porta hepatis when obstructive jaundice has been confirmed by ultrasound.
- Endoscopic or percutaneous cholangiography is useful for further assessment and therapy if obstruction is identified.

Summary

An algorithm summarizing the investigation of a patient with jaundice is shown in Fig. 12.1.

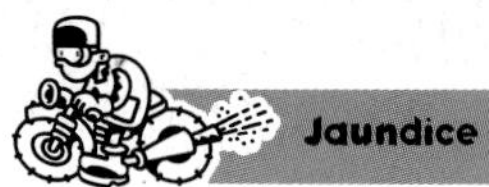

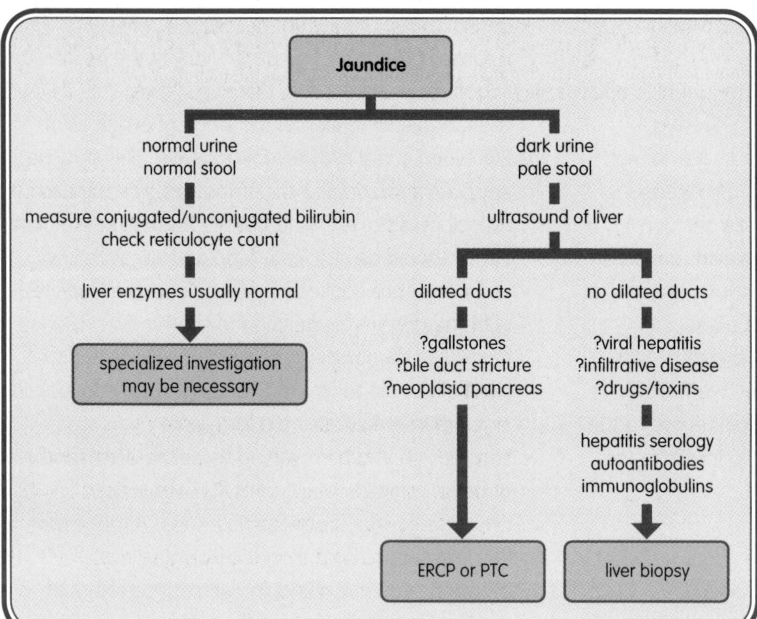

Fig. 12.1 Algorithm for the investigation of a patient with jaundice.

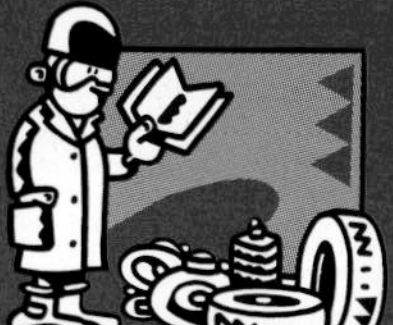

13. Abnormal Liver Biochemistry

Patients are commonly referred to the gastrointestinal clinic for investigation of abnormal liver biochemistry discovered during investigation of other complaints. The four enzymes involved are:

- Alanine aminotransferase (ALT or SGPT in older texts).
- Aspartate aminotransferase (AST or SGOT in older texts).
- Alkaline phosphatase (AlkPhos).
- Gamma-glutamyl transferase (GGT).

Often these tests are referred to as liver 'function' tests. This is misleading because the elevation of liver enzymes does not reflect hepatic function.

Abnormal liver enzymes in the absence of jaundice may be commonly due to:

- Acute or chronic liver disease.
- Cirrhosis.
- Drugs, including alcohol.
- Liver metastasis.
- Cardiac causes such as acute myocardial infarction, cardiac failure, and constrictive pericarditis.
- Bony metastasis or Paget's disease can cause elevation of AlkPhos, as can pregnancy.
- Hypothyroidism or pernicious anaemia occasionally present with abnormal liver enzymes.

HISTORY OF THE PATIENT WITH ABNORMAL LIVER BIOCHEMISTRY

Patients are usually asymptomatic when referred to outpatient clinics, or tests may have been carried out for vague symptoms such as malaise or fatigue. Hence, it is important to interpret these enzymes in order to avoid further unnecessary tests or to direct appropriate investigation. The following points usually help.

Drug history

Prescribed medication is the most common cause of abnormal liver biochemistry in the general population, apart from alcohol:

- Antibiotics such as erythromycin or co-amoxiclav can cause raised transaminases for several weeks after their cessation.
- Many anti-arthritis drugs and anti-epileptic drugs can induce liver enzymes.

Alcohol

Alcohol is often the first thing that comes to mind in relation to liver disease. However, as an aetiological agent, it accounts for less than 20% of patients with liver disease attending outpatients.

There is no specific pattern to liver enzymes with alcohol use:

- GGT is easily induced and the most common liver abnormality to be seen.
- On its own, GGT is of little significance, its most useful role is indicating that a raised AlkPhos is of liver origin.
- An AST to ALT ratio of 2 or more is said to be specific for alcoholic hepatitis, but it is not a sensitive indicator.

Past medical history and surgical history

A history of biliary tract surgery, including cholecystectomy, is particularly relevant. Otherwise, history should concentrate on those aspects discussed in Chapter 12.

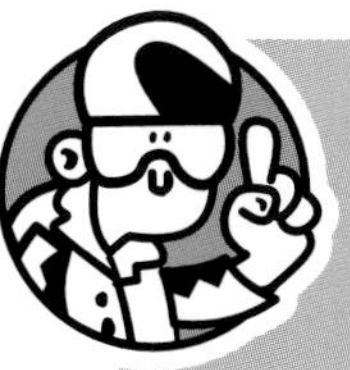

Beware of patients with a past history of malignancy because they may present with either bony or liver metastases resulting in raised AlkPhos.

EXAMINING THE PATIENT WITH ABNORMAL LIVER BIOCHEMISTRY

A general physical examination is clearly important, but in particular, signs of liver disease should be sought as discussed in Chapter 12.

Other medical conditions can also be associated with raised liver enzymes:

- Hypothyroidism.
- Pernicious anaemia.
- Congestive cardiac failure.
- Lymphoma.
- Hypercholesterolaemia or diabetes mellitus.

INVESTIGATING ABNORMAL LIVER BIOCHEMISTRY

The investigation largely depends on the pattern of abnormality produced by the elevated enzymes. The following is only meant as a guide and in clinical practice often it is difficult (sometimes impossible) to decipher the 'picture' of abnormality presented.

Liver chemistry tests

These tests may aid diagnosis:

- The combination of all four liver enzymes being raised makes it more likely that significant liver pathology is present.
- A predominantly hepatitic abnormality is suggested if AST, ALT, and GGT are the most prominently raised enzymes. These may be only slightly elevated in certain conditions such as hepatitis C, haemochromatosis, or alpha-1-antitrypsin deficiency.
- A predominantly cholestatic abnormality is suggested by raised AlkPhos and GGT with or without elevation of serum bilirubin. In this situation, think of intrahepatic or extrahepatic cholestasis. The most common causes in the absence of jaundice are drugs, cholangitis, and primary biliary cirrhosis. Antimitochondrial antibodies may be helpful.

Drug-induced abnormalities do not require further investigation other than cessation of the offending drug (including reducing alcohol intake) and repeating the biochemistry 8–12 weeks later to ensure that it has returned to normal.

Imaging

Ultrasound of liver is essential to exclude bile duct dilatation, liver metastasis, and hepatic congestion.

Biopsy

Liver biopsy may be necessary if no other explanation is found for the abnormal liver biochemistry. It can also be performed to establish the underlying cause of cirrhosis if suspected on ultrasound.

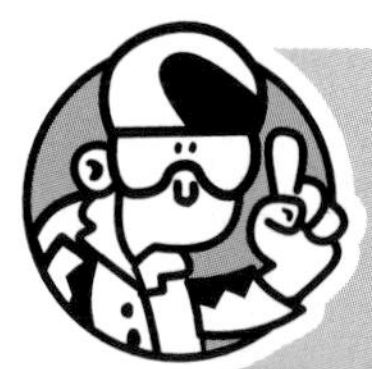

Cirrhosis is a histological diagnosis which cannot be made on ultrasound scanning alone, although there are features such as irregular margins and nodules that may suggest the diagnosis. Metastatic disease is occasionally confused with cirrhosis on ultrasound scans.

Exceptions to consider

Note the following:

- Raised GGT alone is highly suggestive of alcohol consumption or drugs that induce hepatic enzymes such as anticonvulsants, hence, further investigation is usually unnecessary.

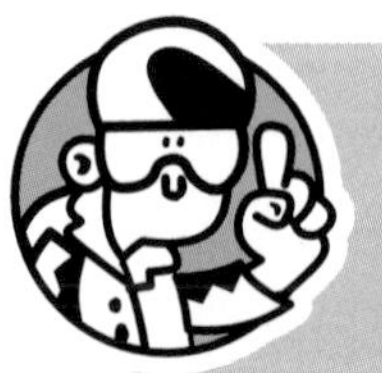

Remember that alkaline phosphatase of bony origin will be elevated with bone growth. Young adults commonly have apparently raised alkaline phosphatase for this reason. Young patients with Gilbert's unconjugated hyperbilirubinaemia may have raised alkaline phosphatase of bony origin, and this is not an indication for extensive liver investigations.

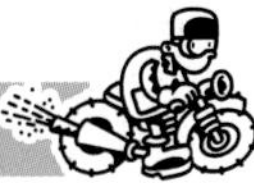

- Raised AlkPhos alone may suggest a non-hepatic origin, such as bone, placenta, or very occasionally intestine. Isoenzymes can be measured if necessary.
- AST is also produced by heart and striated muscle. It can be raised in myocardial infarction, hypothyroidism, and pernicious anaemia, hence its sole elevation should alert one to other medical conditions.
- ALT is much more specific for liver disease. A minor elevation on its own is probably of no consequence, but if raised in association with AlkPhos, it is usually an indication for further investigation including liver biopsy.

Summary

An algorithm summarizing the investigation of a patient referred with abnormal liver enzymes is shown in Fig. 13.1.

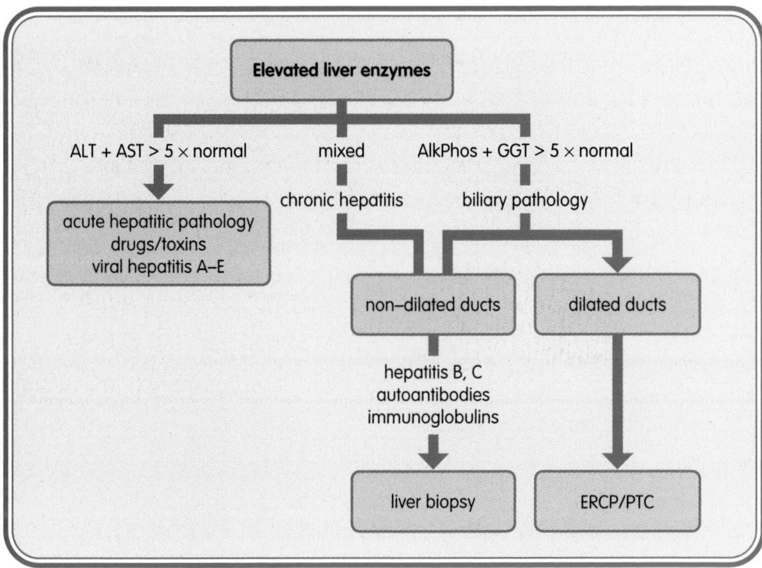

Fig 13.1 Algorithm for the investigation of a patient referred with abnormal liver enzymes. (ERCP, endoscopic retrograde cholangiopancreatogram; PTC, percutaneous transhepatic cholangiogram.)

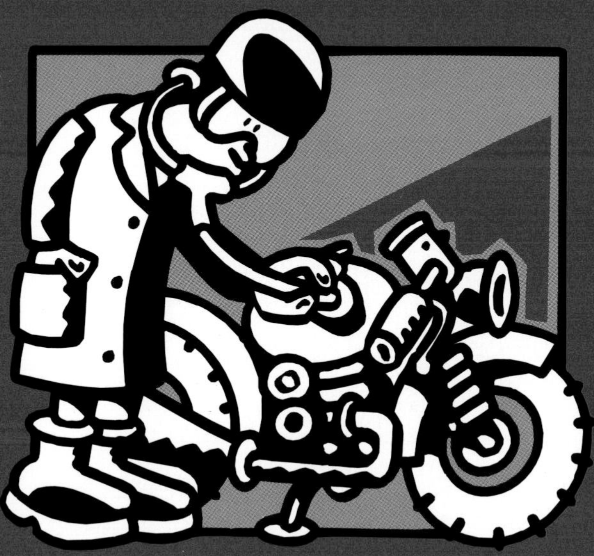

HISTORY, EXAMINATION, AND COMMON INVESTIGATIONS

14. Taking a History

Some of this section is a rewritten version or based on the clinical section of Mosby's Crash Course title Gastrointestinal System, by Elizabeth Cheshire.

Preliminaries

Introduce yourself, be polite, listen carefully, and look interested, even if you have been up all night!

Give patients the time and the opportunity to tell you what you need to know and put them at their ease as many symptoms are embarrassing.

Maintain eye contact (even if patients don't) and watch carefully for clues on how ill they look. Are they agitated or distressed? Are they in pain, can you notice any tremors or involuntary movement? Have they lost a lot of weight (cachexia)? Is there a pale, pigmented, or jaundiced complexion?

Look around the bedside for clues, e.g. inhalers, oxygen, a walking stick or frame, cards from family and friends, sputum pots, reading material and glasses, special food preparations, etc.

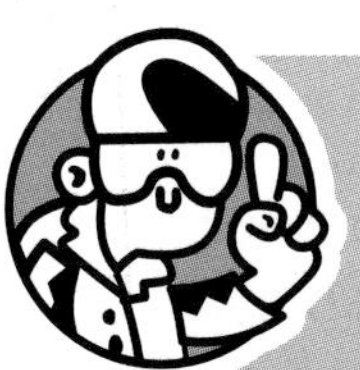

The purpose of taking a history is to arrive at a differential diagnosis. Some information is background and may not be immediately obvious or useful, but can often be vital later on.

THE STANDARD STRUCTURE OF A HISTORY

You are less likely to leave things out if your history is structured. It is possible, and usually better for communication, to have the structure in your head and acquire the information in the context of a conversation with the patient, rather than running though a checklist with pen poised.

Description of the patient

This should be a brief description giving details of the patient's age, sex, ethnic origins, and occupation. It should allow others who have not met the patient to picture him or her in their mind.

Presenting complaint

What prompted the patient to seek help? This will usually be a specific or particular symptom, but may be difficult to identify immediately. Your task is to focus on the symptoms and crystallize them into problems that can be addressed.

Note down the sites of pain (Fig. 14.1).

History of presenting complaint

This is a complete description of the problem that brought the patient to see you, including:

- How and when the symptoms started.
- The speed of onset—was it rapid, or slow and insidious?
- The pattern of symptoms, their duration and frequency—are they continuous or intermittent? How often do they appear?
- If the symptoms include pain, you should describe it fully! Relevant features are site, severity, character (sharp, crushing, gnawing, etc.), radiation, frequency, periodicity, associated features, precipitating and relieving factors, relationship to meals, posture, and alcohol.
- Why has the patient come to the doctor this time? What's different?
- Find out the extent of any deficit. Is there any loss of function, anything the patient can't do or any movement he or she can't make? Is speech and vision normal?
- Is there anything else the patient thinks may be relevant, however trivial?

Past medical history

Has the patient had any medical or surgical contact in the past? Ask specifically about operations, previous transfusions, drugs, especially antibiotics, allergies, and previous investigations.

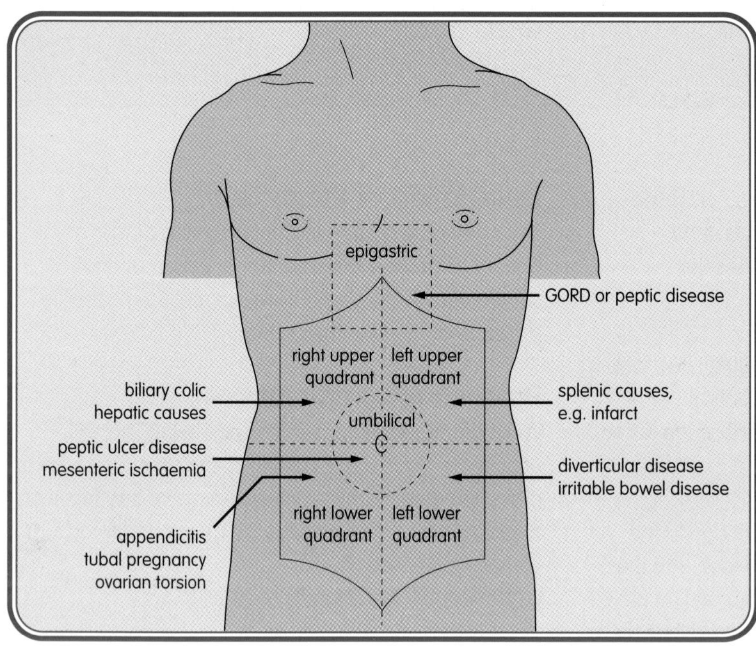

Fig. 14.1 Sites of pain and possible significance.

Obstetric and menstrual history should also be recorded.

Drug history

Ask about all drugs, including contraceptive pills and over-the-counter medicines, as well as medicines that have been prescribed.

Non-steroidal anti-inflammatory drugs are commonly taken as over-the-counter medicines and can cause ulcers.

Lots of people say they are allergic to drugs when what they have actually had was an adverse effect, e.g. diarrhoea after taking penicillin. It is important to establish whether they really are allergic as you may be denying them the best treatment, but do not give them anything they say they are allergic to unless you are confident they are not!

Family history

Ask about the causes of death of close relatives, especially parents and siblings. Practice drawing quick sketches of family trees (Fig. 14.2). Is there a specific family history pertinent to the suspected diagnosis?

Social history

The purpose of this assessment is to see the patient in the context of their environment and gain some idea of how the illness affects this particular patient, what support the patient has and whether he or she can reduce any health risks.

It should include information about the patient's:

- Marital status.
- Children and other dependants.
- Occupational history (including previous occupations): this is especially relevant regarding exposure to toxins, musculoskeletal disorders, and psychiatry.

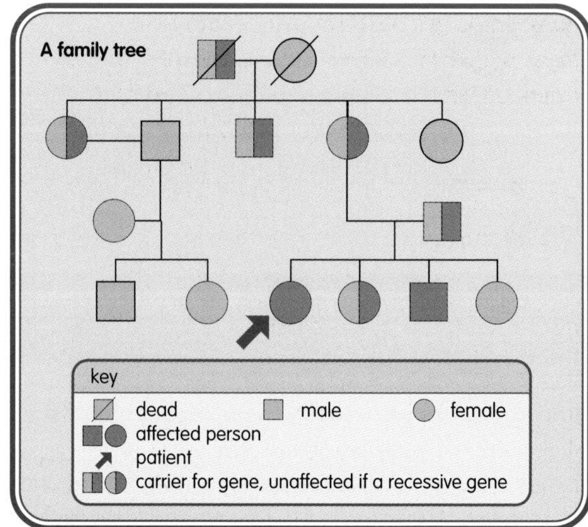

Fig. 14.2 Example of Mendelian recessive inheritence depicted in a family tree. Arrow indicates the propositus, or individual who brought the pedigree to notice.

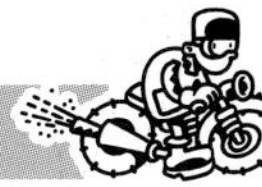

- Hobbies that may result in exposure to toxins or other risk.
- Accommodation: put yourself in the patient's position. Will he or she be able to cope at home? Are there stairs, lifts, bath, shower, etc.?
- Diet—is it adequate? High cholesterol? Vegetarian?
- Exercise—does he or she take any? Is it appropriate?

Is there any risk behaviour?

Consider the following:

- Ask about alcohol—record as units per day or week (Fig. 14.3).
- Ask about smoking (record as number of cigarettes or ounces of tobacco).
- Be tactful but thorough in asking about illicit or recreational drug use.
- Industrial toxins are important in claims for compensation.
- A history of travel to certain regions of the world may be relevant.
- In addition to occupation or hobby, exposure to animals can be important.
- Sexual practice or orientation may be important for some conditions.

Review of symptoms (functional enquiry)

The purpose of this review is to go through the organ systems logically and ensure nothing is forgotten. In addition, it often gives information into the cause or effect of the presenting complaint.

This can be very brief and some of the important questions to ask are listed. If the patient has any of these problems, clearly it is important to take a relevant extended history.

Gastrointestinal tract

Ask about:

- Abdominal pain.
- Indigestion.
- Nausea and vomiting.
- Heartburn.
- Dysphagia.
- Haematemesis and melaena.
- Jaundice.
- Abdominal swelling.
- Change of bowel habit.
- Diarrhoea.
- Rectal bleeding or pain.
- Weight loss.

(For a full discussion of these symptoms, refer to Part I.)

Cardiovascular system

Ask about chest pain:

- Related to exertion or posture.
- Relieved by rest.
- Are there any palpitations or postural syncopal attacks?

Intermittent claudication is a sign of peripheral vascular disease. Ask patients how far they can walk before the pain comes on.

Breathlessness can be a manifestation of cardiac disease.

- Orthopnoea refers to the patient being breathless when lying flat due to increased hydrostatic pressure in the lungs in the context of cardiac failure. It is usually measured in terms of the number of pillows required for sleeping.

1 unit (10 g approx):
1/2 pint beer
measure of spirit or sherry
1/2 glass wine
daily maximum: 3 units males; 2 units females (or 21 and 14 per week)
• beer contains approximately 5% alcohol (i.e. 5 g/100 ml), i.e. 250 ml or 1/2 pint is 1 unit
• wine is usually about 12% alcohol: 750 ml standard bottle is 9 units, 1 unit per 1/2 glass
• spirits are often 40% alcohol: 25 ml measure is 1 unit

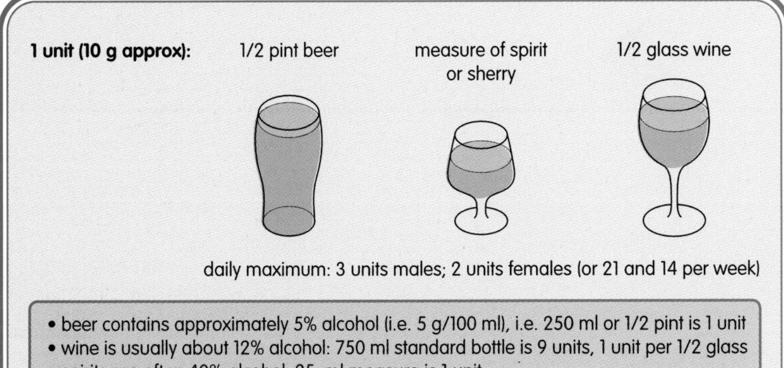

Fig. 14.3 Alcohol measures and recommended limits. Try to work out the units of alcohol for yourself. One unit of alcohol is in fact 8g, but when working out measures it is rounded up to 10g to simplify the calculations.

- Paroxysmal nocturnal dyspnoea—the patient wakes up from the lying down position gasping for air for reasons similar to those for orthopnoea.

Respiratory system

Any chest pain? Is it 'pleuritic'? Has there been any wheeze, cough, or haemoptysis? If there is sputum, enquire about colour, nature, and amount.

Endocrine and reproductive system

Has there been:

- Any polyuria or polydipsia (indicative of diabetes, hypercalcaemia)?
- Any heat or cold intolerance with mood change and/or weight change (suggestive of thyroid disease)?
- Any fatigue with pigmentation and dizzy spells (possibly Addison's disease)?
- Any erectile/fertility (male) or menstrual/fertility (female) problems?

Genitourinary tract

Is there any dysuria, nocturia, hesitancy, dribbling or incontinence, genital discharge?

Central nervous system

Did the patient ever suffer with:

- Headache?
- Speech or visual disturbance?
- Dizzy spells?
- Fits or blackouts?
- Loss of power or sensation in any area?

Joints

Has there been pain or swelling in any joint, or any back pain?

Skin

Is there a skin rash, itchiness (pruritus), or lumps or bumps?

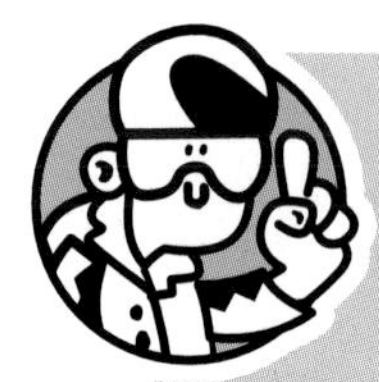

Try to formulate an impression or differential diagnosis based on the history before proceeding to examination.

15. Examination of the Patient

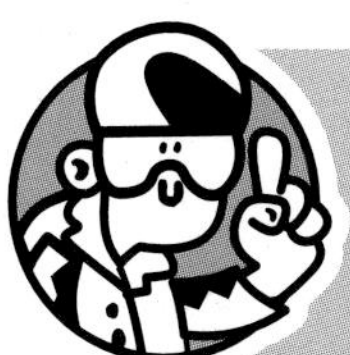

The purpose of the clinical examination is to find evidence in support of or against the differential diagnosis you are considering after taking the history. It should be thorough enough so as not to miss other possibilities that you had not considered and to consider causes and effects of each putative diagnosis.

Examination preliminaries

The main purpose of a general inspection is to determine how ill the patient is. Bear this in mind as you introduce yourself and take a history; if the patient is very ill, do not waste valuable time asking questions that can wait until later.

During the examination:

- Look at the patient's facial expression: is he or she comfortable, in obvious distress, looking furtive, receptive, hostile?
- Assess the patient's body posture and mobility, and his or her weight and size.
- Consider whether he or she is appropriately dressed and behaving appropriately in the circumstances.

Many diseases and conditions do not have a direct effect on the gut. However, always remember that the patient may be receiving medication for a pre-existing condition, and this may affect the dose of drug you are intending to give for his or her gastrointestinal condition (e.g. the patient may already be receiving enzyme-inducing drugs for another condition). Current medication may even be producing the gut symptoms (e.g. diarrhoea caused by antibiotic therapy).

The following examination primer is orientated for gastrointestinal disorders and is not comprehensive. You should read the relevant system in Crash Course for other disorders.

FACE

The face can be a mine of information. Some 'facies' are pathognomonic of certain conditions, e.g. dystrophia myotonica, Graves' disease, and acromegaly, and have a peculiar habit of turning up in examinations. Here, we concentrate on the facial signs of GI disease.

General inspection

Ask yourself the following questions:

- Are there any signs of mania or psychosis (possibly related to steroids, systemic lupus erythematosus [SLE], Wilson's disease, porphyria)?
- Is the patient agitated and not just anxious to see you (possible sign of hyperthyroidism, alcohol withdrawal)?
- Is the general appearance unkempt or neglected (e.g. due to alcohol or depression)?
- Is there excessive skin hair (hypertrichosis can occur with excess steroids, cyclosporin, or minoxidil)?
- What is the skin's colour and its relevance (Fig. 15.1)?

Are there specific skin lesions suggestive of a particular disorder (Fig. 15.2), such as:

- Dermatitis herpetiformis (coeliac).
- Psoriasis (colitis, sometimes liver disease).
- Eczema (atopy).
- Telangiectasia (CREST; Calcinosis cutis, Raynaud's phenomenon, oEsophageal stricture or dysmotility, Scleroderma, Telangiectasia).
- Spider naevi (liver disease).
- Pyoderma gangrenosum (ulcerative colitis).

Pigmentation of the skin and its significance in gastroenterology	
Colour	**Possible significance**
Yellow	Jaundice, carotenaemia
Grey	Haemochromatosis
Brown	Addison's
Dusky	Primary biliary cirrhosis, renal failure
Blue	Cyanosis (cardiac, respiratory)
Red	Plethora, carcinoid flush
Blotchy	Vitiligo

Fig. 15.1 Pigmentation of the skin and its significance in gastroenterology.

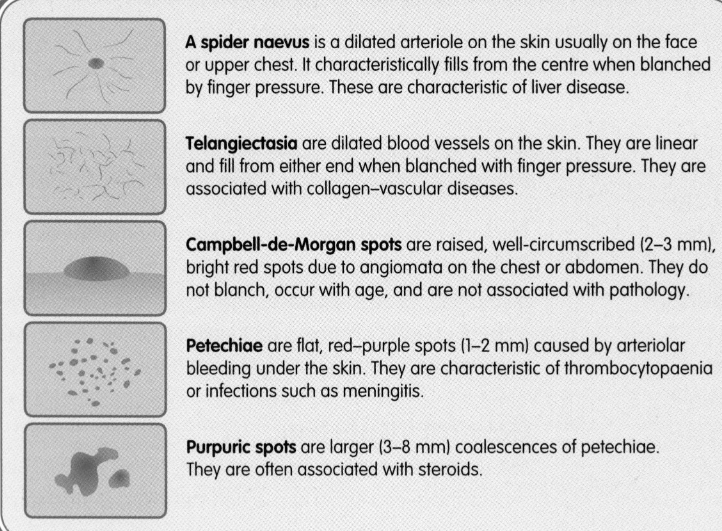

Fig. 15.2 Definitions of common skin lesions found in GI examination.

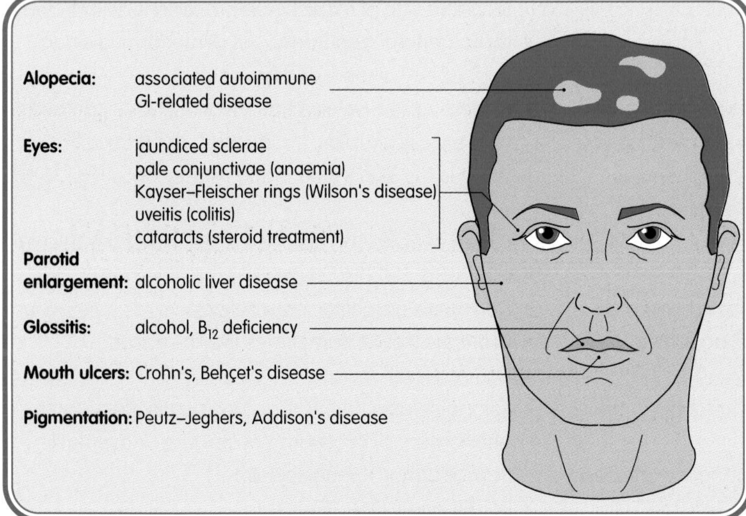

Fig. 15.3 Specific facial features of disease.

Specific examination

Examine the face specifically for particular signs indicative of disease (Fig. 15.3).

HANDS

Examine the hands for particular signs indicative of GI-related disease (Figs 15.4 and 15.5).

Take the pulse, blood pressure, and feel the palms for temperature.

Find out whether there is:

- Any tremor: is it coarse or fine? Does it disappear with voluntary intent?
- A flap indicative of liver failure or CO_2 retention.

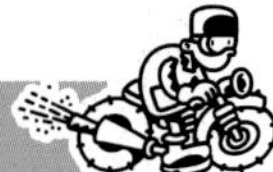

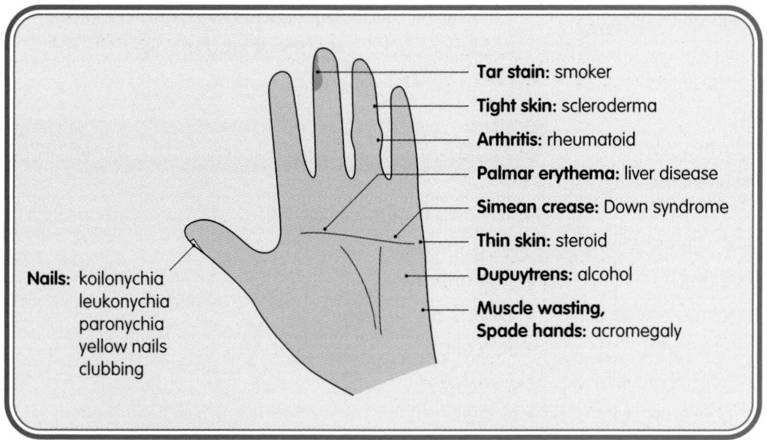

Fig. 15.4 Clinical signs in the hands indicative of disease.

Causes of clubbing of the nails

GI causes	Cardiac causes	Respiratory causes
cirrhosis coeliac disease Crohn's disease ulcerative colitis	bacterial endocarditis congenital cyanotic heart disease atrial myxoma	fibrosing alveolitis suppurative disease (bronchiectasis, empyema) mesothelioma bronchial carcinoma

Fig. 15.5 Causes of clubbing of the nails.

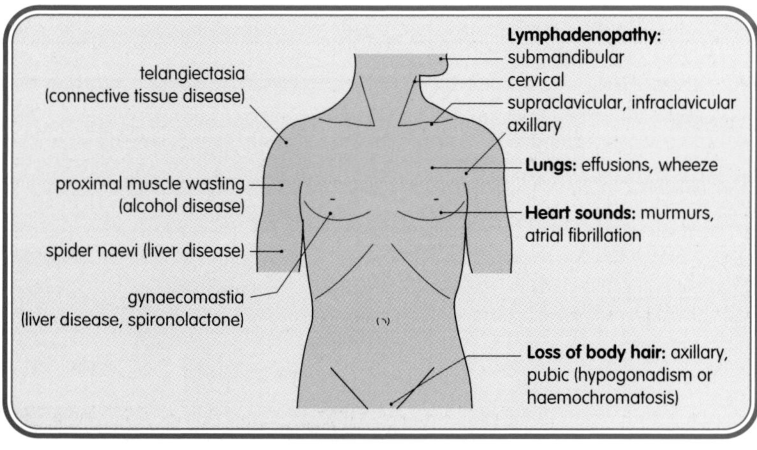

Fig. 15.6 Signs relating to GI pathology to be sought in upper torso. (Afib, atrial fibrillation.)

NECK, THORAX, AND UPPER LIMBS

Examine the neck and upper chest together looking for signs of:

- Liver disease.
- Portal hypertension.
- Metastatic disease.
- Systemic disease (e.g. endocrine) that may produce gastrointestinal symptoms (Fig. 15.6).

Examine the neck, supra- and infraclavicular fossae, and axillae for lymph nodes indicative of metastatic disease or lymphoma.

LOWER LIMB

Proximal myopathy may be a sign of generalized debility or due to biochemical pathology, e.g. alcoholism. Steroids used for chronic inflammatory disease such as colitis may produce proximal muscle weakness.

A patient with arthritis may be taking medication that can cause GI problems [e.g. non-steroidal anti-inflammatory drugs cause gastritis and gastric erosions]. Conversely, the arthritis may be an extra-intestinal manifestation of GI pathology (e.g. arthritis of colitis or chondrocalcinosis associated with haemochromatosis).

Ankle oedema can be due to hypoabluminaemia from liver cirrhosis or chronic diarrhoea, e.g. coeliac disease.

Fig. 15.7 shows a summary of the signs of GI disease in the legs.

BACK

Don't forget to examine the patient's back (Fig. 15.8):

- Are there structural bone problems such as ankylosing spondylitis (associated with colitis) or kyphoscoliosis?
- Tender renal angles from pyelonephritis may be an explanation for abdominal pain. Haemorrhagic pancreatitis may manifest as haematoma in the flanks or back (Grey Turner's sign).

ABDOMINAL EXAMINATION

Warm your hands before you start or you may produce reflex guarding. Inspect for:

- Asymmetry.
- Lumps and bumps.
- Pulsation.
- Peristalsis.
- Scars.
- Distension.

Superficial palpation is to detect tenderness or guarding. Deep palpation is to detect organomegaly and masses: do not hurt the patient!

Percussion is useful to confirm enlargement of liver. Percussion is essential if the abdomen is distended, to differentiate fluid (dull) from air (tympanitic).

You must know how to check for:

- Shifting dullness (dull percussion note becomes resonant when you roll the patient and shift the fluid).
- A fluid thrill (this can transmit 'tapping' from one side of the abdomen to the other).

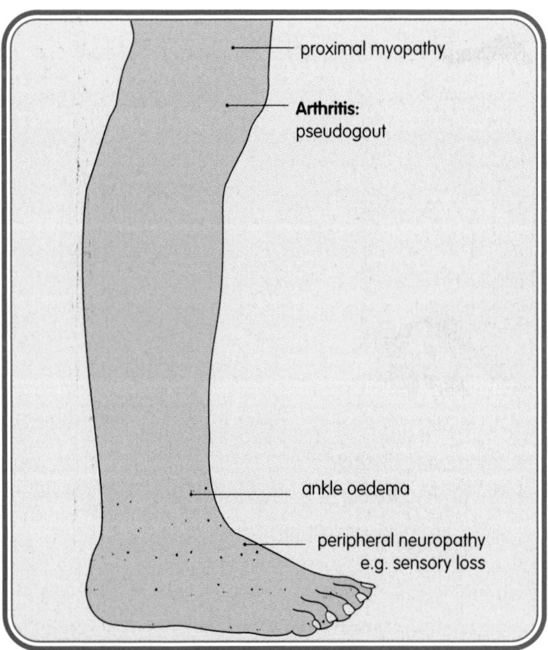

Fig. 15.7 Signs of GI disease in the legs.

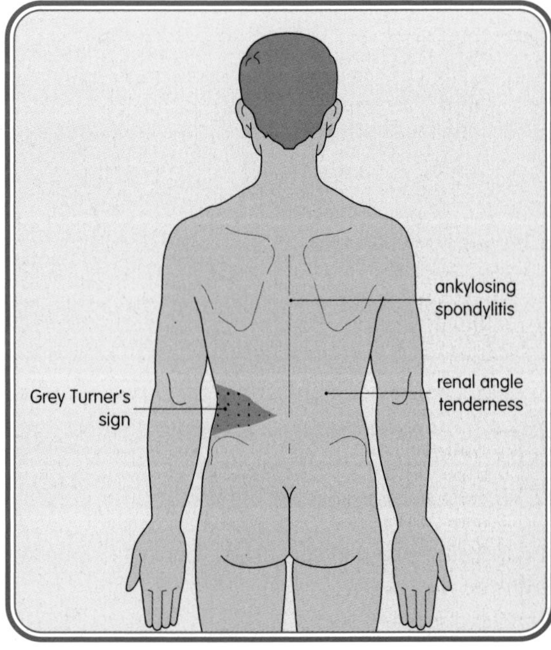

Fig. 15.8 Examine the back for signs of intra-abdominal pathology.

Listen for bowel sounds and bruits. Accentuated auscultation (listening with stethoscope over solid structure while lightly scratching over organ edge) can also be used to confirm liver or spleen enlargement.

Check inguinal, scrotal, and umbilical hernial orifices.

Expected normal findings on examination of the abdomen are shown in Fig. 15.9.

The abnormal abdomen

Any abnormality detected should be characterized carefully. Inspect the abdomen for scars—you need to be aware of their possible significance as, occasionally, the patient is not (Fig. 15.10).

Masses or organomegaly in particular should be measured and commented on as in Fig. 15.11. Causes of common abdominal masses are listed in Fig. 15.12.

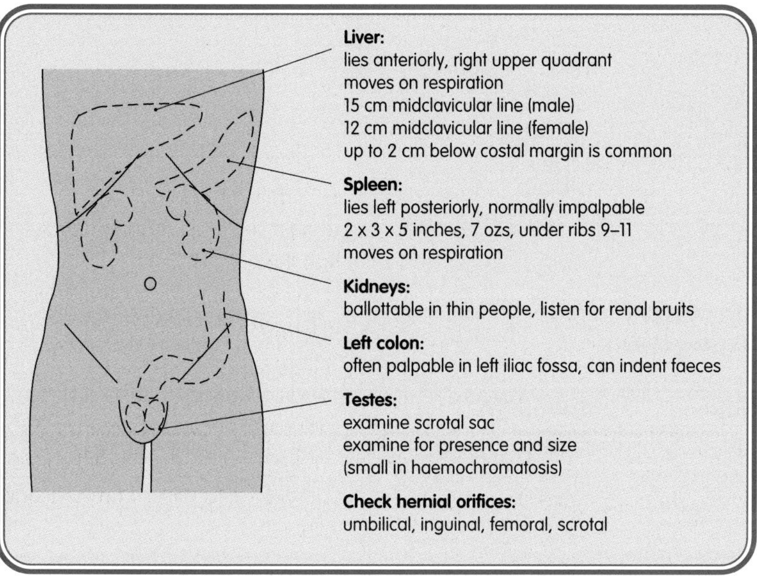

Fig. 15.9 Examination of the abdomen—expected normal findings.

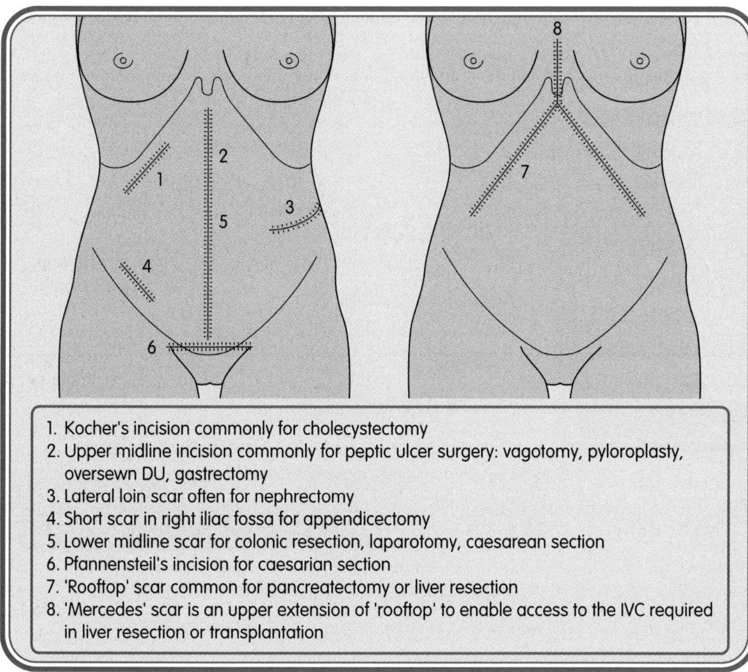

Fig. 15.10 Illustration of common abdominal surgical scars and their possible significance.

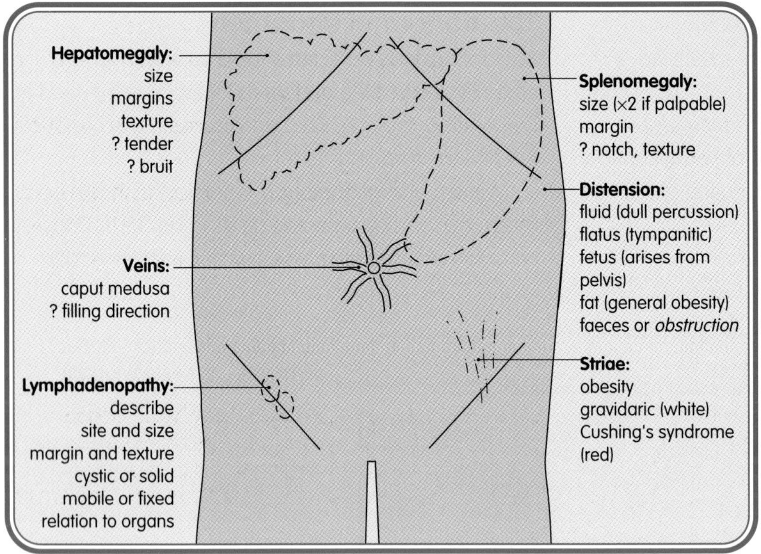

Fig. 15.11 Characterization of abnormal abdominal findings.

Causes of abdominal masses

Right iliac fossa mass	Hepatomegaly	Splenomegaly
Appendix abscess	Cirrhosis (PBC)	Portal hypertension
Ectopic pregnancy	Metastases/neoplasia	Myelofibrosis or CML
Crohn's mass	Hepatitis	Lymphoma
Ileocaecal TB	Alcoholic liver disease	CMV or EBV mononucleosis
Ovarian tumour/tubal pregnancy	Congestion (Budd–Chiari)	Anaemia: sickle cell, PA
Carcinoma caecum	Storage disorders	Storage: Gaucher's
Carcinoid tumour	Riedel's lobe	
Amoebic abscess		

Fig. 15.12 Causes of common abdominal masses. (CML, chronic myeloid leukaemia; CMV, cytomegalovirus; EBV, Epstein–Barr virus; PA, pernicious anaemia; PBC, primary biliary cirrhosis; TB, tuberculosis).

During superficial palpation for guarding and tenderness, look at the face to check for reaction to pain.

RECTAL EXAMINATION

This is a very important part of GI examination, but must be done properly or is not worth doing. Clearly, there are sensitive issues of modesty and cultural code of which you need to be aware. Examination of a patient without consent may constitute an assault, and the more intimate examinations can be an area where failure to communicate your intention can produce difficulties.

Preparation:

- Make sure the patient understands what you want to do and why (consent).
- Have a chaperone or assistant present (same sex as patient if possible).
- Position patient in left lateral fetal position (bottom over edge of couch).
- Use xylocaine or KY jelly on gloved hand.

RECTAL EXAMINATION TECHNIQUE

Inspect the anus for:

- Excoriation (pruritus ani).
- Tags (associated with colitis).

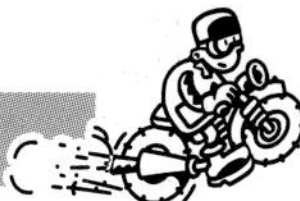

- External haemorrhoids.
- Fistulae (associated with Crohn's disease).

Press gently on the anal orifice with the pulp of your index fingertip and flex the finger through anal canal (Fig. 15.13). Gauge the sphincter tone: if necessary ask patient to squeeze.

Rotate your finger to feel the prostate or uterus anteriorly, the rectal mucosa all around, and assess the consistency of any stool present.

Look at the glove stain for blood or mucus.

Ancillary examinations are often available in clinic to help with diagnosis. These include:

- The guaiac test (Haemoccult) to examine the faecal stain for blood.
- Proctoscopy to examine the anal canal for fissures (painful) or haemorrhoids.
- Rigid sigmoidoscopy to inspect the rectal mucosa and take a biopsy.

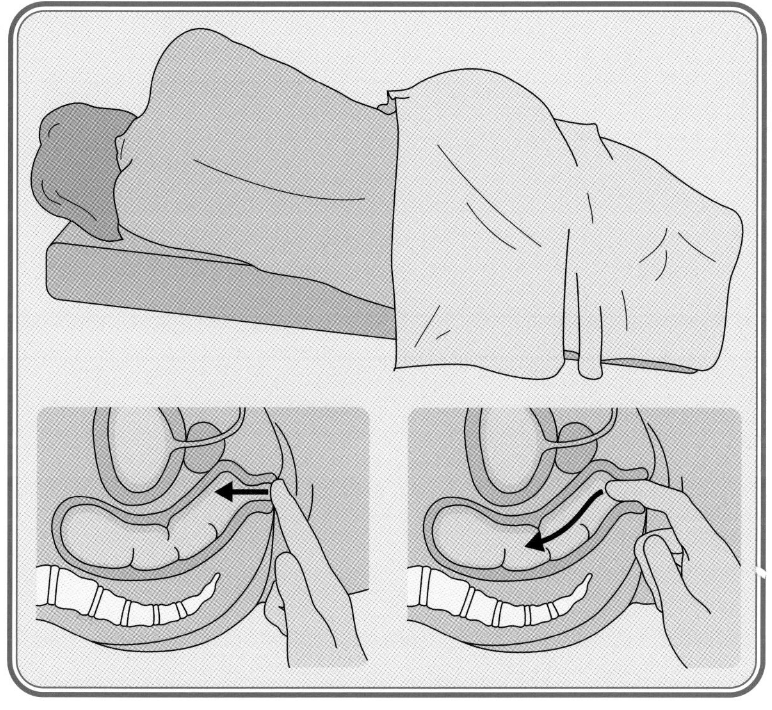

Fig. 15.13 Rectal examination technique: press gently on the anal margin with the pulp of your forefinger and gently rotate inwards.

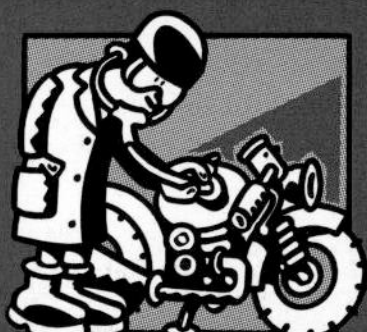

16. Writing Up A Medical Clerking

PURPOSE

The purpose of recording a history and examination in notes is to remind yourself and convey to others what the patient's problems were at the time. Notes must be legible, timed or dated, and signed in order to be used by other professionals. Do not use abbreviations unless they are so well recognized as to be easily understood.

STRUCTURE

Your history and notes will be much easier to follow if they are structured. Follow the same structure used in the history section of the sample medical clerking (see pp. 74–75). This is conventional and has the advantage that your colleagues will know where to look for specific information.

ILLUSTRATION

This can be very useful to document injuries or to convey very concisely the site of pain. Take care if you are using illustrations that, where they convey quantitative rather than qualitative data, they are clear (e.g audible murmur 2/6, diminished muscle power 3/4). Examples are given in Figs 16.1–16.4.

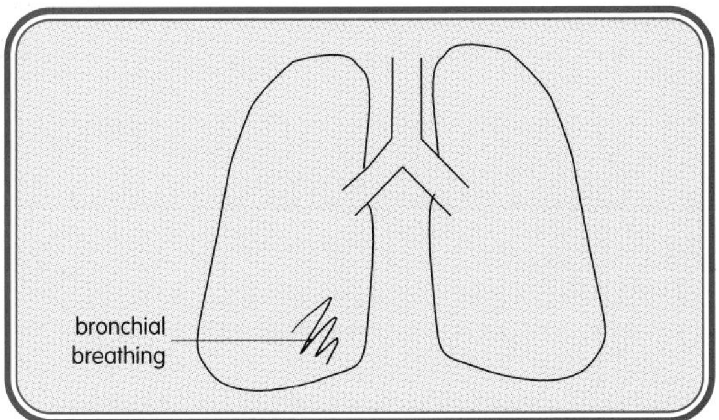

Fig. 16.1 Sample illustration of chest examination: usually the trachea and lung fields are drawn. In the example shown, an area of dullness to percussion in the right lower zone is shown.

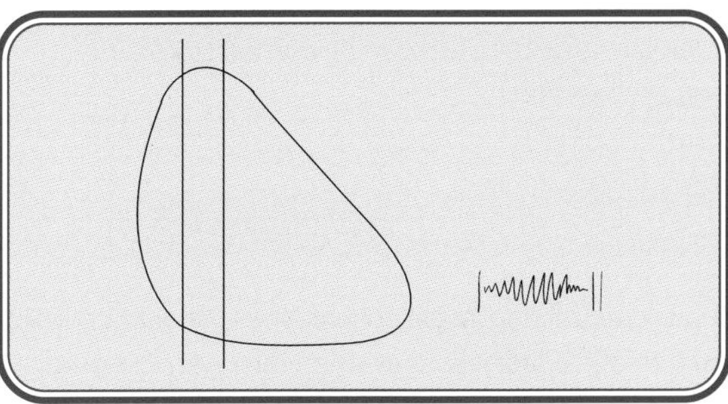

Fig. 16.2 Sample illustration of cardiac examination, showing how a murmur may be represented. In this example, a crescendo–diminuendo murmur was heard in systole (between the first and second heart sounds) and was best heard at the apex.

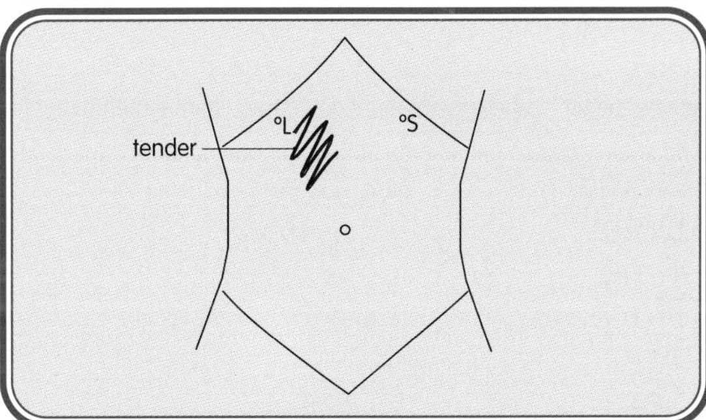

Fig. 16.3 Sample illustration of abdominal examination. In this example, there was an area of tenderness in the right upper quadrant. The degree symbol is often used to denote absence or negative findings, e.g. °L and °S indicate no hepatosplenomegaly found.

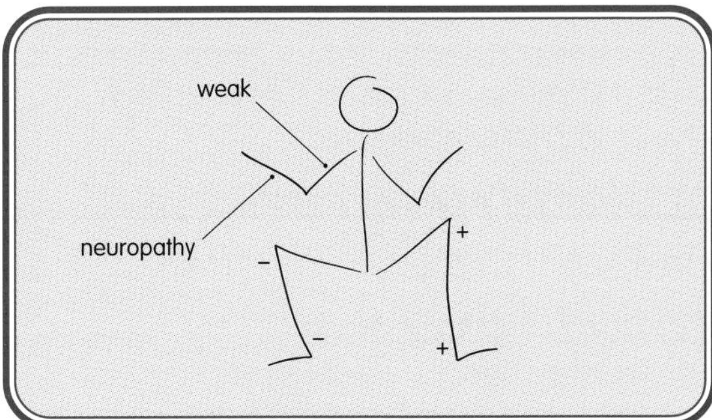

Fig. 16.4 Sample illustration of neurological examination. Reflexes are often represented as present (+), brisk (++) or absent (-). Comments or scores are used to illustrate power or sensory loss.

FORMULATING A DIFFERENTIAL DIAGNOSIS

It is important that you convey your impression at the time of taking a history. The clinical picture may change later, but valuable clues can be gained by recording early impressions.

INVESTIGATION

If you are ordering investigations, these should be listed and dated so that it is clear when they were ordered. It is also very useful if a list of investigations is required, that a summary of results is put alongside the list as they come through.

CONTINUITY

Clinical situations are rarely static. For subsequent entries, it is useful to state briefly the purpose or context of your review, e.g. called to see because complaining of chest pain.

If the clinical notes are extended because the patient has a long or complex history, a frequent update or summary is very useful to keep everyone focused on the problems. Some clinicians find it useful to keep a problem list which is updated daily. The important element throughout is clarity of thought and intent.

SAMPLE MEDICAL CLERKING

An example of a medical clerking is shown below. It highlights some of the points discussed earlier in this chapter.

CHECKLIST	EXAMPLE
Name:	Bea Smith
Date:	1st January 2000
Time:	1015 hrs
Place:	A & E
Age:	26
Sex:	female
Occupation:	Clerical worker
Referred by:	GP

PC (presenting complaint)

c/o Abdo pain LIF, colicky, intermittent
Assoc. diarrhoea 4/day, loose, no blood or mucus
Intermittent constipation 2–3 days per week.
No wt loss/bleeding/jaundice

HPC (history of presenting complaint)

About 6/12.

Relieving/exacerbating factors:

Better after toilet.

Associated symptoms:

Tummy very noisy.

Relevant previous history:

Constipated as a child.

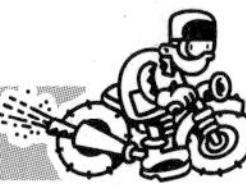

PMH (past medical history)
'98: appendicectomy.

-S/E (systems enquiry)

General
Fatigue lately, appetite unchanged, weight stable, no sweats or pruritus, sleeping well.

CVS
No chest pain/palpitations/oedema.

RS
No dyspnoea/wheeze/cough/sputum

GIT
as above. No nausea/vomiting.

GUS
LMP 3 wks ago. Normal. No GU problems.

NS
No dizziness/headaches/paresis or paraesthesia.

MS
Joints: No aches/swelling

Skin
No rash/pruritus.

Drug history
Taking OCP 5 years.

Diet
Very low res. Chips++, soft veg. irregular meals, no cereal. Coffee++.

FHx (Family history)
M a/w age 56; F rip IHD age 42.
3 sibs: 2m, 1f, no problems
No Hx IBD or CA colon.

SHx (Social history)
Lives with boyfriend. Non-smoker. Alcohol 10 u/wk.
Clerical work. No sports.

O\E (on esamination)
Pleasant 26 yo.
No signs jaundice/anaemia/cyanosis.
No lymphadenopathy or goitre.

p.80/min reg. BP 130/80
Heart sounds: 1,2, nil added
Chest clear A/P, good AE
Abdomen: soft, tender LIF, faeces palpable

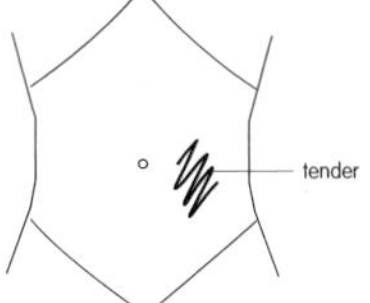

PR and Sig15: normal mucosa, pellet stool.

Imp:
IBS

Plan:
Explain IBS symptoms
Reassure no CA
Invx not necessary, review to reinforce & d\c 3/12.

*Abbreviations used in this example:
GP, general practitioner; OCP, oral contraceptive pill; M, mother; F, father; m, males; f, females; IBD, inflammatory bowel disease; CA, carcinoma; GIT, gastrointestinal tract; GUT, genitourinary tract; LMP, last menstrual period; CNS, central nervous system; CVS, cardiovascular system; Resp, respiratory system; A/P, auscultation & percussion; A/E, air entry; LIF, left iliac fossa; PR&Sig15, per rectal examination & sigmoidoscopy to 15cm above anal verge; Imp, impression; IBS, irritable bowel syndrome; d/c, discharge.

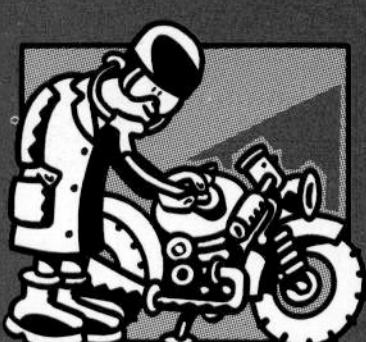

17. Common Investigations

Investigations are used to confirm or refute a differential diagnosis. You ought to be able to justify any test you order on clinical grounds. Brief notes follow to aid interpretation of tests in gastrointestinal disease.

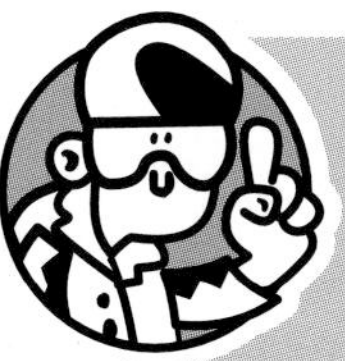

Investigations should be used to confirm or refute the diagnosis arrived at on the history and examination.

ROUTINE HAEMATOLOGY

A full blood count (FBC) is often performed as a routine on every patient and can give important information if interpreted correctly (Fig. 17.1).

A blood film can be very valuable if anaemia is present:

- Cells can appear small (microcytosis) in iron deficiency anaemia.
- Cells appear large (macrocytic) with vitamin B_{12} deficiency.

Reticulocytes may be raised following recent blood loss and can account for a macrocytosis on the FBC result. Target cells (ringed red blood cells) are common in liver disease.

Other haematological investigations can be helpful in gastrointestinal (GI) disease:

- Vitamin B_{12}. If low, consider gastric or ileal resection, or disease (e.g. pernicious anaemia, Crohn's disease), blind loop syndrome, bacterial overgrowth, malabsorption. If high, consider fibrolamellar hepatoma (rare).
- Schilling test: replacing deficient intrinsic factor allows radiolabelled vitamin B_{12} to be absorbed (e.g. gastrectomy, pernicious anaemia: positive test), but has no effect if absorptive mucosa is absent or diseased (e.g. ileal resection, Crohn's disease: negative test) (Fig. 17.2).
- Folate can be low with any chronic debilitating state, malabsorption, excess alcohol, and certain drugs (e.g. sulphonamides, cholestyramine, anticonvulsants).
- Erythrocyte sedimentation rate (ESR)—non-specifically raised in inflammatory and malignant diseases. Limited usefulness.

Routine haematology tests

Parameter	Level	Inference
HB	Low	?Dietary iron deficiency, malabsorption, or blood loss (achlorhydria, gastrectomy, coeliac disease)
WCC	Low High	Viral infection (e.g. hepatitis) Bacterial infection, colonic inflammation, alcoholic hepatitis, steroids
Platelets	Low High	Portal hypertension and hypersplenism Inflammatory disease (e.g. Crohn's)
MCV	Low High	Iron deficiency Reticulocytosis (recent bleed), macrocytosis (B_{12} deficiency or alcoholic liver)

Fig. 17.1 Routine haematology tests in GI disease.

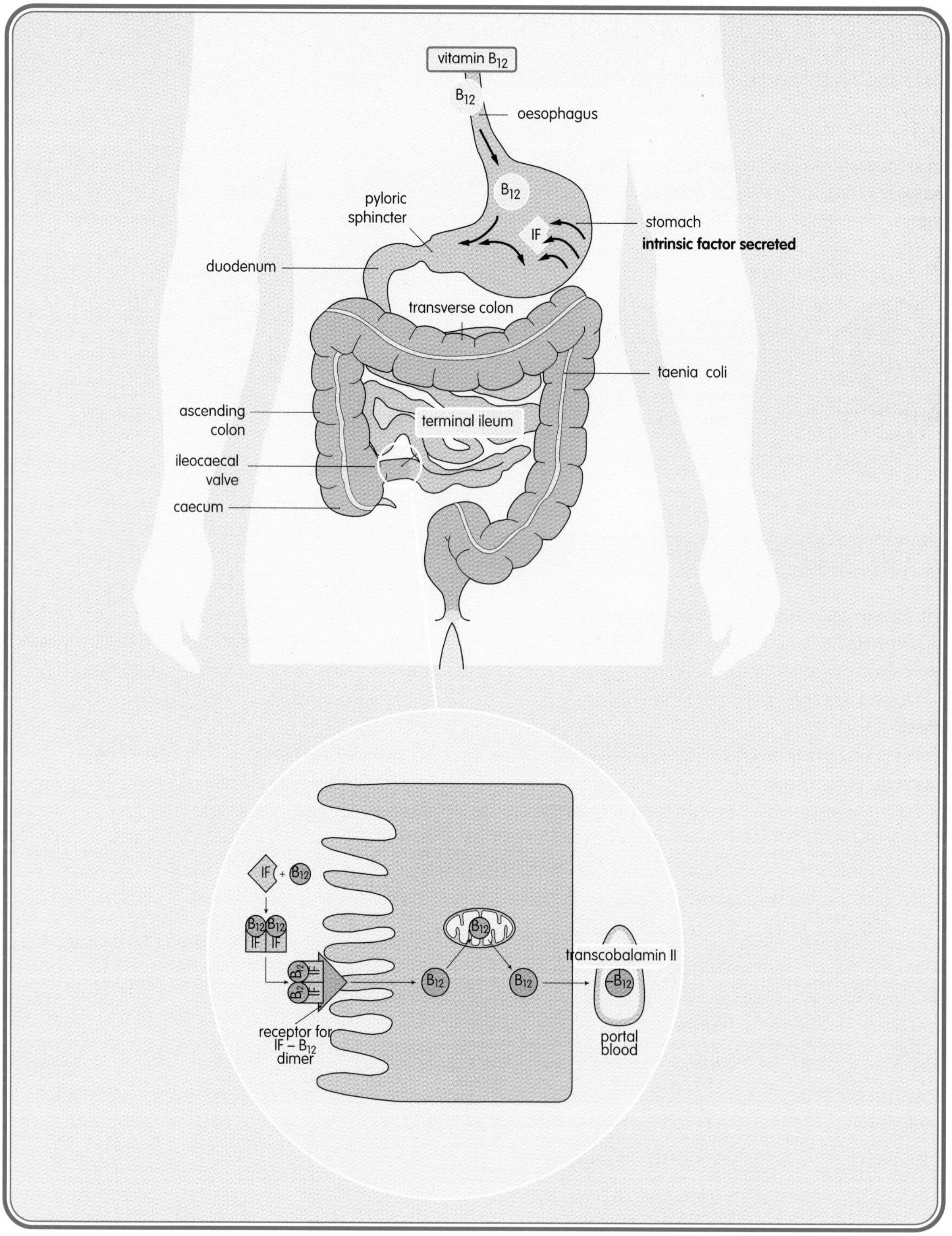

Fig. 17.2 Schematic representation of Schilling test: radiolabelled vitamin B_{12} is given orally and absorption is assessed by its appearance in the urine. Dietary vitamin B_{12} combines with intrinsic factor (IF) secreted by the stomach and can then be absorbed in the terminal ileum. Lack of IF causes pernicious anaemia and can be identified by the Schilling test. A positive test (correction of B_{12} malabsorption with IF) indicates a gastric cause. A negative test may indicate terminal ileal disease.

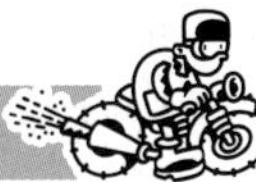

BIOCHEMISTRY

Urea and electrolytes are commonly recommended as a routine test for most patients. Sodium is commonly slightly low in many sick patients due to the syndrome of inappropriate anti-diuretic hormone (ADH) secretion. Some inference about GI pathology can be made from routine biochemistry (Fig. 17.3).

C-reactive protein

C-reactive protein (CRP) is an acute-phase protein and correlates with inflammatory activity in some diseases (e.g. in Crohn's).

Amylase

Amylase:

- Is raised non-specifically in many causes of abdominal pain.
- Is commonly raised without pain following endoscopic retrograde cholangiopancreatography (ERCP).
- Should be moderately raised (>500 IU/L) in acute pancreatitis.
- Is usually normal in chronic pancreatitis.

Arterial blood gases

Patients who are ill from any cause develop metabolic acidosis, often with compensatory respiratory alkalosis (hyperventilation). Following a paracetamol overdose, pH is a particularly useful prognostic measurement.

Alcohol

Alcohol measurement can be useful in determining occult causes of coma or abnormal liver enzymes in patients presenting acutely.

ENDOCRINE AND METABOLIC TESTS

Thyroid function

Thyroid disease does not usually cause GI problems, but may accentuate symptoms such as diarrhoea (hyperthyroidism) or constipation (hypothyroidism) from other causes. Hyperthyroidism needs to be excluded as a cause of weight loss (in children, it can cause weight gain!).

Catecholamine levels

A 24-hour urinary vanillylmandelic acid (VMA) is used to diagnose adrenaline and noradrenaline excess produced from adrenal medullary tumours. These may present with GI symptoms of weight loss, nausea, vomiting, and altered bowel habit. Associated features are flushing and cardiovascular abnormality (arrhythmias and hypertension).

Routine biochemistry

Parameter	Level	GI significance
Urea	Low High	Malabsorption or liver disease Slightly (up to 14 mmol/L): dehydration (nausea, vomiting, Addison's) Moderate (up to 20 mmol/L): profound dehydration, GI bleed (protein load) Severe (more than 20 mmol/lL): renal failure, hepatorenal syndrome
Sodium (Na)	Low	Common in diarrhoea, vomiting, alcoholic liver disease, diuretics
Potassium (K)	Low High	Common in diarrhoea, vomiting, alcoholic liver disease, loop diuretics Possible renal failure, diuretics especially spirononlactone
Calcium (Ca)	Low High	Correct for albumin, common in coeliac disease Associated with malignant disease, hyperparathyroidism
Magnesium (Mg)	Low	Commonly in malnutrition, malabsorption, alcoholic diseases
Creatinine	High	Renal failure (all causes)

Fig. 17.3 Routine biochemistry and its significance in GI disease.

Cortisol

An absent or impaired cortisol response following adrenocorticotrophic hormone is useful to diagnose Addison's disease. This can present with nausea, vomiting, weight loss, or diarrhoea. Acute adrenal failure may present as severe abdominal pain, mimicking an acute abdomen.

Gut hormone profile

Serum gastrin

Serum gastrin is raised slightly in patients with *Helicobacter pylori* infection, peptic ulcer disease, or in patients on long-term treatment with proton pump inhibitors (PPIs). It is markedly raised in gastrinomas. These amine precursor uptake and decarboxylation (APUD) tumours arise most commonly in the pancreas, but also in the mucosa of the duodenum or antrum. They present with peptic ulcers, diarrhoea, and weight loss.

Urinary 5-hydroxyindole acetic acid (5HIAA)

5-HIAA is a breakdown product of serotonin (5-HT) produced by argentaffin cells. Primary carcinoid tumours arise in the small intestine or rectum. The syndrome due to 5-HT excess occurs when the tumours metastasize to the liver, and comprises abdominal pain and watery diarrhoea. Associated features are facial flushing and respiratory wheeze.

Vasoactive intestinal peptide

Vasoactive intestinal peptide is produced in excess by rare pancreatic tumours and causes severe watery diarrhoea.

Glucagon

Glucagon is produced in excess by alpha cell tumours of the pancreas, producing diabetes mellitus and a skin rash.

Somatostatinomas

Somatostatinomas produce diarrhoea and weight loss with diabetes mellitus.

Porphyrins

These are intermediate metabolites in the haem biosynthetic pathway. Enzyme absence or deficiency in the pathway results in their accumulation leading to:

- Neuropsychiatric disorder.
- Hypertension.
- Photosensitive skin rashes.

Gastrointestinal presentation is common with abdominal pain, vomiting, and constipation. Excess porphobilinogen is found in urine. Red blood cell porphobilinogen deaminase and aminolaevulinic acid synthase, the most common enzyme deficiencies, can be measured (Fig. 17.4).

Nutrient elements

Iron

Serum iron is subject to too much fluctuation to be useful on its own. When compared with its binding capacity (total iron binding capacity; TIBC), the percentage saturation of transferrin can be derived:

- Values below 20% are considered iron deficient.
- Values above 50% are probably iron overloaded.

Ferritin

Ferritin reflects body iron stores in adults and is a useful tool for investigating iron overload. However, as an acute-phase protein, it is elevated in any cause of inflammation and this can cause confusion:

- It can be raised in rheumatoid disease despite anaemia.
- It may be raised in alcoholic hepatitis, in which it may be difficult to differentiate from haemochromatosis.

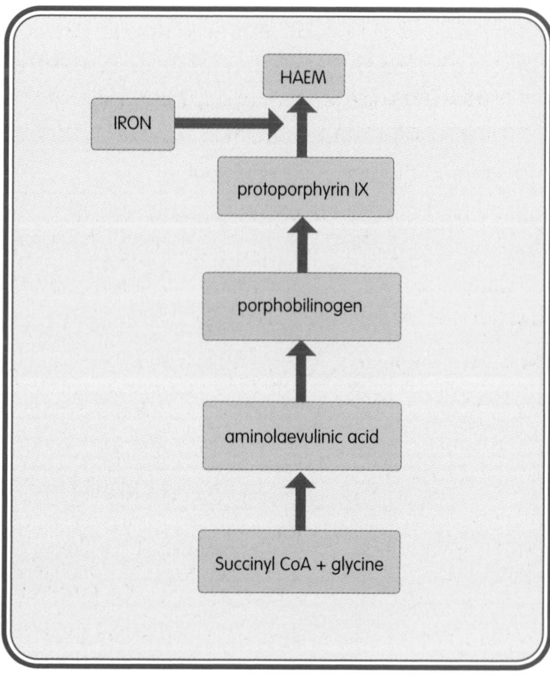

Fig. 17.4 Haem biosynthetic pathway.

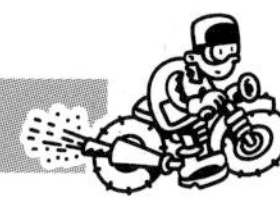

Caeruloplasmin

A plasma protein that binds copper, caeruloplasmin is reduced in most cases of Wilson's disease, but this is not sufficient to make a diagnosis. Serum copper should also be elevated and 24-hour urinary copper excretion increased.

Zinc

Zinc is low in alcoholic liver disease; its deficiency can cause an enteropathy as well as skin rashes.

LIVER ENZYMES AND LIVER FUNCTION TESTS

Liver enzymes

Elevated liver enzymes in serum signify hepatic injury of some kind, but give no information about liver function. For this, routine measurement of metabolites made or excreted by the liver are very useful. Dynamic function tests are also available, although rarely used.

Use Figs 17.5 and 17.6 to help you to work out how to interpret liver enzyme levels.

The pattern of elevation may give some clue about the disease process. This is easiest to understand by reference to the hepatic lobule in Fig. 17.6:

- A predominant or disproportionate rise in alkaline phosphatase and gamma glutamyl transferase indicates biliary tract pathology such as obstruction or biliary cirrhosis.
- A predominant rise in transaminases usually indicates a parenchymal processs such as hepatitis.

Tests of liver function

Standard blood tests

Prothrombin time is a sensitive test of hepatic synthetic function because it reflects interaction of all the clotting factors made by the liver. It is sometimes expressed as international normalized ratio (INR) against a control.

In cholestatic syndromes, prothrombin time may also be abnormal because absent bile reduces absorption of vitamin K from the intestine. In this situation, the INR will correct with parenteral vitamin K but not in parenchymal liver disease. Albumin depletes rapidly in chronic debilitating or inflammatory conditions. It is made in the liver (half-life = 20 days) and is low in chronic liver disease and malabsorption.

Bilirubin in serum can be conjugated or unconjugated:

- Unconjugated elevation (clinically, acholuric jaundice) occurs in haemolytic disorders or with deficiencies of conjugation enzyme, e.g. Gilbert's disease, Rotor syndrome).
- Conjugated hyperbilirubinaemia indicates cholestasis or loss of hepatocyte function.

Causes of jaundice include:

- Hepatitis (viral and alcoholic).
- Drugs, e.g. phenothiazines, anticonvulsants, some antibiotics such as clavulanic acid and flucloxacillin.
- Poisons, e.g.carbon tetrachloride (CCl_4).
- Chronic liver diseases such as primary biliary cirrhosis (PBC) or primary sclerosing cholangitis (PSC).
- Extrahepatic bile duct obstruction (choledocholithiasis and benign or malignant bile duct strictures).

Elevation of liver enzymes	
Liver enzymes	**Significance**
AST (aspartate transaminase)	Very high (thousands) in acute hepatitis or necrosis Moderate (approx. 500) in chronic active inflammatory disease Mild (<300) in portal tract damage, focal hepatitis Also present in muscle (raised in myocardial infarction)
ALT (alanine transaminase)	As for AST, but more specific to liver In alcoholic hepatitis usually less than AST by ratio of 2
Alkaline phosphatase	Highest in cholestatic syndromes (portal tract disease or bile duct obstruction). Remember other sources: bones (especially young), placenta (females), intestine (rare)
Gamma glutamyl transferase	Very labile enzyme, often mildly elevated Highest levels in portal tract disease and alcoholics

Fig. 17.5 Elevation of liver enzymes and their significance.

It is often forgotten that gluconeogenesis and glycogenolysis (the mechanisms for maintaining blood glucose levels) take place in the liver.

Profound hypoglycaemia can occur in some acute liver diseases (e.g. fulminant hepatic failure, Reye syndrome) and occasionally with alcoholic binges. Glucose tolerance is impaired in chronic liver diseases.

Immunoglobulins are commonly elevated in chronic liver disease, but not usually in obstructive jaundice or in drug-induced cholestasis.

The mechanisms of elevation are poorly understood, however:

- In cirrhosis, this may involve antigens from the gut bypassing the liver and producing an antibody response predominantly of the IgG and IgM class.
- In alcoholic liver disease, a decline in Kupffer cell activity may explain the rise in IgA because of reduced clearance.
- High IgG is usually associated with chronic active hepatitis and IgM with primary biliary cirrhosis.

Dynamic and metabolic liver tests

These are based on the principle that certain substances are either metabolized or excreted by the liver and their products can be measured after administration as a bolus (Fig. 17.7).

They are mainly useful as research tools and for evaluating response to new treatments. Some of the more commonly used tests are described briefly below.

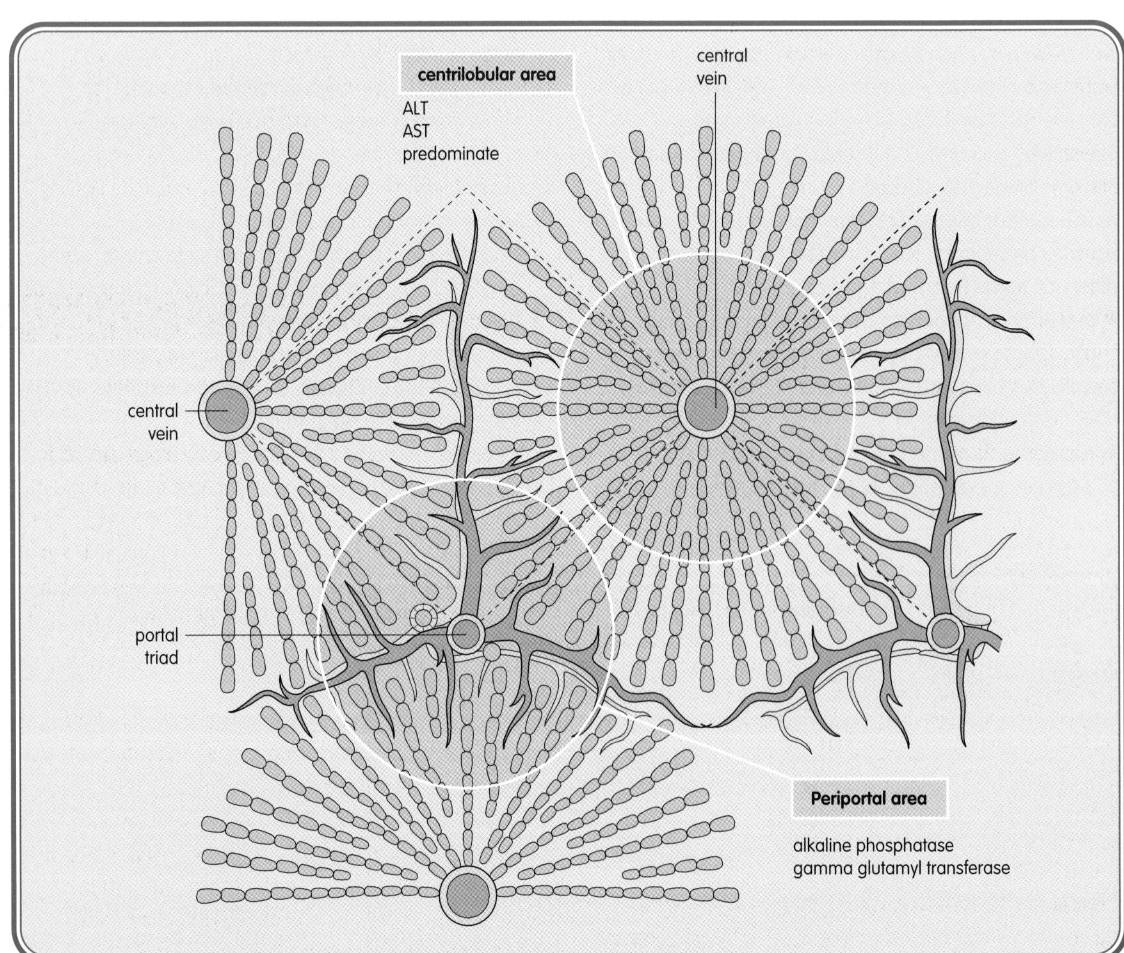

Fig. 17.6 Liver enzymes predominate in different areas of the liver lobule and their relative proportions in serum give a clue about the pathological process in the liver. (ALT, alanine transaminase; AST, aspartate transaminase.)

Bromosulphthalein (BSP) excretion

This organic anion is rapidly taken up by the liver and bound by Y and Z proteins before being excreted. The 45-min BSP percentage retention following an intravenous bolus infusion can detect subtle changes in hepatic dysfunction in mild disease, but is not now much used clinically. Changes in serum albumin and hepatic blood flow affect the result. Delayed excretion (a second peak) is pathognomonic of Dubin–Johnson syndrome.

Indocyanin green

This is another organic anion which is more avidly bound to plasma protein and more actively extracted by the liver. It is safer, easier to measure (including dichromatic earlobe densitometry), and less susceptible to variability than BSP, but less useful in detecting subtle changes in function. It reflects hepatic blood flow very well and is mostly employed for this purpose. Normal in Dubin–Johnson syndrome.

Bile acids

Bile acids more specifically reflect excretory hepatic function than serum bilirubin. They are sensitive and specific, and can be used to detect subtle dysfunction or differentiate liver disease from congenital hyperbilirubinaemias or haemolysis. A bile acid challenge test has been devised for even greater sensitivity. In practice their measurement offers little advantage over enzyme estimation in combination with measurements of protein and bilirubin.

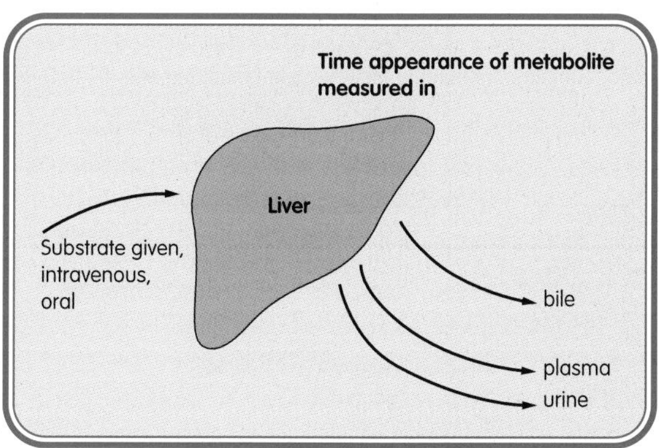

Fig. 17.7 Principal of dynamic liver function tests: a known amount of substrate is given and its metabolite(s) measured at set time points in plasma or urine. Metabolism is a function of hepatic functional mass and blood flow.

IDA excretion (HIDA, DISIDA scans)

Imino-iodoacetic acid (IDA) derivatives are taken up by hepatocytes and excreted in bile. They can be tagged with ^{99}Tc to evaluate excretory function and gall bladder concentration of bile. They can be useful in difficult cases of intrahepatic bile duct stasis.

Metabolic challenge tests

These rely on functional hepatic mass to produce or excrete a metabolite.

Antipyrine clearance, aminopyrine breath test, and caffeine or lignocaine clearance have been used to investigate and test microsomal function. They correlate well with hepatic dysfunction but offer little advantage over measurement of prothrombin time, serum albumin, or the Child–Pugh score.

Galactose tolerance test

Galactose is rapidly phosphorylated in hepatocytes and eliminated. After an infusion or bolus, the rate of elimination can detect subclinical cirrhosis and distinguish parenchymal from obstructive liver disease. It offers no advantages clinically over routine tests.

LIVER BIOPSY

Ultimately, for the assessment of liver pathology a liver biopsy will be required.

The usual indications are to help in diagnosis or to assess the severity of inflammation and fibrosis in established disease to guide treatment and prognosis.

The procedure is undertaken usually with a slicing or suction needle percutaneously under local anaesthetic. A Menghini hollow, wide-bore needle inserted into the liver with suction via a syringe may be used as an alternative.

Sub-costal or shoulder tip pain is common. More serious complications include bile leak or haemorrhage. Perforation of a viscus is rare (mortality 1:1000).

If coagulation is abnormal (>4 seconds prolonged) or thrombocytopaenia significant (<80 000), a biopsy can be obtained with a long flexible needle via the jugular and hepatic veins or by laparoscopy under direct vision. The standard vital stains used are haematoxylin and eosin and reticulin to demonstrate fibrosis.

TESTS OF PANCREATIC FUNCTION

Pentagastrin

These tests are now rarely used. Following an overnight fast, gastric juice is aspirated via a nasogastric tube (the basal acid output or BAO). Pentagastrin, a synthetic gastrin analogue is given to stimulate maximal acid output (MAO) and the aspiration repeated.

- A high BAO results from high gastrin levels (now known to be due to *Helicobacter* infection) or very high levels in Zollinger–Ellison syndrome.
- A low MAO indicates atrophic gastritis or achlorhydria.

Lundh test

Following a fatty meal, duodenal content is aspirated and assayed for trypsin and lipase. The levels are low in chronic pancreatitis. Variations of this test are also undertaken with secretin or cholecystokinin provocation.

Para-aminobenzoic acid (PABA)

Para-aminobenzoic acid (PABA) is a peptide hydrolysed by chymotrypsin causing release of free PABA which is excreted in the urine. A less than expected amount of PABA in the urine following an oral load is diagnostic of pancreatic insufficiency.

Fat malabsorption

Fat malabsorption can be determined by detecting a high proportion of unabsorbed fat following a test meal (3-day faecal fat collection) or detecting a lower than expected amount of $^{14}CO_2$ in exhaled air following an oral dose of ^{14}C-labelled triglyceride (e.g. ^{14}C trioleine). To confirm that this result is due to pancreatic insufficiency, this is often compared and expressed as a ratio to $^{14}CO_2$ following an oral dose of fatty acid (e.g. ^{14}C oleic acid).

Pancreolauryl test

Fluorescein-conjugated dilaurate is hydrolysed by pancreatic esterase; the released fluorescein is absorbed and detectable in urine. False positives may occur if bacterial esterases are present.

BREATH TESTS

The general principle of these tests is that a substrate is metabolized when the relevant enzyme is present in the gut lumen, resulting in release of CO_2 or hydrogen which are absorbed by diffusion and exhaled in the breath. Normally, breath hydrogen is undetectable, so elevation is consistent with bacterial hydrolysis. To detect CO_2 by this process, either ^{13}C or ^{14}C is used in the substrate (Fig. 17.8).

Lactulose

Lactulose is hydrolysed by bacterial enzymes causing the release of hydrogen. Once bacteria in the oral cavity are neutralized with an antiseptic mouthwash, an early rise will indicate bacteria in the proximal small intestine beyond the acid stomach. A late rise, due to bacteria resident in the colon, is normal.

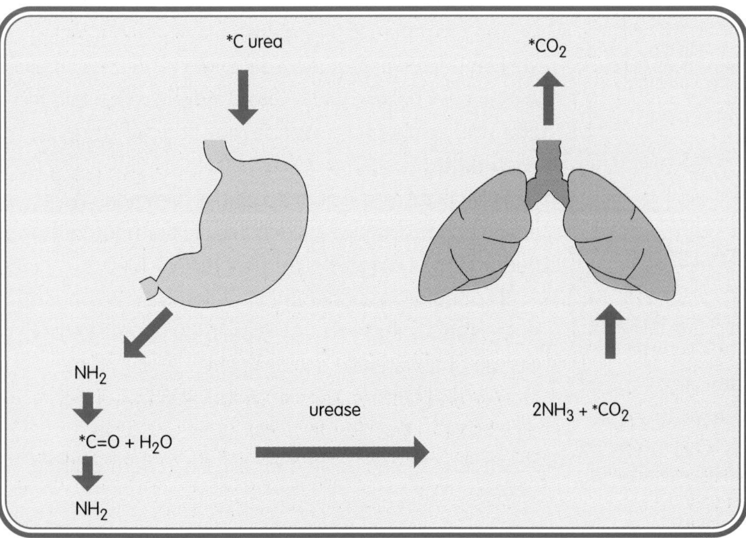

Fig. 17.8 Schematic representation of the biochemical basis of gut breath tests. The example shown is the urea breath test in which ^{13}C or ^{14}C urea is given orally. If urease is present in the stomach, the urea is split into ammonia and radiolabelled CO_2 which can be detected in the exhaled breath. *C indicates that C is radiolabelled.

Lactose

Lactose is cleaved by disaccharidase, allowing its constituent sugars to be absorbed. Failure to detect a rise of plasma glucose following an oral load of lactose indicates disaccharidase deficiency. Avoidance of dairy produce usually alleviates the associated diarrhoea.

D-Xylose

D-xylose is a synthetic sugar absorbed, like all sugars, from the proximal small intestine. Measurement of serum xylose following an oral load has been used as a test for malabsorption but is too sensitive and non-specific to be clinically useful.

Urea

Urea labelled with ^{13}C or ^{14}C and given orally is cleaved to ammonia and radiolabelled CO_2, which is detectable in exhaled breath if urease is present in the stomach. This enzyme is present on the coat of *Helicobacter pylori* and the test identifies patients with current gastric infection.

Glycholic acid

Glycholic acid is a bile salt which can be conjugated to ^{14}C glycine. Bacteria, if present in the small intestine, deconjugate the bile salt and the glycine is metabolized, releasing $^{14}CO_2$ which is absorbed and exhaled in expiration.

MOTILITY PHYSIOLOGY

Oesophageal manometry

This is undertaken for the investigation of non-cardiac chest pain if dysmotility is suspected or in the assessment of gastro-oesophageal reflux disease or non-mechanical dysphagia.

A tube with either solid-state or water-pressure transducers at intervals along its length is passed nasogastrically and peristaltic swallow waves are recorded (Figs 17.9 and 17.10).

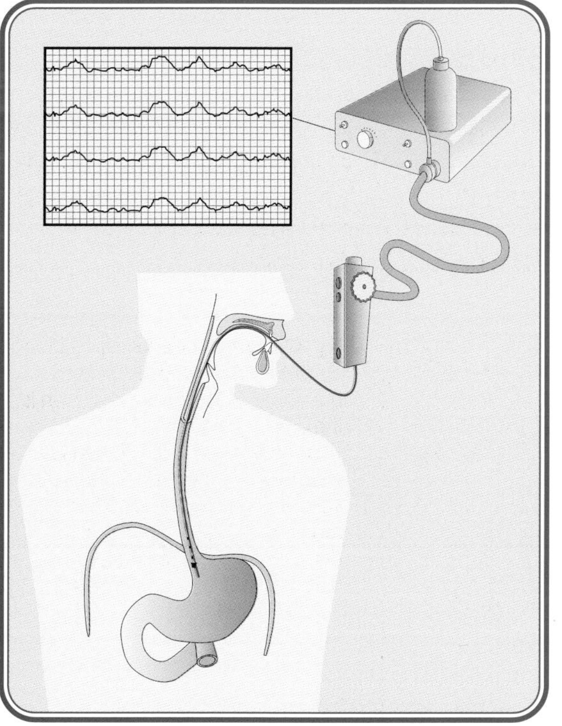

Fig. 17.9 Measurement of oesophageal motility. A probe is passed nasogastrically with several transducers at 1 cm intervals. These pick up sequential pressure waves as the peristaltic swallow travels down the oesophagus. This is represented by the waveforms shown in Fig. 17.10.

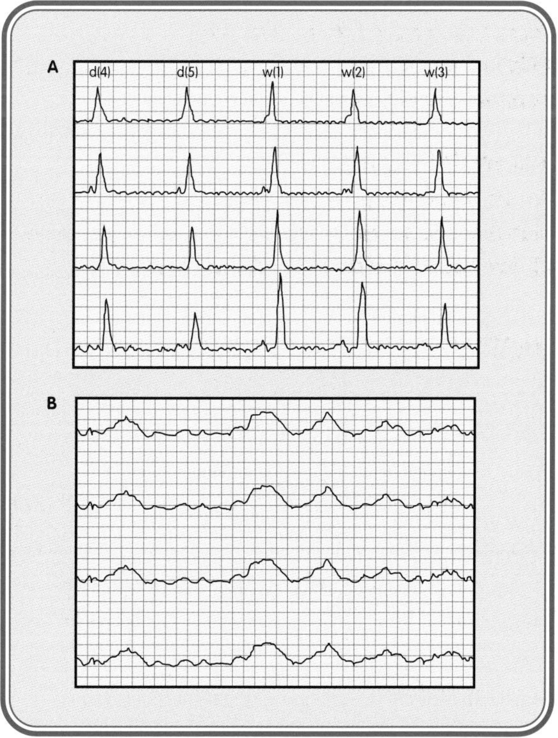

Fig. 17.10 (A) Oesophageal motility showing normal peristalsis and (B) from a patient with achalasia where the peristalsis is uncoordinated The lower sphincter also fails to relax in achalasia (not shown in this tracing)

- Uncoordinated peristalsis with failure of the lower oesophageal sphincter to relax is diagnostic of achalasia.
- High pressure waves (nutcracker oesophagus) may indicate oesophageal spasm.
- Diffuse hypomotility is common in scleroderma.

Ambulatory oesophagogastric pH

This is often undertaken is combination with manometry in the assessment and management of reflux disease. The patient wears the tube attatched to a small solid state recorder for 24 hours and the result analysed by a computer (Figs 17.11 and 17.12).

The transducer is placed 5 cm above the oesophagogastric junction where the pH is normally above 4, and detects reflux of acid when the pH drops below 4. Results are expressed as the number of reflux episodes and total time below pH 4 in the oesophagus (normally <5%).

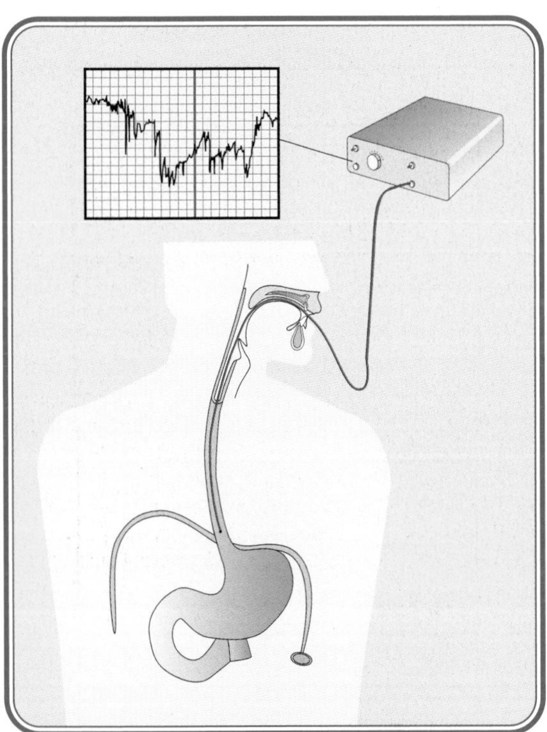

Fig. 17.11 Method for assessing oesophageal pH: a nasogastric tube with a probe sensitive to hydrogen ions is placed 5 cm above the gastro-oesophageal junction. pH here should be greater than 4. Dips below this identify episodes of gastro-oesophageal acid reflux. This is represented by the waveforms shown in Fig. 17.12.

Anorectal manometry

This is undertaken for the investigation of faecal incontinence or chronic constipation. A narrow tube with pressure transducers is passed across the anus and measures resting tone and squeeze–relaxation activity. The patient can be instructed by a biofeedback mechanism to improve anal sphincter tone and defaecation technique.

SEROLOGY TESTS

A large variety of tests are based on the interaction of antibodies with antigen in radioimmunoassay kits and enzyme-linked immunosorbent assay (ELISA) kits (Fig. 17.13). Their principal use is to screen for infection, tumours, or immunoinflammatory disease when those conditions are suspected by the clinical presentation or the results of other tests.

These are useful confirmatory tests, but are much less useful and often confusing if used as screening tests. Here, they are classified according to their clinical implications in gastrointestinal pathology.

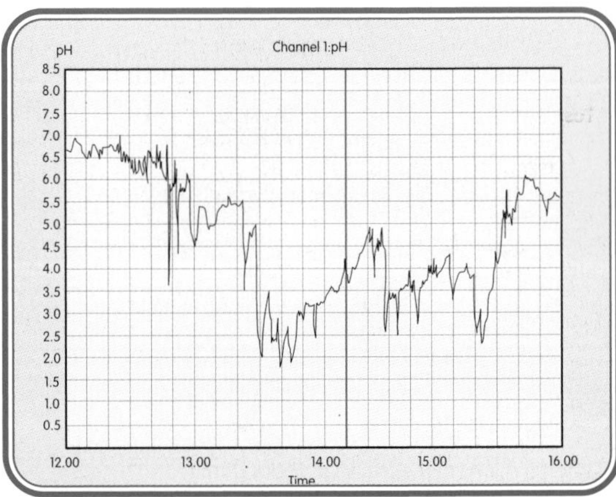

Fig. 17.12 Example of 24-hour pH recording from a patient with significant acid reflux. pH dipping below 4 indicates acid reflux from the stomach.

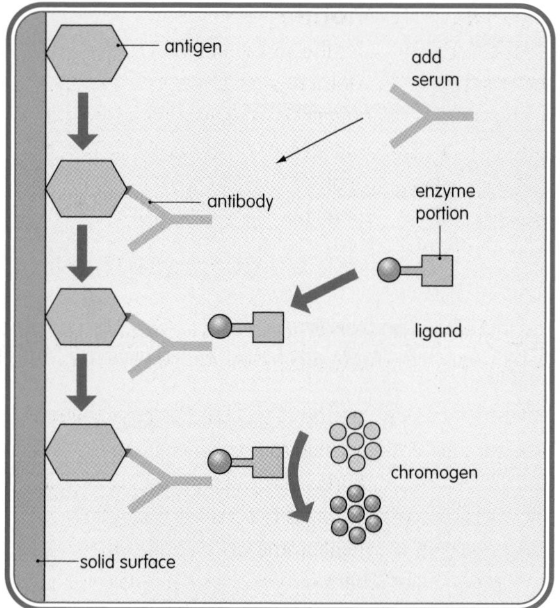

Fig. 17.13 The principles of ELISA. A solid surface is labelled with antigen (the solid phase). The patient's serum is added and if the specific antibody is present, it is held by the antigen and can be detected by a labelled antibody sandwich technique with a colouring agent.

Markers of autoimmune disease

Antibodies to various nuclear components are found in a number of diseases (Fig. 17.14), but also in up to 20% of the normal population.

More specific antibodies to double-stranded DNA are found in 50% of patients with systemic lupus erythematosus (SLE), and speckled pattern anti-nuclear factor (ANF) in mixed connective tissue disease.

- Smooth muscle antibodies are found in 60% of cases or autoimmune chronic active hepatitis. Anti-liver–kidney microsomal (LKM) antibodies are found in a subgroup of these patients with a more protracted course of disease.
- Gastric parietal cell antibodies are found in 90% of patients with pernicious anaemia.
- Rheumatoid antibody is found in 70% of patients with rheumatoid-like arthritis and is the determining factor for seropositivity which tends to run a more severe course.
- Anit-neutrophil cytoplasmic antibody (ANCA) antibodies are found in a variety of connective tissue diseases, but the p-ANCA variety is found more commonly (in 70% of cases) in primary sclerosing cholangitis.
- Endomysial antibody is found in 60% of cases of coeliac disease, but it is not sensitive enough to be very useful clinically.
- Alphagliaden antibody was initially thought to be a good marker of coeliac disease, but is only present in about 50–70% of cases.

Common autoantibodies

Test	Significance	Application
Anti-mitochondrial Ab	PBC	When biliary enzymes raised
Anti-smooth muscle Ab	AICAH	When ALT raised
Anti-LKM Ab	AICAH	When ALT raised
Anti-nuclear Ab	CAH	When ALT raised
Anti-dsDNA Ab	SLE	Abnormal LFTs
Anti-endomyseal Ab	Coeliac	In chronic diarrhoea/malabsorption
Anti-gliaden Ab	Coeliac	In chronic diarrhoea/malabsorption
Anti-neutrophil cytoplasmic Ab	Ulcerative colitis	In blood diarrhoea

Fig. 17.14 Common autoantibodies and GI disease. (PBC, primary biliary cirrhosis; AICAH, autoimmune chronic active hepatitis; SLE, systemic lupus erythematosis; ALT, alanine aminotransferase; LKM, liver–kidney microsomal antibody.)

Markers of infection		
Test	**Significance**	**Application/comment**
Hepatitis AIgM	Indicates acute or recent infection	Use for acute presentation of hepatitis
HBsAG (surface antigen)	Indicates current or chronic infection or the carrier state. Becomes negative after the virus has been cleared	Used to screen in acute hepatitis and blood donors
Anti-HBs	Indicates immunity to hepatitis B virus	May appear in this situation or following vaccination
HBcIgM (core antigen)	Indicates recent infection	
HBeAg (envelope antigen)	Indicates current infection and correlates with viral replication and serum levels of hepatitis B virus DNA	Used to confirm infection if HBsAg positive
Anti-HBe	Indicates that immune response has been successful against viral replication	Infectivity is low, virus dormant or cleared
HCV-Ab	Indicates current or past infection with hepatitis C virus	Screening tests are undertaken with an ELISA kit and these are confirmed by RIBA assays. Blood products have been screened only since 1991
HCV PCR	RNA can be detected by PCR or the b-DNA (branched DNA) assay	PCR positivity indicates active viral infection
CMV	Antibody kits are available to determine past or current infection	Is endemic in many countries and does not usually pose problems except in the immunocompromised host, e.g. after transplantation
EBV	This is tested by an immunoprecipitation test formerly called the Paul Bunnell or monospot test	Is the cause of infectious mononucleosis
Helicobacter pylori	An antibody test indicating past or current infection with the organism	Should be considered in the investigation of patients with dyspepsia. Its clinical use is limited, as it cannot discriminate past from current infection

Fig. 17.15 Markers of infection.

Markers of infection

These are shown in Fig. 17.15.

Markers for tumours

Examples of markers for tumours may include:

- Alpha-fetoprotein can be mildly elevated in chronic liver diseases. Higher levels are found in the third trimester of pregnancy or in patients with hepatoma.
- Carcinoembryonic antigen (CEA) levels are non-specifically raised in colonic disease. These are high with colonic tumours or metastatic disease. They are usually used as serial measurements following colonic resection.
- CA19.9 is a marker for adenocarcinoma, but is relatively specific in for pancreatic carcinoma.
- CA125 is a marker also for adenocarcinoma, but is relatively specific in for ovarian carcinoma.
- CAM17.1 is the marker for adenocardinoma, but is relatively specific for pancreatic carcinoma.

GENETIC MARKERS

Genetic haemochromatosis

Genetic haemochromatosis has been formerly associated with HLA type A3 and B7 in up to 70% of patients. More recently, a mutation (C282Y) in the 'HFE gene' has been described and is present in more than 90% of patients with this condition (Fig. 17.16). Its role in pathogenesis is not yet known.

Wilson's disease

A variety of genes associated with this condition have been localized to chromosome 13. There is no specific

Markers of infection continued	
Test	**Application/comment**
Leptospira	Should be considered as a cause of jaundice or headache in patients whose occupation takes them into contact with rodent infested areas
Brucella	Should be considered in patients, particularly farmers with pyrexia of unknown origin, or granulomatous liver disease
Entamoeba histolytica	CFT should be considered in patients returning from Africa or Asia with pyrexia, diarrhoea, or pain in the right upper quadrant
Hydatid	Should be considered in any patient with pain in the right upper quadrant, pyrexia of unknown origin, or unexplained liver abscess, who may have been in contact with animals, particularly sheep
Clonorchis	Is endemic in parts of Asia and the fluke worm ends up in the bile duct, sometimes causing obstruction with cast formation. This should be considered in patients with obstructive jaundice from endemic areas
HIV	Indicates exposure to HIV
Toxocara	This protozoan infection is uncommon, but should be suspected in patients with obscure liver disease who are in contact with animals, particularly cats and dogs
Toxoplasma	This protozoan infection is uncommon, but should be suspected in patients with obscure liver disease who are in contact with animals

Fig. 17.14 Markers of infection (continued).

screening test as no single mutation explains most cases. The genetic defect is in an ATP protein which exports copper to the Golgi complex, where it stimulates production of and is bound to caeruloplasmin. Hence, the absence of ATP7 protein is associated with low caeruloplasmin levels.

Cystic fibrosis

The gene responsible for this is a chloride transporter and a marker is available (Δ508).

Alpha-1-antitrypsin

A number of genotypes and corresponding phenotypes exists for alpha-1-antitrypsin. The varieties associated with liver disease included PIZZ and PIMZ (Fig. 22.10).

IMAGING

Endoscopy

The principle of endoscopy is shown in Fig. 17.17.

Upper GI endoscopy

Upper GI endoscopy is useful:

- For the investigation of dyspepsia.
- To identify the cause of bleeding or blood loss in patients who present acutely or with iron deficiency anaemia.

Duodenal aspirate is useful for the diagnosis of *Giardia lamblia* or to collect pancreatic juice for the estimation of enzyme activity.

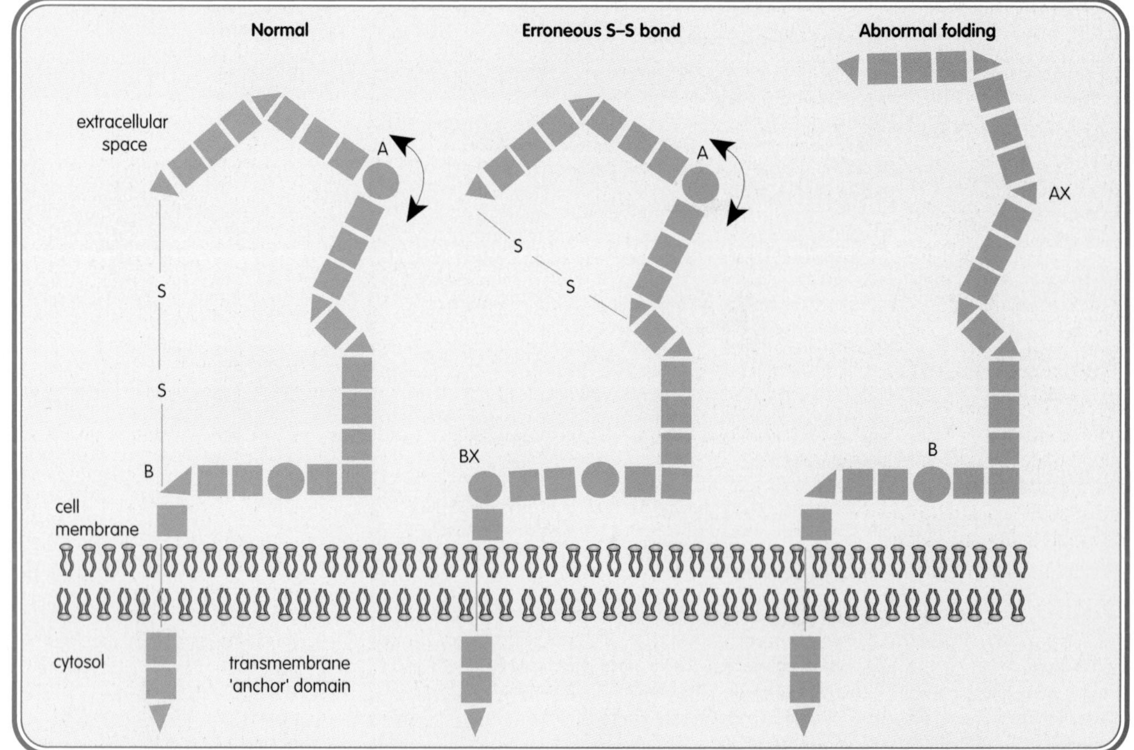

Fig. 17.16 Schematic drawing showing how protein conformational structure and function can change with a single amino acid substitution at sites A or B. Amino acid substitution in turn is due to a single nucleotide substitution or mutation in its coding DNA. Some amino acids allow more flexible conformation (e.g. A) and if substituted will not allow conformational change (AX). Cysteine residues in particular (e.g. B) allow -S–S- bonds to stabilize conformations and can affect ligand binding. If substituted this can also affect conformational possibilities (BX).

Sigmoidoscopy

Sigmoidoscopy is often undertaken in the clinic with a rigid tube and light source to inspect the anorectal margins and rectal mucosa. A biopsy can be taken.

Proctoscopy

Proctoscopy is undertaken with a translucent tube so that the walls of the anus can be inspected while parted. This is useful for anal fissures and haemorrhoids

Flexible sigmoidoscopy

Flexible sigmoidoscopy can also be undertaken to inspect the rectum and the lower sigmoid colon where up to two-thirds of colonic tumours are known to occur.

This is also useful as a prelude to barium enema for complete examination of the colon.

Full colonoscopy

Full colonoscopy is indicated when a lesion has been seen on barium enema which needs biopsy, or in the investigation of acute iron deficiency anaemia or blood loss.

Enteroscopy

Enteroscopy is indicated when a lesion has been seen on barium meal that needs biopsy, or in the investigation of acute iron deficiency anaemia or blood loss.

Endoscopic retrograde cholangiopancreatography

Endoscopic retrograde cholangiopancreatography (ERCP) is undertaken for the diagnosis and treatment of bile duct and pancreatic duct problems. Various interventions can be undertaken including

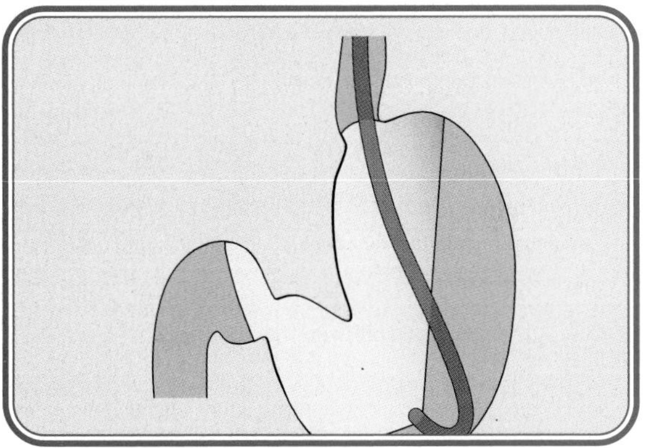

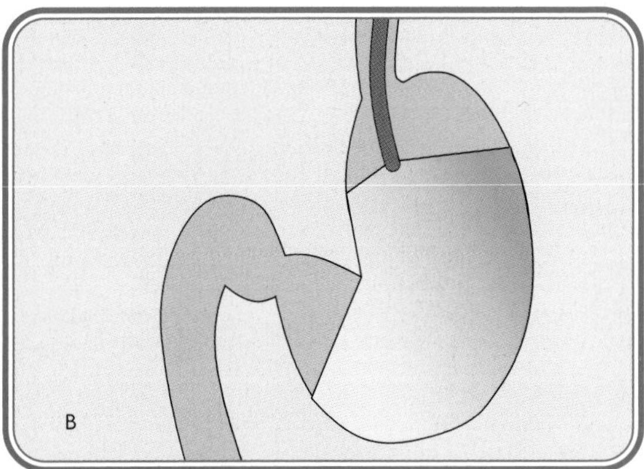

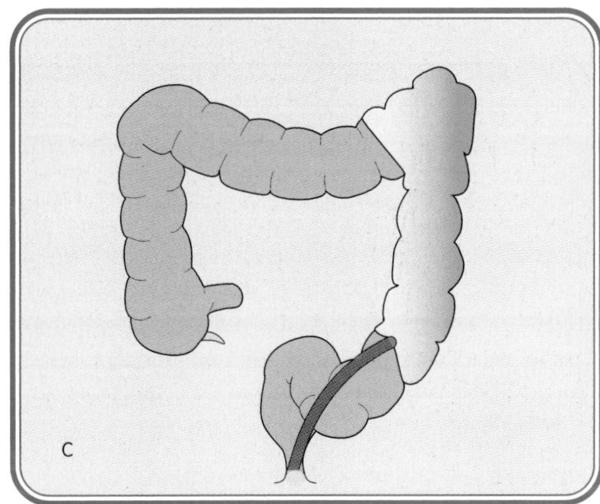

Fig. 17.17 Principle of endoscopy: a flexible tube is passed into the GI lumen and relays video images to the operator. The endoscope can be manoeuvred to see all parts. Specially designed instruments can be used to undertake techniques (e.g. forceps biopsy, polypectomy) through channels in the endoscopy.

sphincterotomy and removal of bile duct stones (choledocholithiasis). For obstructing lesions, an endoprosthesis can be inserted either into the bile duct or pancreas (Fig. 17.18). In the pancreas, further intervention may involve removal of pancreatic duct concretions or passing a stent through the posterior stomach wall into a pancreatic pseudocyst (endoscopic cystgastrostomy).

Endoluminal ultrasound

The principle of ultrasound is shown in Fig. 17.19. Endoluminal ultrasound is an endoscopic examination of the oesophagus, stomach, duodenum, bile duct, pancreas, or rectum with an ultrasound probe on the end of the endoscope. It is useful for:

- Gaining more information on mucosal or submucosal lesions in these areas.
- For differentiating stones from malignant obstruction in the bile duct (Fig. 17.20).

Endoluminal ultrasound is becoming increasingly important for the investigation of pancreatic abnormalities and tumours.

Bile duct manometry

Bile duct manometry is undertaken by passing a pressure transducer on a catheter through an ERCP endoscope. This is undertaken for rare causes of biliary pain thought to be due to biliary dyskinesia.

Pressure waves are obtained as for oesophageal manometry.

Laparoscopy

Laparoscopy is now increasingly undertaken to perform surgical operations such as cholecystectomy. However, its original, and still very useful, indication is for inspection of intra-abdominal organs, including the liver. Ultrasound and biopsy can also be undertaken through the laparoscope.

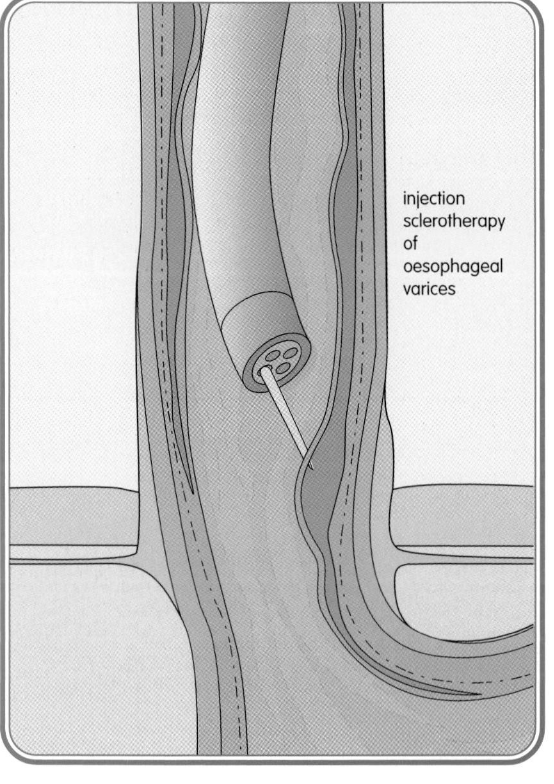

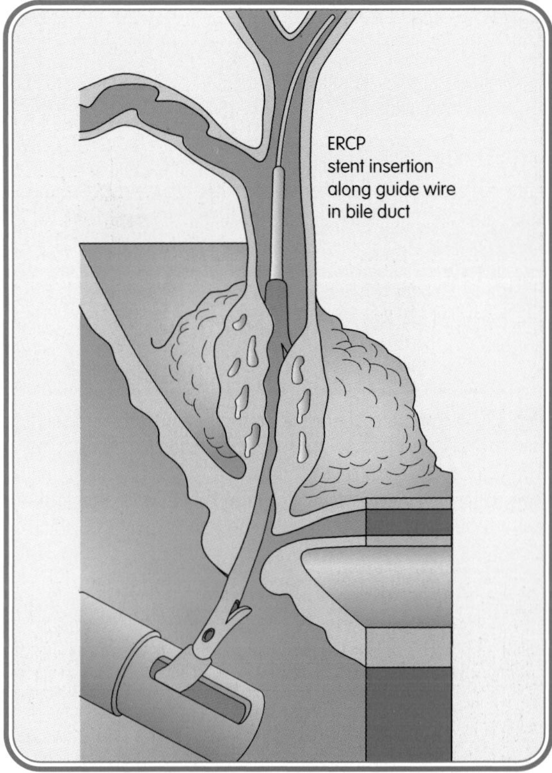

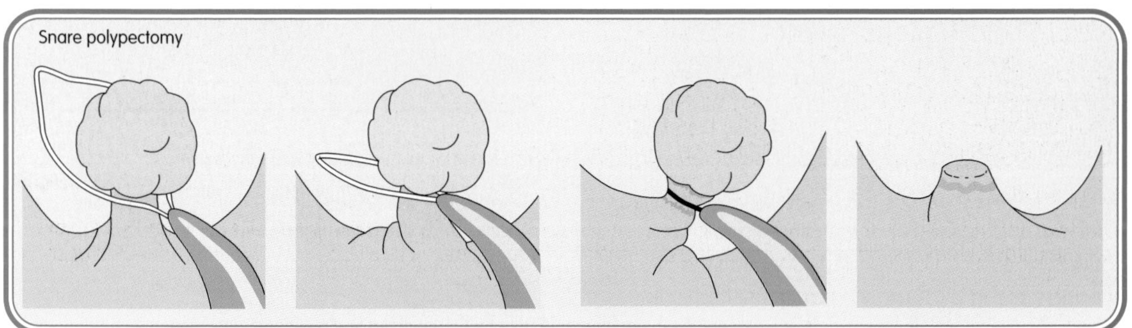

Fig. 17.18 Therapeutic procedures in endoscopy: examples of injection sclerotherapy to oesophageal varices, snare polypectomy with diathermy, and placement of an endoprosthesis across a tumour involving the lower bile duct at ERCP.

Endoluminal biopsy

This is now commonly undertaken endoscopically, during which 2–5 mm pinch biopsies are obtained by forceps.

- In the oesophagus, stomach, and colon, this is used to assess abnormal mucosal appearances (Figs 17.21 and 17.22).
- In the small intestine, it is performed for the investigation of iron deficiency anaemia or malabsorption to exclude coeliac disease.

Complications are rare. The standard vital stain used is haematoxylin and eosin.

Rectal biopsy

This can be obtained endoscopically as described or in a clinic via a rigid endoscope with pinch forceps. Usually used to diagnose or assess colitis or proctitis, rectal biopsies are also obtained for the diagnosis of amyloidosis where a Congo Red stain is used to produce green birefringence in polarized light.

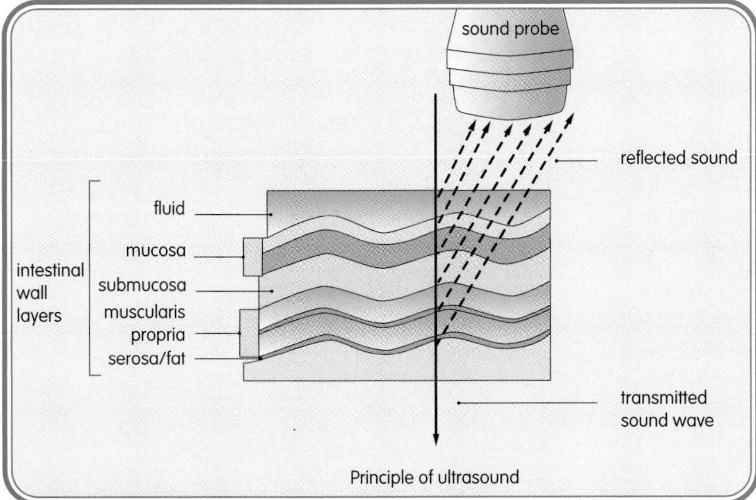

Fig. 17.19 Principle of ultrasound. A sound probe transmits an energy wave through the tissue. At the interface between layers of different density, some sound waves are reflected (echoed) back and can be translated into an image as shown in Fig. 17.20. Ultrasound probes can be used transcutaneously (transabdominal), endoscopically, or even endovascularly.

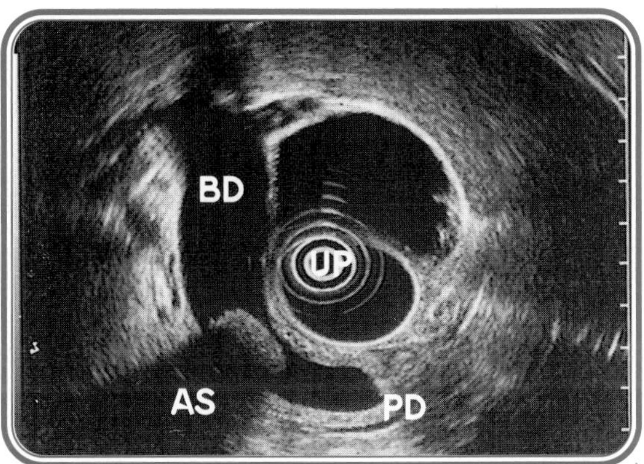

Fig. 17.20 EUS demonstrating a gallstone within the bile duct. An acoustic 'shadow' (AS) is cast behind the stone. Note the ultrasound probe (UP), bile duct (BD), and pancreatic duct (PD).

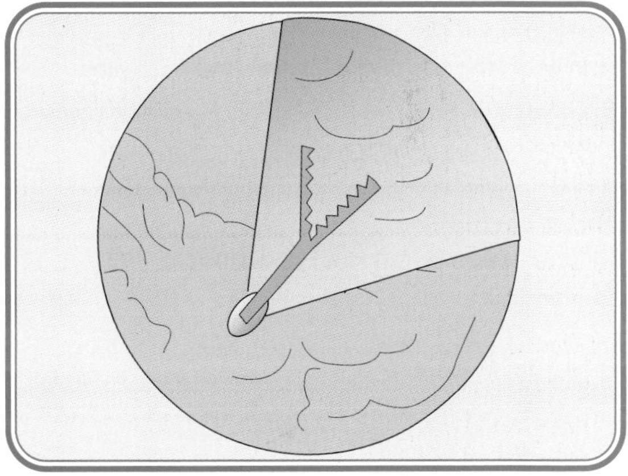

Fig. 17.21 Endoscopic biopsy: a grasping forceps can be used through the endoscopy to obtain pinch biopsies of mucosa.

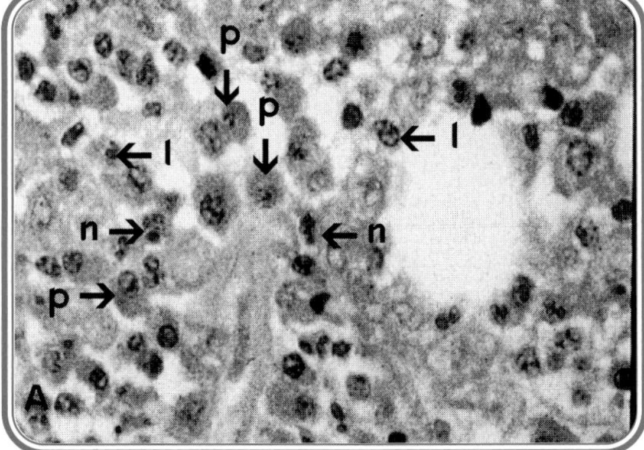

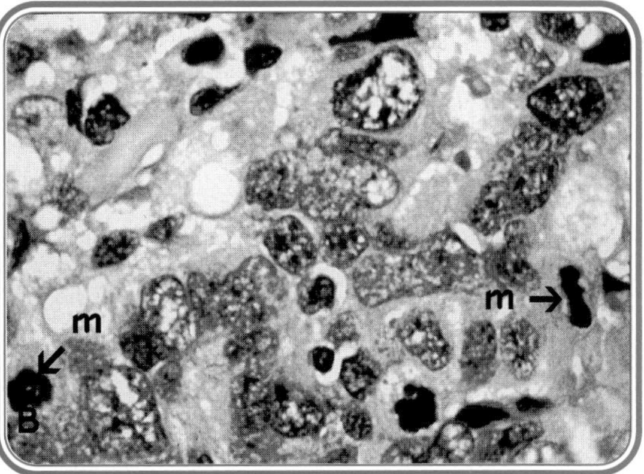

Fig. 17.22 Histological examination is important for identifying the cause of inflammation or for demonstrating malignant transformation in tissue. (A) Acute and chronic inflammation with neutrophils (n), plasma cells (p), lymphocytes (l), and the occasional eosinophil. (B) Large pleomorphic (bizarrely shaped) nuclei with little cytoplasm (increased nuclear:cytoplasmic ratio). Mitotic (m) figures can be seen.

Radiology

Chest X-ray

A chest X-ray is useful in the investigation of liver disorders to assess heart size and concomitant pulmonary disease. In the investigation of patients with an acute abdomen, it is essential to exclude perforation by looking for air under the diaphragm (see Fig. 3.1).

Cirrhosis cannot be diagnosed by ultrasound and if suspected, must be confirmed by liver biopsy.

Plain abdominal X-ray

This is useful in cases of obstruction to look for fluid levels in the bowel (see Fig. 3.2). It is also useful in patients with colitis to assess mucosal oedema and colonic dilatation.

Abdominal ultrasound

This is undertaken in the investigation of abdominal pain, usually to exclude gallstones, or for the investigation of abnormal liver enzymes. It is useful:

- In assessing bile duct dilatation and its causes.
- To screen for hepatic metastases or pancreatic tumours.

Barium swallow

Barium swallow is frequently undertaken in the investigation or assessment of dysphagia. Compared with endoscopy:

- The additional advantage is that peristaltic pressure waves are observed and signs of gastro-oesophageal reflux can be sought.
- The disadvantage is that direct inspection of the mucosa cannot be undertaken and biopsies cannot be obtained.

Barium meal

This is an alternative to endoscopy for the investigation of dyspepsia or abdominal pain depending on local circumstances (Figs 17.23 and 17.24). The disadvantage is that direct inspection of the mucosa cannot be undertaken and biopsies cannot be obtained.

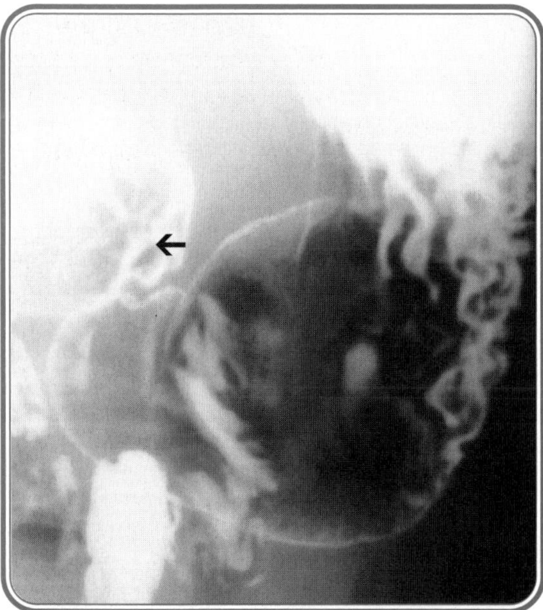

Fig. 17.23 Barium meal demonstration of a duodenal ulcer (long arrow) surrounded by oedema which appears as radiating folds (arrow).

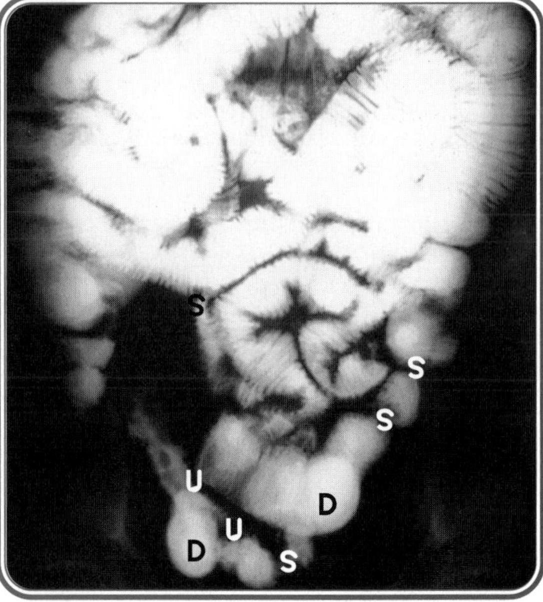

Fig. 17.24 Barium follow-through showing multiple areas of strictures (S), deep ulcers (U), and dilatation (D) resulting from Crohn's disease.

Small bowel enema

This is frequently undertaken in the investigation of either malabsorption or abdominal pain, especially where Crohn's disease is suspected.

Barium enema

Barium enema is frequently undertaken in the investigation or assessment of lower abdominal pain or altered bowel habit (Fig. 17.25). The disadvantage over colonoscopy is that direct inspection of the mucosa cannot be undertaken and biopsies cannot be obtained.

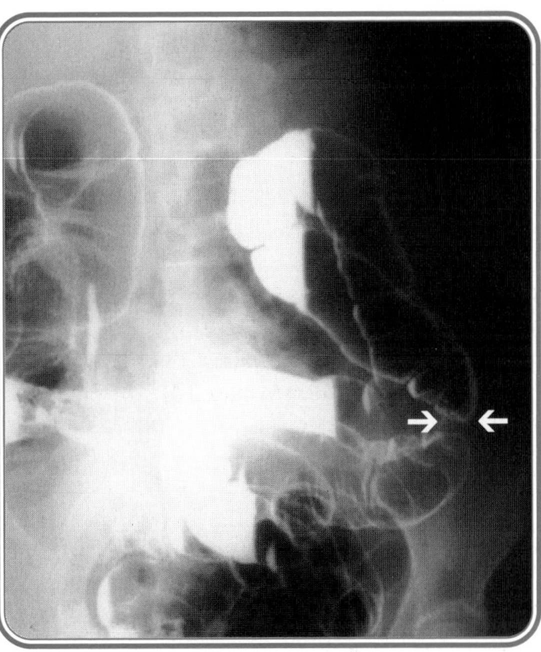

Fig. 17.25 Barium enema demonstrating an 'apple-core' lesion (carcinoma) in the ascending colon (arrows).

Nuclear medicine

White cell scan

The buffy coat of a patient's blood sample is removed and labelled with ^{111}indium. This is then given back to the patient. The white cells accumulate in areas of inflammation and can be detected by a gamma camera.

Octreotide scan

Somatostatin (octreotide is a somatostain analogue) is taken up by neuroendocrine cells in certain tumours (e.g. carcinoid, gastrinoma) and can be detected by gamma camera.

MIBG scan

Metaiodobenzylguanidine (MIBG) is also taken up by neuroendocrine amine precursor uptake and decarboxylation (APUD) cells and will accumulate in areas of high content such as the pancreas, but also in liver tumours and carcinoid disease.

Red blood cell scan

An aliquot of patient's blood is labelled with ^{51}chromium and given back to the patient. In this situation, the leakage or a collection of isotope detected by a gamma camera and located to the lumen will indicate bleeding or red blood cell loss.

Sehcat scan is used to detect bile salt malabsorption.

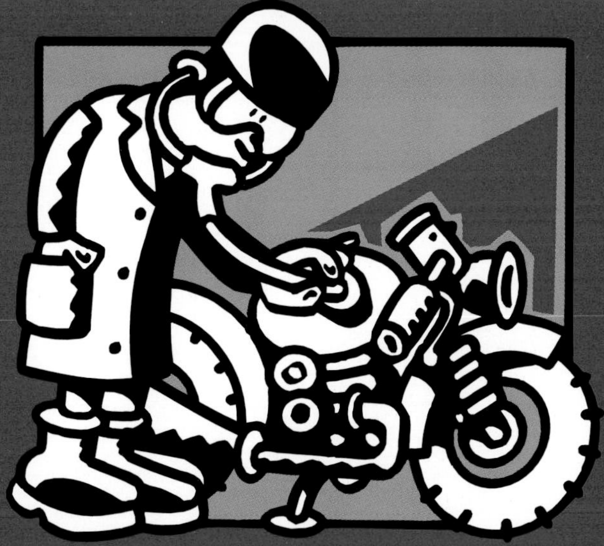

DISEASES AND DISORDERS

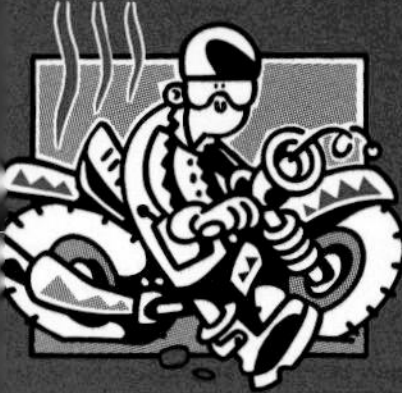

18. Oesophagus

ANATOMY, PHYSIOLOGY, AND FUNCTION OF THE OESOPHAGUS

The oesophagus is a muscular tube composed of two layers:

- An outer longitudinal layer.
- An inner circular muscle layer.

The oesophagus connects the pharynx to the stomach. Striated muscle in the upper portion gradually changes to smooth muscle in the lower part and continues with the muscle layer of the stomach. The lining of the oesophagus also changes from a stratified squamous epithelium to columnar epithelium at the gastro-oesophageal junction.

When a food bolus is propelled into the pharynx by the tongue, the upper oesophageal sphincter (controlled by cricopharyngeus muscle) relaxes, allowing the passage of food into the oesophagus. A primary peristaltic wave starts from the pharynx and continues down along the length of oesophagus. Secondary peristalsis occurs locally due to distension of the oesophagus by a food bolus. The lower oesophageal sphincter (LOS) relaxes prior to peristaltic contractions when swallowing is initiated. The progression of a peristaltic swallow wave can be followed by placing pressure transducers at intervals along the oesophagus (oesophageal manometry; see Figs 17.9 and 17.10).

Preventing regurgitation of the stomach contents back in to the oesophagus is dependent on:

- Gravity.
- LOS pressure.
- The oblique course of the gastro-oesophageal junction.
- The diaphragmatic crura wrapped around the oesophagus.
- The physiological emptying of the stomach contents into the duodenum through the pylorus.

INFLAMMATORY CONDITIONS

Reflux oesophagitis

Incidence

A common condition of which the incidence increases with age. This may be related to the fact that hiatus hernias are found more commonly in elderly people.

Clinical features

A variety of symptoms are associated with the reflux of gastric acid contents to the oesophagus. When the symptoms produce upper abdominal pain, belching, or heartburn, they are referred to collectively as dyspepsia. Otherwise, more specific terms should be used to describe them:

- Heartburn is the most common presenting symptom due to reflux of gastric acid into the oesophagus. This can cause erosive oesophagitis. It worsens on stooping forward and is relieved by antacids. Correlation between symptoms and extent of oesophagitis is poor.
- Chest pain can be due to spasm of the distal oesophageal muscle or from inflammation. It characteristically radiates to the back between the shoulder blades. It may mimic cardiac pain because it can also be relieved by sublingual nitrates. Acid reflux occasionally can cause coronary arterial spasm producing angina pectoris.
- Vomiting of blood (haematemesis) can present in association with severe oesophagitis.
- Iron deficiency anaemia can occur due to insidious blood loss from chronic inflammation.
- Cough due to early morning bronchospasm and nocturnal cough may occur as a result of reflux with microaspiration into the trachea. There is some evidence that acid in the oesophagus can precipitate reflex bronchospasm. There is a high prevalence of reflux in asthmatics and an increased prevalence of bronchospasm in patients with reflux.

Diagnosis and investigation

Endoscopy

This may show the varying grades of oesphagitis and in severe cases, ulceration. However, normal endoscopy does not exclude reflux oesophagitis.

Twenty-four hour intraluminal pH monitoring

This is probably the most accurate way of detecting reflux disease because there is a reasonable correlation between low pH (<4) occurring within the 24-hour period and symptoms of reflux (see Figs 17.11 and 17.12).

Barium swallow

This is still used, but is only significant when a free reflux of barium is demonstrated. The presence of a hiatus hernia alone has no diagnostic relevance in reflux oesophagitis.

Aetiology and pathogenesis

A reduction in tone of the LOS is the main factor contributing to acid reflux. This normally occurs when the patient lies down or if there is raised intra-abdominal pressure (e.g. pregnancy, obesity, weight lifting, chronic constipation). Reduction in the resistance of the oesophageal mucosa to acid and delayed gastric emptying will also predispose to acid reflux. Drugs such as non-steroidal anti-inflammatory and anticholinergic drugs may also aggravate symptoms of reflux.

Alcohol and smoking have also been implicated in its pathogenesis: smoking reduces LOS tone and alcohol stimulates gastric acid production.

A sliding-type hiatus hernia, where the gastro-oesophageal junction lies above the diaphragm, is associated with oesophageal reflux. However, its presence alone is not diagnostic because not all patients with hiatus hernia will develop symptoms.

Complications

Stricture

Stricture occurs after long-standing acid reflux, causing stricture of the lower oesophagus, producing symptoms of dysphagia.

Barrett's oesophagus

Columnarization of squamous epithelium (metaplasia) occurs with chronic reflux. Cells that develop other abnormal features may become dysplastic with potential for malignant transformation. This may be prevented or possibly even reversed by antireflux therapy.

Prognosis

Over 50% of patients will have significant improvement with only conservative treatment.

Aims of treatment

Treatment is mainly for symptom control. Barrett's oesophagus should be treated and surveillance for development of dysplastic features should be undertaken by endoscopy.

Treatment

Treatment may include:

- Conservative treatments, such as weight reduction, cessation of smoking, and reduction in alcohol consumption, will help symptoms in mild cases. If reflux is mainly nocturnal, then raising the head of the bed may be of benefit. Regular meals and avoidance of fatty food is important.
- Antacids, such as magnesium trisilicate or alginate-containing compounds (Gaviscon), coat the mucosa and will abolish symptoms in most mild cases.
- H_2-receptor antagonists, e.g. cimetidine or ranitidine, work by reducing acid production in the stomach.
- Proton pump inhibitors, e.g. omeprazole is a potent inhibitor of acid production. It, or other proton pump inhibitors, is the drug of choice for severe symptoms and Barrett's oesophagus because it inhibits almost all acid production from the stomach. Patients with severe reflux may require long-term treatment.
- Prokinetic drugs, e.g. cisapride, can enhance gut motility, probably by increasing the release of acetylcholine. Cisapride improves gastric emptying and also increases LOS pressure.
- Surgery. Tightening the lower oesophagus by wrapping the fundus of the stomach around it (fundoplication) is reserved for patients who are symptomatic despite conforming with treatment. Patients should be carefully selected. Too tight a wrap results in dysphagia.

Barrett's oesophagus

Incidence

About 15% of patients with prolonged reflux of acid into the lower oesophagus have Barrett's oesophagus.

Aetiology and pathogenesis

Prolonged irritation causes the transformation (metaplasia) from squamous epithelium to columnar-type gastric epithelium, which is covered by mucin (Fig. 18.1). Metaplastic change is occasionally followed by

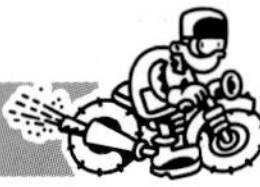

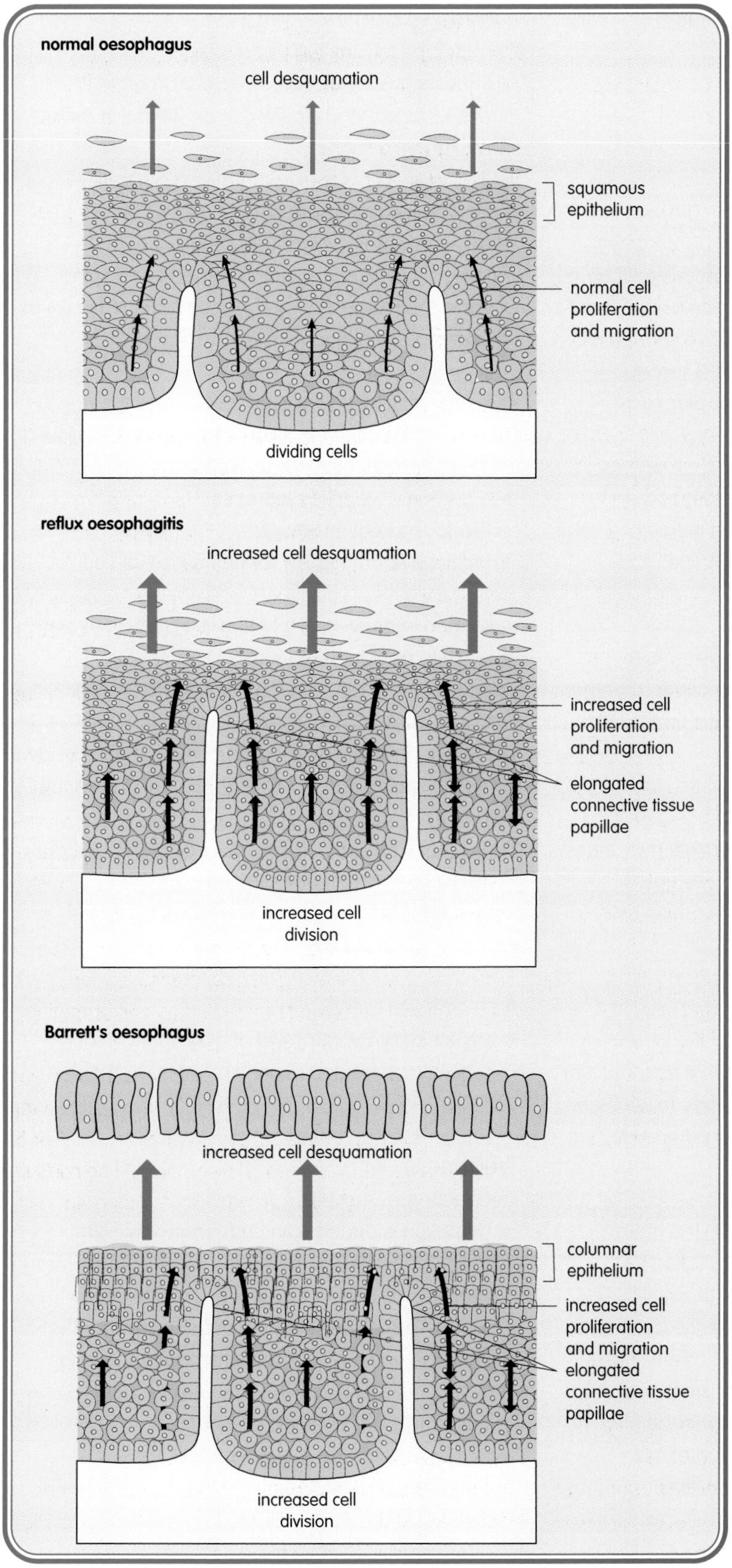

normal oesophagus

cell desquamation

squamous epithelium

normal cell proliferation and migration

dividing cells

reflux oesophagitis

increased cell desquamation

increased cell proliferation and migration

elongated connective tissue papillae

increased cell division

Barrett's oesophagus

increased cell desquamation

columnar epithelium

increased cell proliferation and migration

elongated connective tissue papillae

increased cell division

Fig. 18.2 Changes in Barrett's mucosa: the normal squamous epithelium is replaced by columnar epithelium. Cells with abnormal nuclear material constitute dysplastic change and herald malignant transformation.

dysplastic change predisposing to malignant transformation.

Clinical features

The clinical features are the same as for reflux oesophagitis.

Diagnosis and investigation

Seen at endoscopy, where normal squamous epithelium is replaced by columnar epithelium (metaplasia). Barrett's oesophagus manifests endoscopically as a change of colour, from pink to slightly orange, and of texture. Histological examination will confirm the diagnosis.

Complications

Barrett's oesophagus predisposes to adenocarcinoma of the oesophagus. This tumour has an increasing prevalence throughout the developed world.

Prognosis

Adequate treatment with a proton pump inhibitor abolishes symptoms of reflux and may allow columnar epithelium to return to normal squamous epithelium, thus avoiding premalignant change.

Treatment

Proton pump inhibitors such as omeprazole may be given long-term to prevent recurrence. Repeated endoscopies may be required to monitor dysplastic change if present.

Oesophageal strictures

Incidence

Benign strictures secondary to reflux are becoming less common among the reflux population because of the availability of H_2 antagonists and proton pump inhibitors.

Clinical features

Dysphagia, or difficulty in swallowing, is the main presenting symptom. This can be progressive from solids to liquids as fibrosis worsens.

Weight loss can be marked because the patient may have difficulty maintaining the required caloric intake. The patient may often give a history of preceding reflux that disappeared before the onset of dysphagia as the stricture prevented reflux. Symptoms can mimic malignant stricture, making diagnosis difficult.

Diagnosis and investigation

Consider the following investigations:

- Endoscopy can show extensive scarring of the oesophagus, and biopsy can be helpful in excluding malignant disease.
- Barium swallow is an alternative if the patient cannot tolerate endoscopy. A smooth diffuse stricture can be seen usually without shouldering.
- Imaging by endoluminal ultrasound or a spiral computed tomography (CT) scan may be necessary to exclude malignant infiltration (Fig. 18.2).

Aetiology and pathogenesis

Long-standing acid reflux causes permanent scarring and fibrosis. Other causes include:

- Ingestion of caustic substance.
- Previous radiotherapy.
- Previous sclerotherapy for oesophageal varices.

Prolonged intubation of a nasogastric tube can also give rise to benign strictures.

Complication

There is an increased incidence of malignant change in benign strictures, but this may reflect the underlying pathology.

Prognosis

Once a stricture has formed, the condition is likely to remain throughout life.

Aim of treatment

Purely for symptomatic relief of dysphagia. Reflux should also be treated to prevent worsening of the condition.

Treatment

Treatment may include:

- Dilatation is undertaken endoscopically with graduated tubes of increasing sizes inserted through the affected part of the oesophagus to widen the lumen. The procedure may need to be repeated because narrowing of the lumen recurs over a period of time. Endoscopic balloon dilatation is an alternative which is probably safer.
- Surgery—required if dilatation fails to control symptoms of dysphagia.

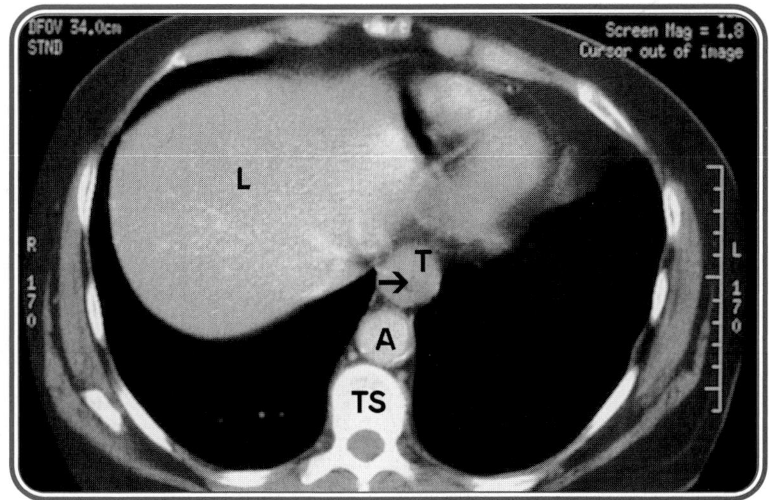

Fig. 18.2 Computed tomography (CT) scan demonstrating malignant infiltration from an oesophageal stricture. Only a pinhole lumen remains of the oesophagus (arrow), which is surrounded by tumour (T). (A, aorta; L, liver; TS, thoracic spine.)

NEOPLASIA

Carcinoma of oesophagus

Incidence

Occurs in approximately 10 out of 100 000 people in the UK. A higher rate is seen in parts of China and Africa, possibly related to local diet.

Clinical features

Dysphagia is the most common presenting symptom, and is progressive from solids to liquids.

Other features include:

- Weight loss—due to anorexia as well as dysphagia.
- Anaemia due to ulceration of the lesion is common, and may cause insidious blood loss, resulting in iron deficiency anaemia.
- Pain on swallowing (odynophagia) occurs in advanced stages; local infiltration by the tumour causes diffuse pain over oesophageal area.
- Dyspnoea and cough, due to aspiration of pharyngeal secretions. In advanced cases, this may be due to oesophagotracheal fistulae or tracheal encasement.

Diagnosis and investigation

Consider the following investigations:

- Endoscopy—the investigation of choice because it allows direct visualization of the lesion and an opportunity for biopsy and histological confirmation.
- Barium swallow—reserved for patients who cannot tolerate an endoscopy, or those suspected of having a high-level stricture. Malignant strictures characteristically have a shouldered appearance (see Fig. 2.3B).
- Endoscopic ultrasound and spiral CT scan of thorax—used for staging if surgery is under consideration. Commonly, this is precluded by the frailty of the patient or concomitant medical conditions .

Aetiology and pathogenesis

Rarely seen under age of 50 years. Two histological types are seen:

- Squamous carcinoma.
- Adenocarcinoma.

Squamous carcinoma:

- 90% of cases: over half occur in lower third of oesophagus.
- Higher incidence in China, which may suggest a dietary aetiology.
- More common in men, particularly with high alcohol intake and cigarette smoking.
- Predisposing factors include achalasia, Plummer–Vinson syndrome, and tylosis (hyperkeratosis of palms and soles inherited as an autosomal dominant condition).

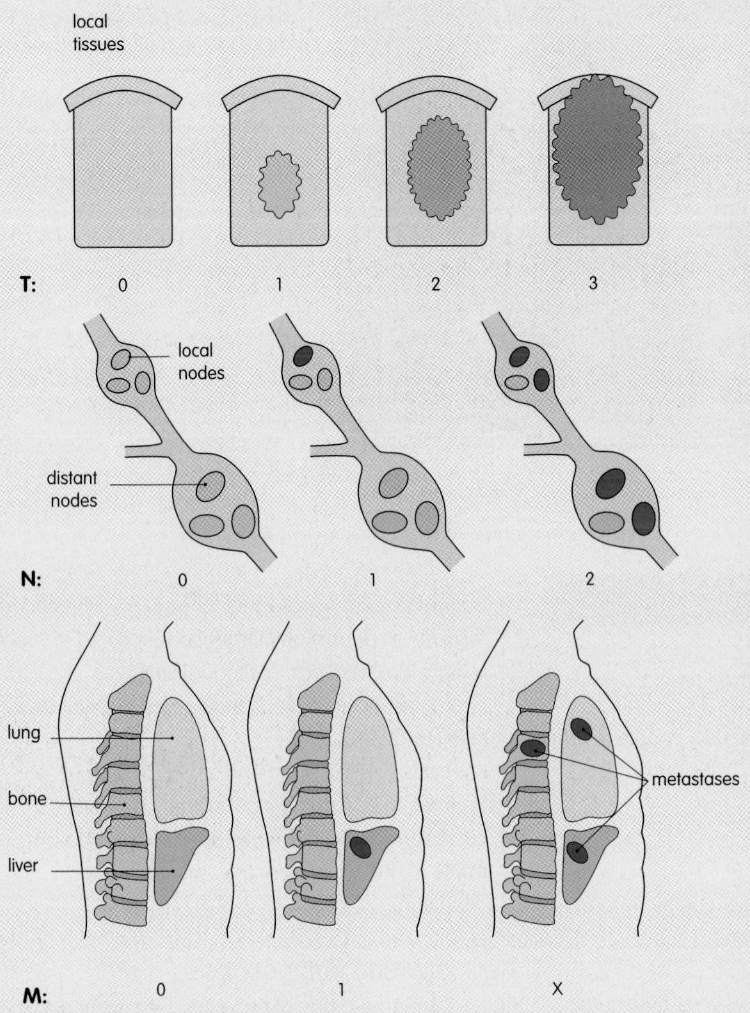

local tissues

T: 0 1 2 3

local nodes

distant nodes

N: 0 1 2

lung

bone

liver

metastases

M: 0 1 X

T = graded 0–4, refers to the primary tumour according to its depth of involvement
TO = no evidence of primary tumour

N = 0–2, refers to lymph nodes involved; increasing score indicates higher numbers of lymph node involvment

M = 0 or 1 refers to presence and absence of metastases. The example shown might be for carcinoma of the colon

Fig. 18.3 Graphic illustration of the TNM classification of mucosal malignant disease.

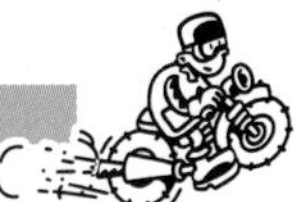

Adenocarcinoma:

- Usually as a result of malignant transformation of Barrett's oesophagus.
- Occasionally it arises as an extension from adenocarcinoma of gastric cardia.

Complications

The tumour may erode:

- Through the oesophagus and into a bronchus, resulting in an oesophageal–bronchial fistula producing recurrent pneumonia.
- Into the aorta, resulting in rapid exsanguination.

Prognosis

Poor, with an overall survival of 2% at 5 years.

Treatment

Mainly palliative because curative treatment is rarely possible due to late presentation of the disease. Consider:

- Surgery—provides the only possible cure but carries an operative mortality of 10%. Less than 40% of patients are suitable for surgical resection at presentation, but these patients are often elderly and frail, and associated medical conditions often preclude radical surgery.
- Radiotherapy—reduces the bulk of the tumour and may relieve dysphagia. Fistula formation is more common after radiotherapy treatment.
- Laser therapy—high-energy thermal laser ablation is used to burn through the bulk of tumour and restore oesophageal lumen. An alternative for smaller tumours is photodynamic therapy, using a lower energy laser light in combination with a chemical photosensitizer which is selectively taken up by tumour tissue. Repeated administration of either modality may be required.
- Endoscopic placement of a plastic or expanding metal hollow stent (endoprosthesis) across the obstructing lesion can give palliative relief of dysphagia. This carries a risk of perforation in 10% of patients.

TNM classification of tumours

The approach to management of many malignant tumours depends on their stage. In addition, a comparison of treatment strategies is heavily reliant on making sure that like is compared with like.

An internationally accepted classification for tumours is the TNM staging system. This system varies for different organs and tissues but follows the general principle shown in Fig. 18.3:

- 'T' refers to the extent of the tumour itself: T0 usually indicates no detectable tumour, T1 is confined to mucosa, and T3+ is infiltrating deeper layers or surrounding structures depending on the site.
- Similarly, 'N' refers to lymph node involvement, N0 meaning no node involvement, N1 is usually confined to local nodes and N2+ is confined to more distant nodes specified for that tumour type.
- Very distant nodes are usually classified as 'M' for metastatic. M0 means no metastases detected, Mn indicates distant spread, again 'n' having a specific meaning for each tumour type.

Thus, T4N2M2 is a tumour with:

- Extensive local infiltration.
- Distant lymph node involvement.
- Metastatic spread to other sites.

ANATOMICAL AND FUNCTIONAL PROBLEMS

Pharyngeal pouch and oesophageal diverticulum

Incidence

Usually found coincidentally on barium meal performed for other reasons.

Clinical features

The main features are:

- Asymptomatic.
- Rare cause of dysphagia.
- Can cause regurgitation of food.

Diagnosis and investigation

Barium swallow demonstrates the size and location of the lesion (Fig. 18.4).

Aetiology and pathogenesis

Probably related to dysmotility of cricopharyngeus muscle and inferior constrictor forming a mucosal outpouching (pharyngeal pouch). Diverticulae may also occur in the mid-oesophagus due to traction by

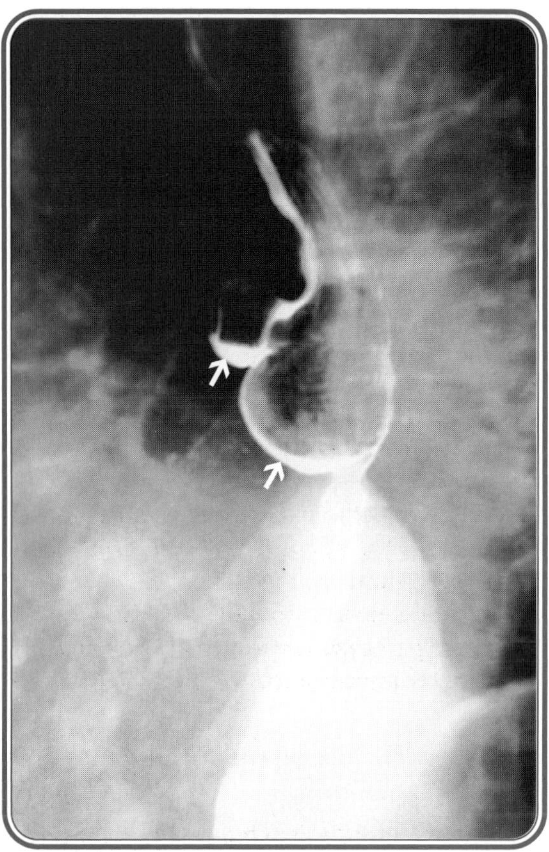

Fig. 18.4 Lateral view of oesophageal diverticulum (arrows) in the upper oesophagus seen on barium swallow. Note the fluid levels.

mediastinal lymph node inflammation (traction diverticulum), or just above the lower oesophageal sphincter (epiphrenic diverticulum).

Complications

Rarely any. Perforation may occur when endoscopy is performed for investigation of dysphagia because the pouch may be mistaken for the oesophageal lumen.

Treatment

Surgical resection for pouches that are problematic.

Oesophageal webs

Incidence

Oesophageal web is often a coincidental finding on barium meal. Those associated with iron deficiency anaemia are rare.

Clinical features

Usually the patient is asymptomatic, but high level dysphagia may occur when tough fibrous food is swallowed without care. A chronic cough may be present due to the aspiration of pharyngeal secretions.

Anaemia may present as part of the Plummer–Vinson syndrome (see below).

Diagnosis and investigation

- Barium swallow—demonstrates narrowing of the oesophagus by fibrous tissue. Proximal part of the oesophagus may be distended with barium.
- Endosopy—webs may be difficult to see, especially those in the postcricoid area.

Aetiology and pathogenesis

Unknown aetiology. Different clinical outcome depending on site of the web. Two types are commonly recognized:

- Postcricoid web.
- Lower oesophageal web.

Postcricoid web:

- Is also know as Plummer–Vinson or Paterson–Brown–Kelly syndrome.
- Is associated with iron deficiency anaemia and atrophic glossitis.

Lower oesophageal web:

- Is also known as Schatzki ring, where there is a small, fibromuscular band that originates from the diaphragm.
- Is often associated with a hiatus hernia.

Complications

There is an increased risk of developing postcricoid carcinoma of the pharynx associated with Plummer–Vinson syndrome.

Treatment

Dilatation of the obstruction is rarely needed.

Iron may be required if iron deficiency anaemia associated with Plummer–Vinson syndrome is present.

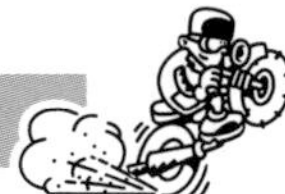

Achalasia

Incidence

Achalasia is a rare condition with a prevalence of approximately 1:100 000.

Clinical features

These include:

- Intermittent dysphagia—usually a long history with both liquids and solids. Presentation in childhood is rare.
- Regurgitation—common; may result in aspiration pneumonia if it occurs at night-time. Dysphagia can sometimes be overcome by drinking large quantities of fluid, hence increases risk of aspiration.
- Chest pain—this is common and is typically retrosternal and occasionally severe, due to non-peristaltic contraction of oesophageal muscles. Often mistaken for cardiac pain, especially when dysphagic symptoms are mild.

Diagnosis and investigation

The following investigations should be considered:

- Chest X-ray—may show a double cardiac shadow with a fluid level behind the heart. Aspiration pneumonia may also be present.
- Barium swallow—dilatation of the oesophagus is seen with a narrowed lower portion (beak appearance) due to lack of relaxation by the lower oesophageal sphincter (Fig. 18.5). Reduced peristaltic contraction is also seen.
- Endoscopy—usually passes through the narrowing part without resistance, and is therefore often missed. Biopsy is taken to confirm the diagnosis and exclude underlying malignancy.
- Motility studies—are used to confirm lack of peristalsis along the oesophagus and failure of relaxation by the lower oesophageal sphincter (see Fig. 17.10B).
- Endoscopic ultrasound—may be helpful in excluding submucosal malignant infiltration.

Aetiology and pathogenesis

Unknown aetiology. Characterized by lack of peristalsis and failure of relaxation by the lower oesophageal sphincter after swallowing.

Histology shows a reduction of Auerbach plexus ganglia cells in the oesophageal walls.

Infection with *Trypanosoma cruzi* (Chagas disease or American trypanosomiasis) will produce a similar appearance.

Complications and prognosis

There is an increased risk of developing oesophageal carcinoma (up to 10% higher than normal population). Reflux oeosphagitis is a major complication after treatment.

Treatment

Treatment may include:

- Dilatation with high pressure balloons—this is undertaken endoscopically and is successful in over two-thirds of cases.
- Surgical division of muscle fibres at lower end of oesophagus (cardiomyotomy)—can now be done laparoscopically.
- Calcium antagonists, e.g. nifedipine, reduce oeosphageal spasm and may be used by elderly patients who are unsuitable for procedures.

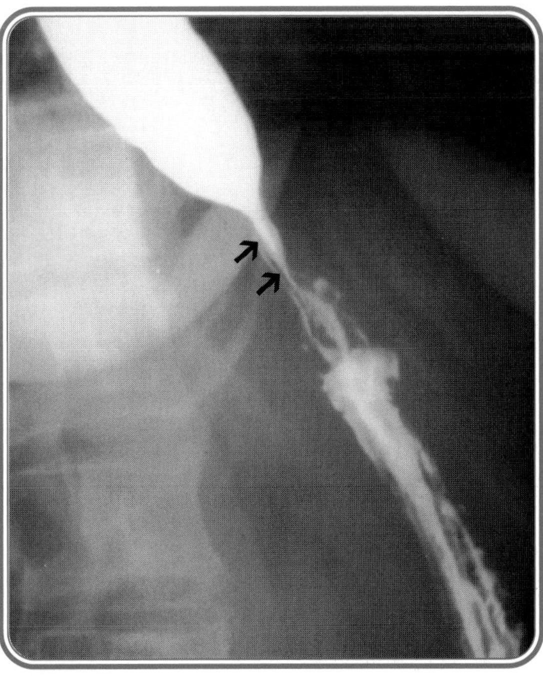

Fig. 18.5 Barium swallow showing bird's beak appearance of achalasia.

Oesophageal spasm

Clinical features

Chest pain is retrosternal and severe, and often radiates to the back. It can be relieved by nitrates, hence, it is difficult to distinguish from cardiac pain. Dysphagia can occur due to marked contraction of oesophageal muscles.

Diagnosis and investigation

The following investigations may be used:

- Barium swallow—characteristically demonstrates a 'corkscrew' appearance due to uncoordinated contraction of oesophageal muscles (see Fig. 1.5). However, similar changes may be seen in elderly people without any symptoms.
- Motility studies—show diffuse contraction of oesophageal muscle without progression of peristalsis. Pressures can be very high ('nutcracker' oesophagus).

Aetiology and pathogenesis

Unknown aetiology. After swallowing, the oesophagus contracts diffusely in an uncoordinated fashion without peristalsis, hence the onset of dysphagia and chest pain.

Complications

Formation of diverticula is commonly associated with oesophageal spasm. Cricopharyngeal spasm is closely related to formation of pharyngeal pouches.

Treatment

Drugs such as antispasmodics, calcium channel antagonists, or nitrates may be of help. Surgery, such as myotomy, may be required in exceptional cases.

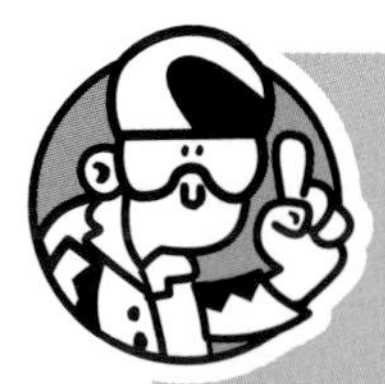

Oesophageal and cardiac pain can be difficult to distinguish. Exercise electrocardiogram and coronary angiography may be necessary, as well as 24-hour oesophageal pH and motility studies.

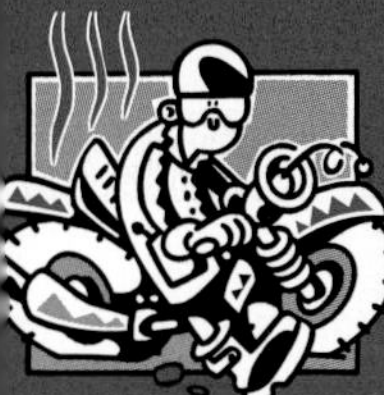

19. Stomach

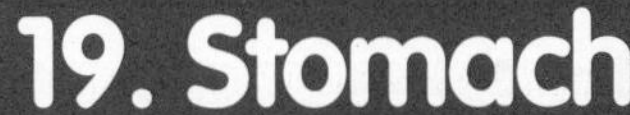

ANATOMY, PHYSIOLOGY, AND FUNCTION OF THE STOMACH

The stomach is divided into:

- An upper portion known as the fundus.
- The body of the stomach.
- The antrum, which extends to form the pyloric region, where the pyloric sphincter is found (Fig. 19.1).

Three muscle layers form the stomach: outer longitudinal, middle circular, and inner oblique. The thickened circular layer at the pyloric area forms the pyloric sphincter.

The upper two-thirds of the stomach contains:

- Parietal cells which secrete acid (hydrochloric acid).
- Chief cells which secrete pepsinogen.

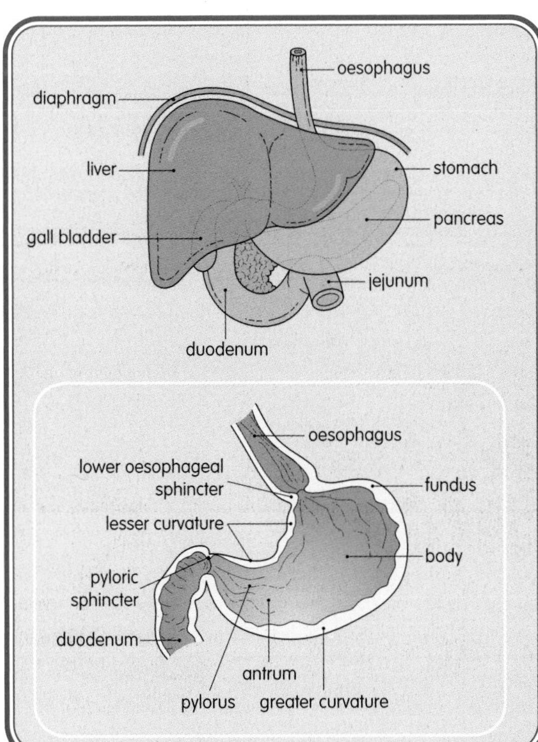

Fig. 19.1 Anatomical relations of the stomach.

The antrum secretes gastrin from G-cells which stimulates acid production.

Acid secretion consists of three different phases (Fig. 19.2):

- Cephalic-mediated via the vagus stimulated by sight or smell of food.
- Gastric distension of the stomach by food directly stimulates secretory cells.
- Intestinal hormones are released as food is passed into small intestine, stimulateing acid release.

A low pH in the stomach is required to activate enzymes required for digestion and to act as a barrier to bacteria. Other functions of the stomach include secretion of intrinsic factor and, of minor importance, absorption of glucose and amino acids.

As the stomach is the port of entry to the body, ingestion of unsuitable material can cause problems. These manifest as nausea, vomiting, or pathologically, as acute gastritis. Other entities are categorized according to pathological mechanisms.

ACUTE GASTRITIS

Incidence

A very common condition with a variety of causes.

Clinical features

These include:

- Nausea and vomiting are the most likely presenting symptoms, together with indigestion.
- Acute gastrointestinal bleed if gastritis is severe.
- Asymptomatic.

Diagnosis and investigation

Often made on clinical grounds, e.g. history of non-steroidal anti-inflammatory drugs (NSAIDs), heavy alcohol consumption, etc.

Endoscopy appearance can vary from superficial erosions to haemorrhage secondary to acute ulceration.

Aetiology and pathogenesis

The pathological appearance is that of an acute inflammatory infiltrate in the superficial mucosa, predominantly of neutrophils. Occasionally, superficial ulceration can be seen. Drugs such as aspirin and other NSAIDs reduce the production of prostaglandin and interfere with cytoprotection. Alcohol damages the mucosal mucus layer and causes gastritis. *Helicobacter pylori* can also cause acute gastritis, but is more commonly associated with chronic gastritis.

Superficial ulceration can develop in acutely ill patients, e.g. acute renal failure, liver disease, sepsis, etc. The exact mechanism is unknown but may be related to the alteration in the mucus barrier.

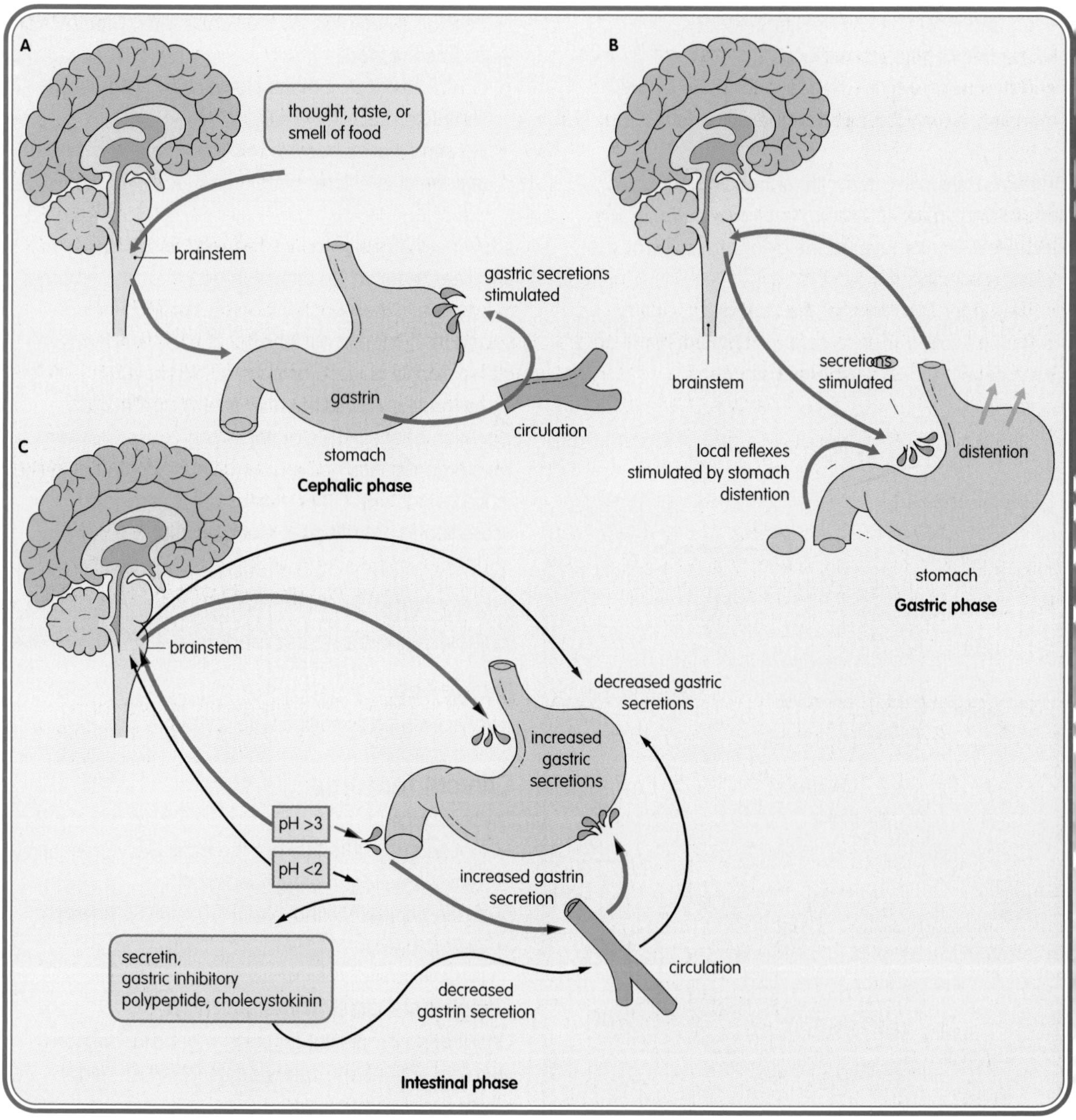

Fig. 19.2 Physiology of acid secretion. (A) Cephalic phase in which taste, visual and olfactory senses act through the brainstem and parasympathetic system to cause gastrin secretion, which in turn stimulates acid production. (B) Gastric phase in which ingested food distends the stomach and stretch receptors act through brainstem reflexes to increase gastric secretions. (C) Food in the intestine has different effects depending upon the pH. At higher pH the pathways are stimulatory and increase gastric secretion further (red lines); at lower pH negative and inhibitory factors come into play to reduce gastric secretion.

Prognosis and treatment

Patients usually recover without any long-term complications. The removal of the offending cause is usually all that is required. An acute GI bleed should be treated in the conventional way. An H_2 antagonist may be of help in some cases.

PEPTIC ULCER DISEASE

Under this heading we include gastritis, gastric ulcer, and duodenal ulcer, which is dealt with here rather than in Chapter 20. These conditions are all associated with *H. pylori* infection.

Helicobacter pylori infection

Incidence

It is estimated that 50% of the population over the age of 50 years are infected with *H. pylori* in developed countries. The incidence is declining with improved sanitation, and there is evidence that most infection is acquired in childhood. In certain parts of the world, e.g. South America, most of the population is infected.

Clinical features

Often patients are found with infection incidentally and have no symptoms. This and the high prevalence of *H. pylori* infection without entities like duodenal ulcer disease in certain populations (e.g. Nigeria) indicate that host factors also have a role in producing pathology and symptoms.

Epigastric abdominal pain described as gnawing and sometimes associated with nausea or vomiting is common. Initially, this can be due to acute gastritis which progresses to chronic gastritis with or without peptic ulcer disease (Fig. 19.3).

Epidemiological data suggest that there is an increased risk of gastric carcinoma, and long-standing gastritis increases the risk of gastric lymphoma.

Diagnosis and investigation

The following investigations may be useful:

- Endoscopy may demonstrate a blotchy mucosal appearance and a biopsy can be taken for urease test, histology, or culture to confirm the presence of *H. pylori.*
- Urease test: an antral biopsy is added to a preprepared urea solution containing a colour reagent. If urease is present, a colour change occurs and is taken to indicate the presence of the bacterium.
- Histology: the bacteria can be detected histologically by routine staining and section.
- Culture: can be achieved in special medium.
- Urea breath test: ^{14}C or ^{13}C radiolabelled urea is given orally and in the presence of *H. pylori* will

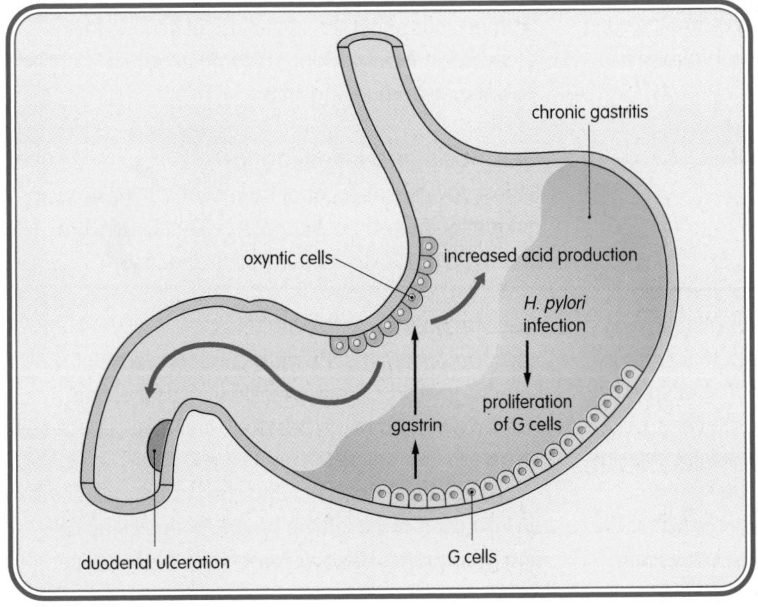

Fig. 19.3 Pathophysiological representation of mechanisms of Helicobacter-induced gastritis.

break down to ammonia and CO_2, which is absorbed and can be measured in the exhaled breath (see Fig. 17.8).

- Serology: a relatively specific antibody can now be measured in serum using an ELISA technique, but its clinical value is limited because it confirms past exposure rather than current infection and it is not helpful in confirming eradication.

Aetiology and pathogenesis

The exact mechanism remains obscure but it is thought that people infected with *H. pylori* have an increased level of gastrin due to G cell hyperplasia in the antrum, which, in turn, predisposes to gastric and duodenal ulceration. There may also be an increase in parietal cell mass and pepsinogen production.

Normal gastric mucosa secretes vitamin C, which is suppressed by *H. pylori*. This may account for the increased incidence of gastric lymphoma and carcinoma that can occur due to loss of reducing activity provided by ascorbic acid.

Most people are infected during childhood and have been associated with overcrowded living conditions. The incidence of infection in many countries is falling as a result of improved living conditions.

Complication

- Acute GI bleed, due to peptic ulcer disease.
- Gastric lymphoma of a particular variety 'Maltoma' has been associated with Helicobacter infection. This is a proliferative disease of the mucosa-associated lymphoid tissue (MALT). Reports of regression following *H. pylori* eradication therapy have been published.

Prognosis

Full eradication is possible for most patients and re-infection rate is low.

Treatment

Different regimens have been described. The most successful regimens currently used involve triple therapy with two antibiotics and a potent antisecretory agent such as a proton pump inhibitor. The antibiotics used are a combination of amoxycillin, clarithromycin, and metronidazole. Currently, this type of triple therapy regimen, employed as a twice-daily dose for 7 days, achieves eradication in more than 80% of patients. The favoured regimens are subject to change continually, making more specific recommendations difficult.

An older triple therapy regimen involved bismuth, metronidazole, and tetracycline for 1 week followed by bismuth alone for 4 weeks. This was usually poorly tolerated because bismuth is unpleasant to take orally.

Any patient receiving metronidazole must avoid alcohol because the drug can inhibit acetaldehyde dehydrogenase and produce unpleasant histamine-induced symptoms if this metabolite builds up.

Chronic gastritis

Incidence

- Can be a progression of acute gastritis.
- *Helicobacter pylori* gastritis is by far the most common aetiological factor.
- Autoimmune gastritis is associated with other autoimmune diseases.

Clinical features

- Most cases are asymptomatic.
- Symptoms are similar to those of acute gastritis, but occurring over a period of time.
- Pernicious anaemia due to loss of intrinsic factor secretion for vitamin B_{12} absorption occurs in patients with autoimmune gastritis.

Diagnosis and investigation

Endoscopy reveals an atrophic mucosa. Intrinsic factor autoantibodies and antiparietal cell antibodies are positive in patients with pernicious anaemia.

Aetiology and pathogenesis

Helicobacter pylori is the most common cause of chronic gastritis. Chronic ingestion of alcohol and NSAIDs may also be contributory, and reflux of bile has also been implicated.

There is loss of parietal and chief cells together with an infiltration of the lamina propria with plasma cells and lymphocytes. Chronic atrophic changes cause intestinal metaplasia.

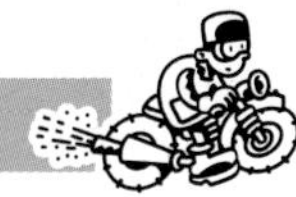

Autoantibodies to parietal cells and intrinsic factor cause achlorhydria and pernicious anaemia with atrophic changes seen in the stomach.

Complications

Intestinal metaplasia predisposes to malignancy.

Treatment

The aim is to treat the underlying cause:

- Eradication therapy for *H. pylori*.
- Vitamin B_{12} is given intramuscularly if pernicious anaemia is present.

For patients requiring NSAIDs, prophylaxis with antisecretory drugs or prostaglandin analogues (misoprostol) may be required.

Gastric ulcer

Incidence

More commonly seen in elderly people, gastric ulceration is less common than duodenal ulceration by a ratio of 1:4. Peak incidence occurs between 50 and 60 years of age.

Clinical features

Epigastric pain can be the main presenting feature. Classically, pain with gastric ulcer is associated with food, whereas duodenal ulcers tend to cause symptoms at night or with an empty stomach and are relieved by food. However, in the majority of cases, the discriminating value of these histories is poor and not helpful in the diagnosis.

Relief by antacids is usually reported.

Associated features include: nausea, heartburn, anorexia, and weight loss. These symptoms also occur with gastric carcinoma. Iron deficiency anaemia is common. Acute GI bleed, perforation, or erosion can occur.

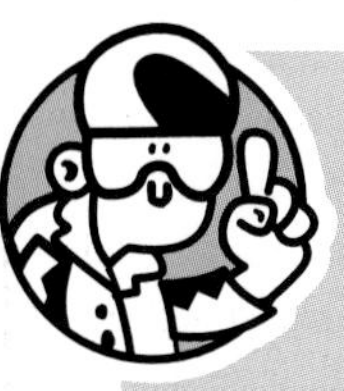

Frequently patients have no pain associated with gastric ulcer, particularly those associated with NSAIDs.

Diagnosis and investigation

Investigations include:

- Endoscopy—the investigation of choice as biopsy makes it possible to differentiate benign from malignant ulcers. During an acute bleed from a vessel, an injection of adrenaline may halt the bleeding.
- Barium meal—will also demonstrate gastric and duodenal ulceration, but biopsies cannot be taken to exclude underlying malignancy.

Aetiology and pathogenesis

The exact aetiology is unknown, but there is an association with NSAIDs, and inhibition of acid usually provides resolution of the ulcer. However, some patients with gastric ulcers have normal or low acid output, especially ulcers occuring at the lesser curve. Theories include:

- A possible defect in the mucosal barrier usually maintained by bicarbonate secretion by the gastric epithelium.
- Prostaglandin-mediated cytoprotection has also been postulated to be deficient.

This may account for the higher incidence seen in elderly people because this cytoprotective mechanism diminishes with age.

Prepyloric ulcers are associated with a high acid output and behave more like a duodenal ulcer.

H. pylori infection also contributes to the development of gastric ulceration.

Differences between malignant and benign gastric ulcers are shown in Fig. 19.4.

Complications

Prepyloric ulcers may cause pyloric stenosis, but this is more commonly seen with duodenal ulcers.

Prognosis

Fifty per cent of gastric ulcers recur within 1 year. It has been suggested that long-term antisecretory medication with H_2 receptor antagonists or proton pump inhibitors (PPI) should be used.

Treatment

Treatment should involve:

- Antisecretory medication, e.g. H_2 antagonists, such as cimetidine or ranitidine, or PPIs such as omeprazole, heal most ulcers.

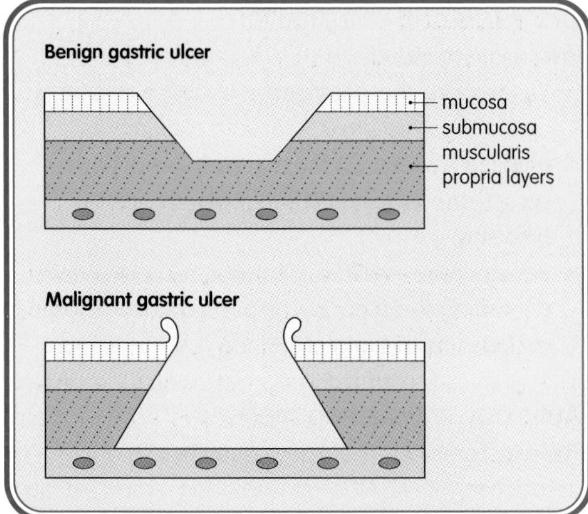

Fig. 19.4 Differences between malignant and benign gastric ulcers. Usually benign ulcers are more superficial. Malignant ulcers have more heaped edges. Multiple biopsy is essential.

- Eradication of *H. pylori*. Bismuth preparation is not very often used because it is unpleasant to take orally. Triple therapy with PPIs and two antibiotics is now more commonly used.
- Sulcralfate, which acts by mucosal protection against action of pepsin, can be useful in resistant cases.
- Avoidance of NSAIDs may be difficult, especially for patients with severe arthritis, but a combined preparation with misoprostol (prostaglandin analogue) is now available to prevent gastric ulceration.
- Discourage smoking because it is linked to increased acid production.

Surgical treatment, such as partial gastrectomy and vagotomy, is now rarely performed, except for patients who have perforated ulcers or have uncontrolled bleeding.

It is essential to review all gastric ulcers endoscopically to ensure healing because this is the only way to be certain they are not malignant.

Duodenal ulcer

Incidence

Approximately 15% of the population will have suffered from duodenal ulceration at some time.

Clinical features

Abdominal pain is mainly epigastric and often intermittent. Classically, duodenal ulcers are said to be be relieved by food or antacids and made worse by hunger. The patient can sometimes point to a specific site of pain in the epigastrium. They can also present with an acute GI bleed.

Diagnosis and investigation

As for gastric ulceration, i.e. endoscopy and biopsy, etc. Tests for *H. pylori* infection should also be done.

Aetiology and pathogenesis

Similar to those of gastric ulceration, i.e. acid production, reduction in cytoprotection, etc. The relationship between *H. pylori* infection and duodenal ulcers is more closely linked because more than 90% of patients with duodenal ulcers are infected with *H. pylori*. The exact pathogenic mechanism remains uncertain.

High acid output states are associated with duodenal ulceration as seen in Zollinger–Ellison syndrome. However over two-thirds of patients have acid secretion within normal limits, which suggests that other factors, such as mucosal barrier and prostaglandin cytoprotection, are involved in its pathogenesis.

Smoking and stress are associated with increased basal output of acid and NSAIDs reduce prostaglandin production, hence predisposing to ulceration.

First degree relatives are at three times the normal risk of developing duodenal ulceration. Blood group O has a 40% increase in risk compared to the general population, especially those who do not secrete group O-related antigen in their gastric mucus glycoprotein.

Complications

Acute GI bleed, especially if there is an erosion of an artery. Gastric outlet obstruction can occur with chronic disease.

Iron deficiency (hypochromic, microcytic) anaemia due to chronic blood loss is unusual in duodenal ulcers and if present, other causes must be sought, such as carcinoma of the colon.

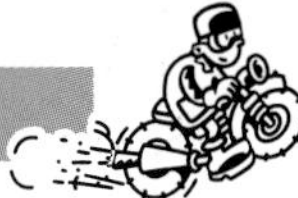

Prognosis

Typically a recurrent disease, approximately 80% of patients relapse within 1 year if no maintenance or eradication therapy is given. Follow-up is not usually necessary in asymptomatic patients.

Treatment

As for those with gastric ulceration.

Eradication therapy should be given in all patients with proven *H. pylori* infection. Some authorities advocate eradication therapy should be given to all patients with duodenal ulceration because the correlation with *H. pylori* infection is so high.

NEOPLASIA OF THE STOMACH

Gastric polyps

Incidence

Rare. Found in approximately 2% of endoscopies.

Clinical features

Majority are asymptomatic. Occasionally they may ulcerate and bleed.

Diagnosis and investigation

Investigations that may be of use include:

- Endoscopy for dyspepsia or abdominal pain often identifies polyps incidentally. If multiple polyps are present, then conditions such as Peutz–Jeghers and familial polyposis coli should be excluded, especially the latter due to its premalignant potential.
- Biopsy will usually confirm the type of polyp present.
- Endoscopic ultrasound may be necessary to exclude submucosal malignant infiltration.

Aetiology and pathogenesis

- Over 90% of polyps are hyperplastic and they are usually harmless.
- Approximately 5% of polyps are adenomas and have similar premalignant potential as those found in the colon.

Rarely, patients with pernicious anaemia have polyps in the fundus, which subsequently turn out to be carcinoid tumours. These may be due to the trophic effects of gastrin secondary to achlorhydria.

Complications

Bleeding and malignant change are the usual complications.

Prognosis and treatment

Resection of the polyp will abolish the malignant risk, hence provide a cure.

Polyps can be removed endoscopically via a snare, but those that are large or sessile may not be suitable, hence multiple biopsies are usually taken and local surgical resection may be required. Hyperplastic polyps are usually left alone unless the patient is symptomatic (Fig. 19.5).

Gastric leiomyoma

Incidence

Most common tumour of the stomach. Autopsy studies have shown the tumour to be present in up to 50% of population over the age of 50 years.

Clinical features

Small tumours are asymptomatic. Larger tumours may ulcerate or bleed causing abdominal pain which can be mistaken for peptic ulcer disease.

Diagnosis and investigation

A leiomyoma is often identified incidentally during an endoscopy carried out for other reasons such as epigastric pain or anaemia.

Aetiology and pathogenesis

A benign tumour of the smooth muscle cells which are submucosal and covered by intact mucosa. Underlying aetiology is unknown.

Treatment

Local resection is curative.

Leiomyosarcoma

Incidence

Accounts for 1% of gastric malignancy.

Clinical features

Similar to those of leiomyoma, except weight loss can be a marked feature. A palpable mass in the epigastrium can be demonstrated in approximately 50% of cases. Larger tumours are more likely to have metastasized at the time of diagnosis to local lymph nodes and lungs.

Treatment
Surgical resection is the treatment of choice.

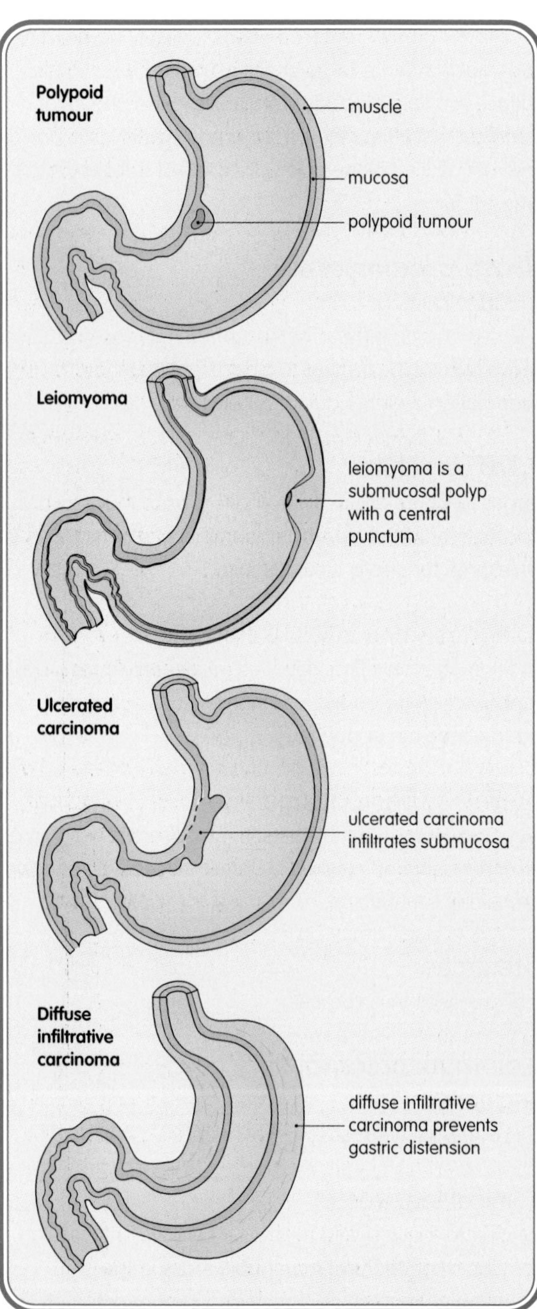

Fig. 19.5 Types of gastric polyps and contrast with leiomyoma and carcinoma.

Ménétrièr's disease
Incidence
Rare.

Clinical features
These include:

- Abdominal pain, vomiting, or bleeding similar to those of chronic gastritis.
- Hypoalbuminaemia due to protein loss from the gastric mucosa.

Diagnosis and investigation
Endoscopy—typical appearance of enlarged thickened folds of mucosa.

Aetiology and pathogenesis
Unknown aetiology. Normal gastric mucosa is replaced by hypertrophied epithelium producing a characteristic appearance. It is not a true 'neoplasia', but can be very difficult to differentiate from infiltrating neoplasms.

Histologically, there is hyperplasia of the mucin-producing glands with glandular proliferation, together with loss of parietal and chief cells (Fig. 19.6). Excessive protein loss occurs through the gastric mucosa via the mucus normally shed.

Complications
The condition is possibly premalignant but the risk is poorly characterized.

Treatment
Treatment includes:

- Antisecretory medication—may be of help to some patients.

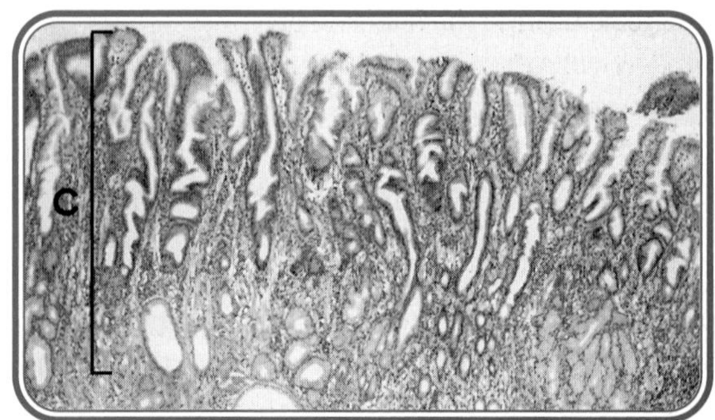

Fig. 19.6 Ménétrièr's disease. The gastric mucosa is grossly thickened due to hypertrophy. Note elongated crypts (C).

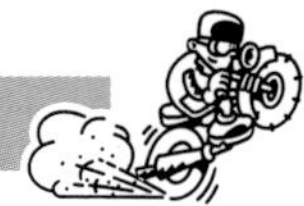

- Partial gastrectomy—may be required to reduce the amount of protein loss.

Gastric carcinoma

Incidence

The frequency of gastric carcinoma increases with age and affects approximately 15 out of 100 000 people in the UK. There is a higher incidence in Japan and the Far East for which dietary factors have been implicated.

Clinical features

These include:

- Abdominal pain similar to that of peptic ulceration, which can be constant and severe if local invasion has occurred.
- Weight loss—often marked and may be the only presenting complaint.
- Nausea, vomiting, and anorexia—these are common features. If the tumour is close to the pylorus, then vomiting can be very marked due to gastric outlet obstruction.
- Anaemia—this occurs as a result of occult blood loss or acute GI bleed.
- Effects of metastases, i.e. to brain, bone, liver, and lung, produce symptoms and variable clinical presentations.

Up to 50% of patients will have a palpable mass at presentation.

Supraclavicular lymph nodes behind the left sternomastoid muscle (Virchow's node) can be palpated in one-third of patients.

Diagnosis and investigation

Investigations of use include:

- Endoscopy—this is the investigation of choice. Care should be taken for biopsy of benign-looking gastric ulcers as negative biopsies can occur. It is essential to repeat endoscopy on any patients with a 'benign' gastric ulcer.
- Barium meal—in the investigation of dyspepsia, barium meal may show a gastric ulcer, or a diffuse infiltrative type of gastric cancer may be seen as a rigid, contracted stomach.

In proven or suspected cases, chest X-ray, liver ultrasound, and computed tomography (CT) scan may be necessary if surgery is contemplated.

Aetiology and pathogenesis

Chronic gastritis leading to metaplasia is a strong risk factor and may be due to *H. pylori* infection. Epidemiological studies show an increased incidence in lower socioeconomic groups which may also be related to *H. pylori* infection.

Dietary factors have been implicated, especially nitrites, which are converted by bacteria at neutral pH to nitrosamines—known to be carcinogenic in animals. Pernicious anaemia is also associated with an increased risk of gastric carcinoma, and this may be partly due to achlorhydria and hence neutral pH in the stomach.

Patients with previous partial gastrectomy are at an increased risk after 20 years.

Genetic predisposition has been described with an increased incidence in people with blood group A.

Gastric polyps are rare, but malignant changes can occur in them and they should be removed.

Two histological types of gastric cancer have been described:

- Glandular adenocarcinoma, similar to that seen throughout the intestine with well-differentiated glandular formation or acini which secrete mucin.
- Diffuse, spreading-type adenocarcinoma with a fibrous stroma giving a fibrotic appearance to the stomach (linea plastica or 'leather-bottle' stomach).

Prognosis

Carcinomas that are confined to the mucosa (rare) have a 90% 5-year survival compared with invasive lesions, which have less than 10% 5-year survival. Early detection appears to be possible in screening programmes such as those in Japan, where gastric carcinoma is common.

Treatment

This includes:

- Surgery—this is the only treatment that can offer a cure. This ranges from partial gastrectomy to radical resection with local lymph node clearance, but is only suitable for patients without widespread metastases.
- Chemotherapy and radiotherapy—these are not usually of use but may be helpful for control of symptoms due to tumour bulk.
- Symptom control with opiate analgesia and antiemetics—can be difficult to achieve.

Gastric lymphoma

Incidence

Accounts for 5–10% of all gastric malignancy in UK.

Clinical features

Same as for gastric carcinoma.

Diagnosis and investigation

Endoscopy and biopsy.

Aetiology and pathogenesis

Nearly all are of non-Hodgkin's B cell type arising from mucosal-associated lymphoid tissue (MALT) rather than a primary lymph node tumour. These tumours are associated with *H. pylori* infections.

Prognosis

Very good, with 80–90% survival depending on the type of lymphoma. Complete excision of the tumour is curative.

Treatment

Treatment options include:

- Surgical resection of the tumour—this is usually required.
- Eradication therapy for *H. pylori*, which can produce regression of certain types.
- Chemotherapy and radiotherapy postoperatively, which may be necessary for metastatic disease.

FUNCTIONAL AND ANATOMICAL DISORDERS

Gastroparesis

Clinical features

Vomiting and nausea are the main symptoms. Weight loss may ensue if the patient avoids eating.

Diagnosis and investigation

Investigations include:

- Barium meal—demonstrates distension of the stomach with markedly reduced passage of barium into the duodenum.
- Radioisotope scan—this is an alternative to barium meal.

Aetiology and pathogenesis

Characterized by reduced motility of the stomach.

Causes include vagotomy or autonomic neuropathy complicating diabetes mellitus. In some cases, no identifiable cause is found.

Complications

Are those associated with prolonged vomiting, i.e. hypokalaemia, aspiration pneumonia, etc.

Treatment

Prokinetic agents such a metoclopramide are often used to enhance gastric emptying. In severe cases, a motilin analogue such as erythromycin may be required.

Gastric outlet obstruction

Incidence

Affects up to 3% of patients with duodenal or prepyloric ulceration.

Clinical features

These include:

- Vomiting—this is the main complaint. Classically, the vomiting is projectile and contains undigested food.
- Pain—which is unusual because the ulcer would have started to heal or scarring has already occurred.
- Succussion splash—may be demonstrated due to distension of stomach with fluid.

Diagnosis and investigation

Investigations should include:

- Barium meal—to demonstrate slow or absent passage of barium into the small intestine.
- Endoscopy—which may also identify the obstruction.

Electrolyte disturbance such as marked metabolic alkalosis can occur because of prolonged vomiting.

Aetiology and pathogenesis

Mainly occurs as a result of long-standing peptic ulcer disease affecting the prepyloric, pylorus, or duodenal area, resulting in scarring and narrowing of the gastric outlet. Gastric outlet obstruction affecting the pylorus is known as pyloric stenosis, which is not to be confused with the congenital type due to hypertrophy of the fibromuscular layer.

Occasionally, the obstruction may be a result of oedema due to an ulcer and this is usually transient.

Gastric outlet obstruction can also be due to external

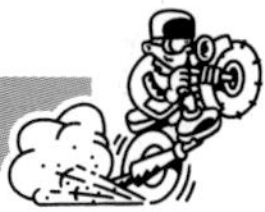

compression from lymph nodes or pancreatic carcinoma, or due to underlying gastric malignancy.

Complications

Those associated with prolonged vomiting, i.e. aspiration pneumonia, electrolyte imbalance, etc.

Treatment

Management should include:

- Correction of electrolyte imbalance and metabolic alkalosis with intravenous fluids.
- Nasogastric tube to aspirate gastric contents and prevent further vomiting.
- Surgical intervention is required unless the obstruction is due to oedema.

POSTGASTRIC SURGERY COMPLICATIONS

The need for gastric surgery to manage peptic ulcer disease is now a rare occurrence but patients who have had surgery previously commonly present with symptoms.

Recurrent ulceration

Incidence

Occurs in approximately 5% of patients after gastric surgery. More common in those with duodenal ulcer.

Clinical features

Similar to those found with duodenal ulceration.

Anaemia and perforation appear to be more common than with primary peptic ulcers.

Diagnosis and investigation

Endoscopy preferred to barium meal due to distorted anatomy.

Aetiology and pathogenesis

As a result of continuing acid production patients with partial gastrectomy without vagotomy are at a higher risk of developing recurrent ulceration compared with patients who had a highly selective vagotomy (only branches to the stomach are severed).

Retained antrum after a Billroth II resection (Fig. 19.7) may be the cause for recurrent ulceration. The antrum may not have been completely resected and continues to produce gastrin because its usual inhibition mechanism is lost (low pH in the antrum inhibits gastrin production). A similar picture may be seen with Zollinger–Ellison syndrome, but this can be distinguished by a lack of gastrin suppression following intravenous administration of secretin.

Treatment

Treatment options:

- H_2 antagonists or proton pump inhibitors are drugs of choice.
- Surgery may be required for retained antrum.

Afferent loop syndrome

Incidence

A rare complication.

Clinical features

Abdominal pain usually occurs up to an hour after meals, associated with distension, nausea, and vomiting. Symptoms are relieved by vomiting.

Diagnosis and investigation

Diagnosis can be difficult, but HIDA scan (see p. 83) may demonstrate bile stasis in the afferent loop.

Aetiology and pathogenesis

Thought to be due to partial obstruction and hence distension of the afferent loop of bowel resulting in incomplete drainage of bile and pancreatic secretions which are stimulated by eating.

Treatment

Surgical revision of the loop is usually required.

Dumping syndrome

Clinical features

Two types have been described:

- Early dumping: usually occurs within 30 minutes after a meal and causes palpitations, lightheadedness, postural hypotension, and sometimes abdominal discomfort.
- Late dumping: typically occurs between 90 minutes and 3 hours after a meal. Similar symptoms of lightheadedness, palpitation, hypotension, and sweating. Syncope may also be seen.

Diagnosis and investigation

Often made on clinical grounds alone. Measurement of serum glucose, electrolytes, and blood pressure during an attack is usually sufficient for diagnosis.

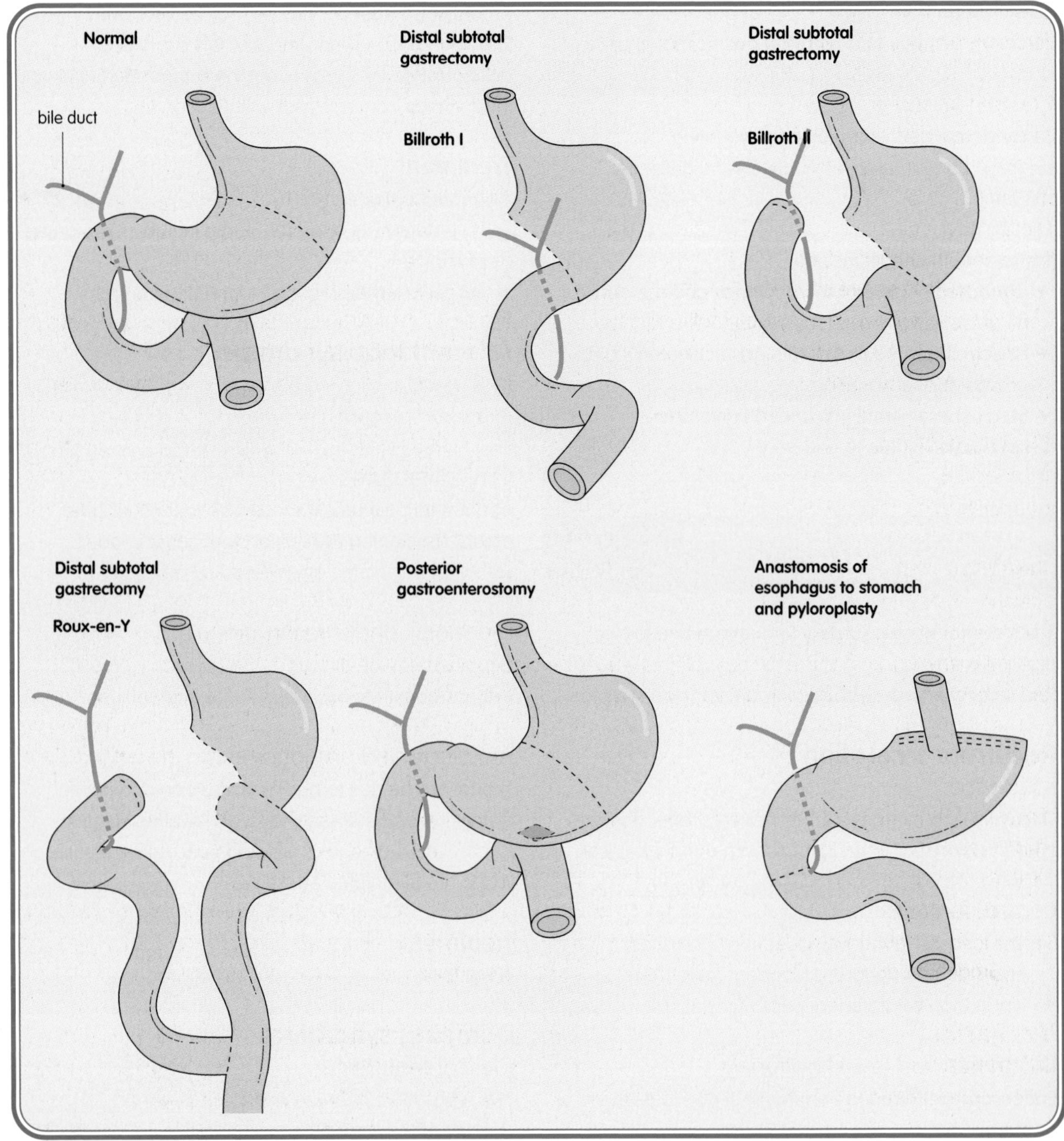

Fig. 19.7 Types of gastrectomy. These not only remove acid-secreting mucosa but also alter the normal anatomy and motility to produce a variety of symptoms. Some re-routing of the duodenum is usually necessary with gastrectomy in order to preserve its relationship to the bile duct.

Aetiology and pathogenesis

Early dumping syndrome is thought to be caused by a vasovagal response to a rapid emptying of gastric contents into the small intestine, resulting in a depletion of intravascular volume secondary to the change in osmotic gradient. Hypokalaemia is noted during such an attack. However, fluid and potassium replacement does not appear to abolish these attacks and there may be some other underlying mechanism involving a complex release of gut hormones.

Late dumping syndrome appears to be caused by hypoglycaemia due to an excessive release of insulin.

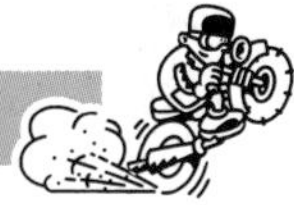

This is thought to occur following transient hyperglycaemia secondary to a rapid emptying of carbohydrate-rich substances in the small intestine. A glucose tolerance test shows an acute hyperglycaemic phase followed by hypoglycaemia.

Treatment

Dietary advice such as small frequent meals may be all that is required in mild cases.

Symptoms in severe cases are very difficult to control. Some have derived symptomatic relief from octreotide (somatostatin analogue) injections but the cost has restricted its use in clinical practice.

Diarrhoea

Incidence

Can affect up to 50% of patients after gastrectomy.

Aetiology and pathogenesis

The exact mechanism is unknown, but patients with truncal vagotomy are affected more commonly.

Other aetiological factors include bile salts and bacterial overgrowth especially in Polya gastrectomy.

Loss of pyloric regulatory emptying mechanism may contribute to diarrhoea.

Treatment

Note that:

- Bile salt diarrhoea can be treated with cholestyramine.
- Bacterial overgrowth can be confirmed with a hydrogen breath test and treated with antibiotics.

Anaemia

Incidence

Often a late common complication of gastrectomy.

Aetiology and pathogenesis

Iron deficiency anaemia is the most common type to be seen and may be related to a reduced amount of hydrochloric acid which solubilizes iron.

Ascorbic acid is also secreted in the normal stomach and aids iron absorption. Supplementing the diet of patients after gastrectomy with vitamin C can improve the anaemia.

A lack of intrinsic factor and bacterial overgrowth will cause macrocytic anaemia due to vitamin B_{12} deficiency.

Diagnosis and investigation

Underlying GI malignancy, whether in the gastric remnant or in the colon, must be excluded when a patient presents with iron deficiency anaemia.

Tests to perform include:

- Serum B_{12} measurement.
- Hydrogen breath test for bacterial overgrowth causing B_{12} deficiency.

Treatment

Oral iron supplements should be given together with ascorbic acid to aid its absorption.

B_{12} injections are given 3-monthly intramuscularly.

Malabsorption

Incidence

Common, and it may contribute to weight loss seen in over 50% of patients after gastrectomy.

Clinical features

The following features may present:

- Weight loss is usually multifactorial.
- Steatorrhoea occurs in severe cases.
- Anaemia is common, as discussed.
- Osteomalacia occurs due to reduced absorption of vitamin D.

Diagnosis and investigation

Depends on clinical presentation.

Mild malabsorption may unmask a subclinical condition such as coeliac disease and pancreatitis and appropriate investigation should be done.

Aetiology and pathogenesis

No single factor accounts for malabsorption seen. The following causes have all been implicated:

- Rapid gastric emptying.
- Reduced capacity of the stomach.
- Reduced bile concentrations in the intestinal lumen.
- Increased gut transit time.

Bacterial overgrowth causing steatorrhoea and reduced absorption of fat soluble vitamins is probably the most important factor.

Treatment

Replacement of trace elements and deficient vitamins.

Carcinoma

Incidence

There is a two-fold increase in the risk of adenocarcinoma at the site of the anastomosis 20 years after gastrectomy. In the interim the risk of gastric carcinoma is less as the stomach has been removed.

Clinical features

Recurrence of epigastric pain in patients who have previously had surgery.

Diagnosis and investigation

Endoscopy, with biopsy of suspicious lesions.

Aetiology and pathogenesis

Bile reflux and *H. pylori* infection have been postulated as potential aetiological factors.

Treatment

Resection of the tumour is required.

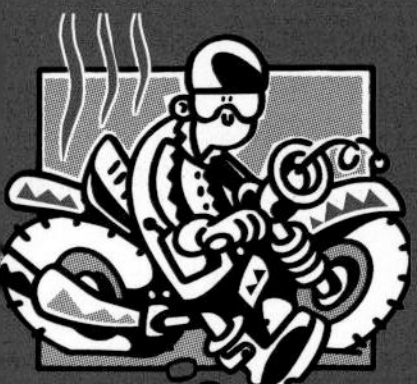

20. Small Intestine

ANATOMY, PHYSIOLOGY, AND FUNCTION OF THE SMALL INTESTINE

The small intestine extends from the duodenum to the terminal ileum where it joins the caecum. The surface area is markedly increased by mucosal folds in the form of villi and microvilli. Each villus contains a core of blood vessels and lymphatic lacteals (Fig. 20.1).

Its main function is absorption of nutrients, i.e. carbohydrate, protein, fat, vitamins, etc. It also secretes IgA locally as part of a defence mechanism against infection.

Absorption takes place via:

- Simple diffusion.
- Active transport (e.g. Na^+/K^+ ATPase for absorption of glucose).
- Facilitated diffusion (a carrier-mediated transport system to allow faster absorption compared with simple diffusion, e.g proteins).

Disease of the small intestine is usually manifest as malabsorption with resultant mineral or vitamin deficiency, weight loss, or diarrhoea.

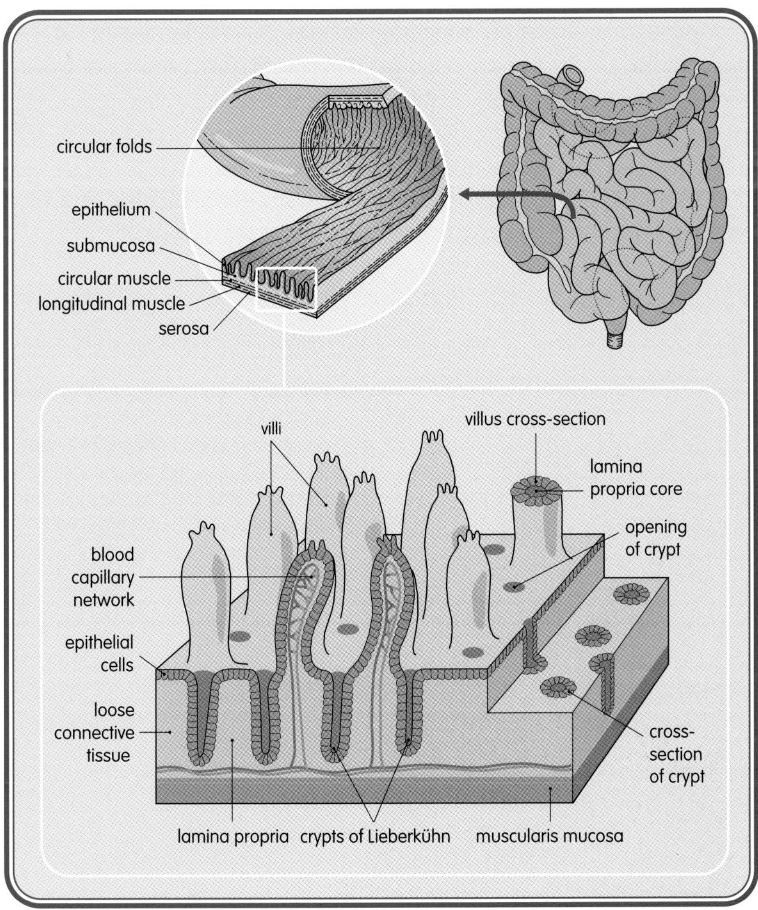

Fig. 20.1 Anatomy of the small intestine with inset showing villous structure.

IMMUNE-RELATED PROBLEMS

Coeliac disease

Incidence

More commonly seen in the west of Ireland, where it occurs in 1 out of 500 compared with an average prevalence in the UK of 1 out of 2000 people. Rarely seen in Black Africans.

Clinical features

Clinical features may include:

- Diarrhoea and steatorrhoea are the most common presentations in adults.
- Abdominal pain and weight loss are associated with general malaise.
- Failure to thrive is the most common presentation in young children.
- Dermatitis herpetiformis is a blistering condition of the skin associated with coeliac disease.
- Hyposplenism is relatively common.
- Howell–Jolly bodies may be seen on a blood film.

Features of mineral and vitamin deficiency may be present, e.g. iron deficiency anaemia, vitamin D deficiency, and osteomalacia.

Diagnosis and investigation

Anaemia can be due to folate or iron deficiency. The blood film will have a dimorphic picture, i.e. both macrocytic and microcytic.

Blood tests may aid diagnosis:

- Biochemistry may show low calcium with or without low phosphate indicative of osteomalacia. Hypoalbuminaemia is seen in severe malabsorption.
- Low urea is usual in any malabsorption.
- Antigliadin or antiendomyseal antibodies can be found in two-thirds of patients.

Duodenal biopsy is the investigation of choice and nowadays is done by endoscopy. Partial or subtotal villous atrophy with increased intraepithelial lymphocytes is diagnostic (Fig. 20.2).

Aetiology and pathogenesis

Due to a gluten sensitivity characterized by villous atrophy of the small intestine, which returns to normal when a gluten-free diet is instituted. Gluten is a high molecular weight compound which is cleaved to alpha, beta-, and gamma gliadin peptides. Alpha-gliadin is said to be toxic to the small bowel and possibly the other forms to a lesser degree.

An immunological basis is likely because of the increased incidence in patients with certain HLA types mainly A1, B8, DR3, DR7, and DQW2. Other autoimmune conditions are also more frequent in patients with coeliac disease.

Viral infections have also been implicated, and the disease may be preceded by an episode of gastroenteritis.

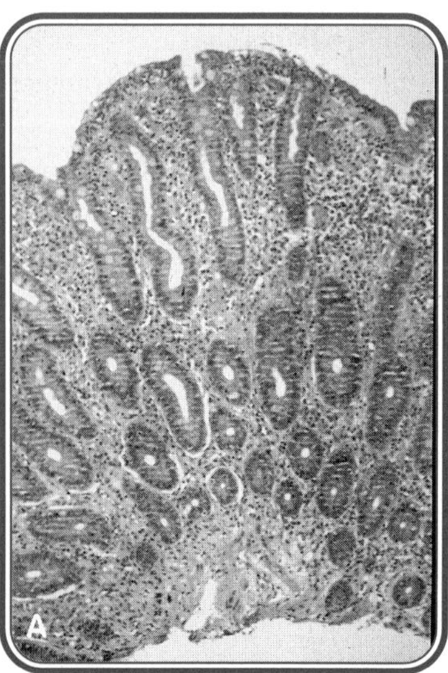

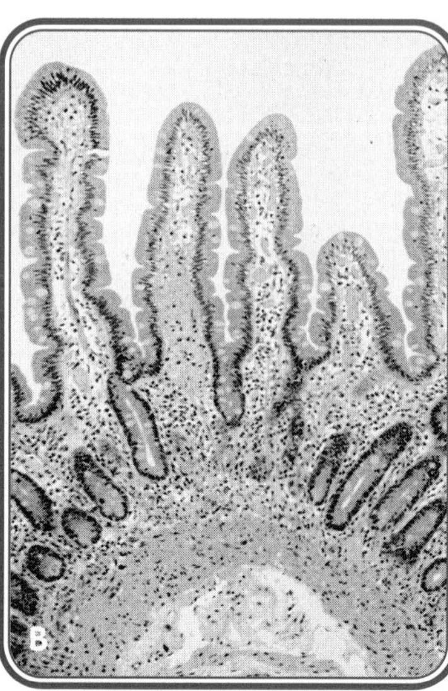

Fig. 20.2 Subtotal villous atrophy in coeliac disease (A) recovers completely with a gluten-free diet (B). Note the increased number of intraepithelial lymphocytes (IEL) and decreased villous height in (A).

Complications

Features of mineral and vitamin deficiency can occur. Severe malnutrition in some cases can result in severe hypoalbuminaemia with ascites and peripheral oedema.

There is an increased risk of developing T-cell lymphoma of the small intestine compared to the normal population but the risk may be reduced by a gluten-free diet. An overall increase in gastrointestinal malignancy is also seen.

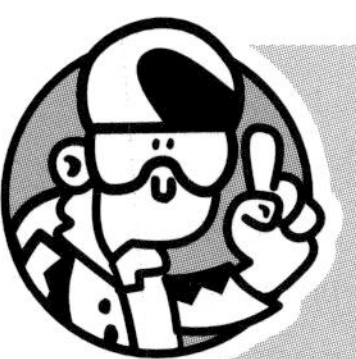

A patient with stable coeliac disease who has recurrence of diarrhoea or weight loss may be unknowingly ingesting gluten or may have developed an intestinal lymphoma.

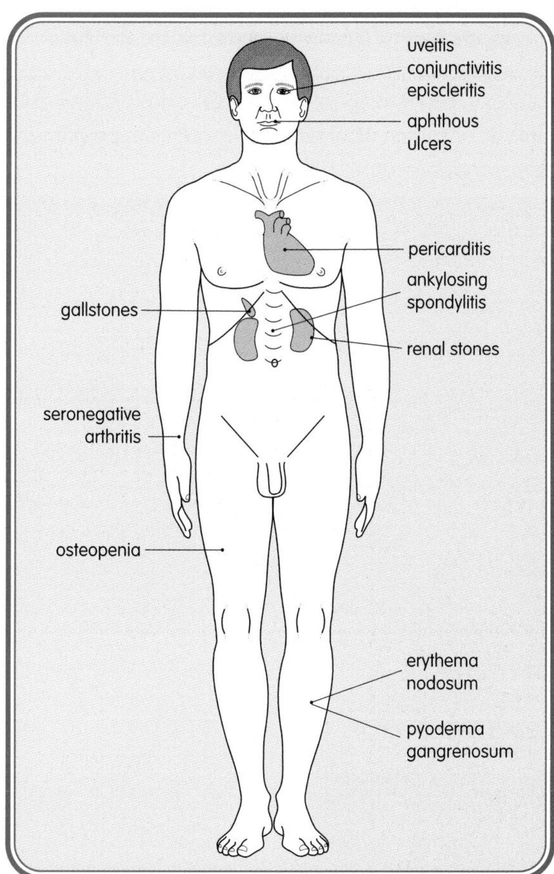

Fig. 20.3 Systemic manifestations of Crohn's disease.

Treatment

Treatment options include:

- Withdrawal of gluten-containing food (e.g. wheat, rye, barley) from the diet will usually provide symptomatic and histological improvement. Non-compliance is usually the cause of relapse or lack of improvement.
- Replacement of deficient vitamins may be needed in the initial stages, but long-term replacement is usually not required.
- Re-introduction of gluten to the diet will result in a reappearance of symptoms and villous atrophy and can be used to confirm the diagnosis in doubtful cases.

Dermatitis herpetiformis will usually resolve with a gluten-free diet. Resistant cases can be treated with dapsone.

Crohn's disease

Incidence

Average of 4 out of 100 000 each year in the UK. Rare in people of Afro-Caribbean origin.

Clinical features

The main symptoms are:

- Abdominal pain.
- Diarrhoea.
- Weight loss.

General malaise, anorexia, and fever are also common. Acute ileitis mimics acute appendicitis with pain in the right iliac fossa.

Extra-gastrointestinal manifestations such as uveitis, oligoarthritis, and erythema nodosum can also be seen (Fig. 20.3).

Diagnosis and investigation

On investigating Crohn's disease, note the following:

- Anaemia is common and can be of normocytic, normochromic type of chronic disease or secondary to iron deficiency/folate due to blood loss/malabsorption. Platelets are increased and reflect inflammatory activity.
- Low albumin levels indicate severe disease. Liver enzymes are less commonly affected compared with ulcerative colitis.
- Blood cultures are important if the patient is septicaemic.

- Stool cultures should be routinely done for patients presenting with diarrhoea.
- Small bowel enema/follow-through is used to visualize the small bowel to locate the affected area and determine extent of disease (see Fig. 17.24).
- Colonoscopy is preferred if diarrhoea is the predominant symptom rather than pain, as colitis is more likely and biopsies can be taken to distinguish from ulcerative colitis.
- Computed tomography (CT) or magnetic resonance (MR) scan of abdomen is helpful if fistula or abscesses are suspected. Magnetic resonance scan may be more sensitive.

Aetiology and pathogenesis

This is a chronic inflammatory condition characterized by the presence of non-caseating granulomas which can affect any part of the bowel from mouth to anus but more commonly seen in the terminal ileum. Another feature is that of 'skip lesions', where normal bowel is seen in-between diseased bowel. Affected bowel wall is usually thickened and narrowed, producing obstruction clinically. Deep ulceration and fissuring is also seen producing a 'cobblestone' appearance endoscopically.

C-reactive protein is elevated during acute attacks, mirroring inflammatory activity in Crohn's disease and is useful for prognosis.

Inflammation affects all layers of the bowel (unlike ulcerative colitis) and there are non-caseating granulomas with chronic inflammatory infiltrates which are typical. Crypt abscesses may also be seen in colonic disease (Fig. 20.4)

The exact aetiology is unknown, but the epidemiology suggests an environmental agent with a genetic predisposition. Up to 10% of patients' relatives have either Crohn's or ulcerative colitis and some investigators say that the two diseases represent a spectrum of a single pathology.

Tobacco smoking is associated with increased risk of Crohn's, whereas non-smokers or ex-smokers are more likely to develop ulcerative colitis.

An infective cause has been postulated, but there is no clear evidence to support such an hypothesis. Similarly, immunological abnormalites have been noted but it is uncertain whether these changes are a primary or secondary event.

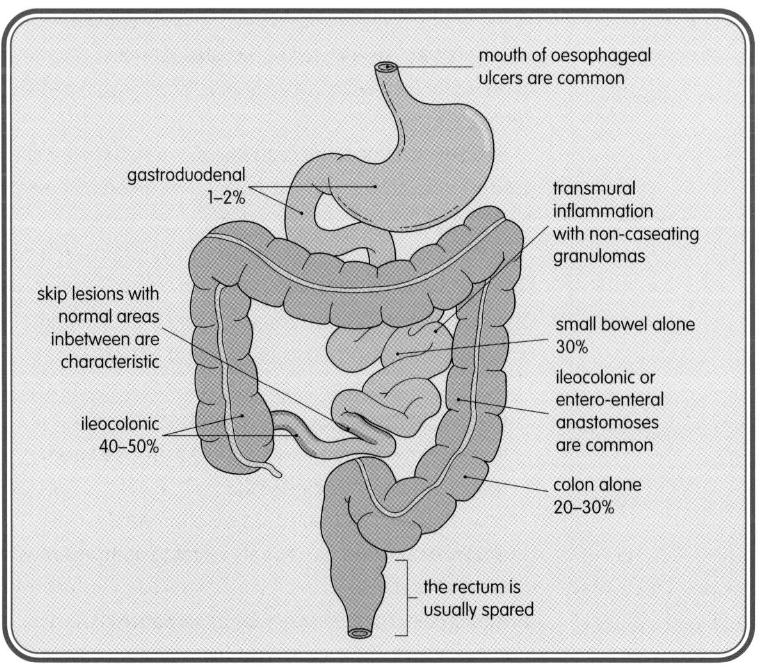

Fig. 20.4 Gastrointestinal features of Crohn's disease.

Complications

Fistulae can form between bowel and bladder (enterovesical), another segment of intestine (entero-enteral), skin (sinus), or vagina (entero-vaginal). There are often very disabling symptoms.

Amyloidosis can occur due to high levels of acute-phase proteins produced during an acute attack. There is an increased risk of developing adenocarcinoma.

Treatment

Corticosteroids

These are used empirically for acute attacks to suppress symptoms, but there is little evidence to suggest that the prognosis improves with treatment. Maintenance steroids should be avoided if at all possible due to the long-term risk of osteoporosis. Localized rectal Crohn's can be treated by steroid suppositories or enemas to reduce the systemic side effects.

Salicylates

Salazopyrine is a 5-aminosalicylic acid (5-ASA) attached to sulphapyridine and is broken down in the colon by bacteria to release the active compound 5-ASA. Unlike ulcerative colitis in which the drug is very effective, the beneficial effect in Crohn's is more uncertain.

Newer compounds such as mesalazine and olsalazine are now available which have fewer toxic side effects because they do not have a sulphonamide component. These compounds may be useful in Crohn's colitis but not in small bowel disease alone.

Antibiotics

Antibiotics to note:

- Metronidazole is used for perianal disease in which anaerobic infections are common and its use often has to be prolonged to be effective. Problems arise due to peripheral neuropathy with long-term use.
- Rifampicin has been used, but is not dramatically effective.
- Quinolones such as clarithromycin are showing promise.

Immunosuppression

Commonly, azathioprine is used as a steroid-sparing agent and can be effective for severe disease. Cyclosporin A has also been given with variable success. The systemic toxicity of these compounds limits their use.

Elemental diets

Enteral or parenteral feeding can induce remission, especially in small bowel disease. The bowel is allowed to 'rest' and hence reduce inflammation and exposure to potential antigens.

Parenteral feeding via a central venous line may be necessary for patients who are severely malnourished or for whom enteral feeding is not suitable, e.g. fistula formation. Unfortunately, over half of the patients relapse when a normal diet is re-introduced.

Surgery

Approximately 80% of patients will require surgery at some point. Usually required because of complications such as fistula, obstruction from strictures, toxic dilatation, or failure to respond to medical treatment, causing ill health.

Extensive resection should be avoided because recurrence of the disease is common.

Alpha chain disease

Incidence

Also known as immunoproliferative small intestinal disease (IPSID). Seen mainly in Mediterranean countries, Africa, South America, and the Far East.

Clinical features

Symptoms include:

- Malabsorption, which is the most common presenting symptom and can be severe.
- Abdominal pain.
- Anaemia.
- Finger clubbing—often seen.

Diagnosis and investigation

IgA alpha chains can be detected in urine and serum. These can also be detected by immunofluorescence of gut mucosa.

Aetiology and pathogenesis

The underlying aetiology is unknown. There is a proliferation of the plasma cells in the lamina propria which produces the heavy or alpha chain of IgA molecules without the light chains, probably as a result of long-standing antigenic stimulation. Subsequently, there is a defect in the IgA secretory function resulting in bacterial overgrowth, villous atrophy, and malabsorption. The disease is associated with low socioeconomic groups in areas where poor hygiene and chronic intestinal infestation are common.

Complication

The condition is considered to be premalignant with progression to small bowel lymphoma of B cell type.

Treatment

In early stages, tetracycline will give some improvement in the condition. Once invasive lymphoma has occurred then surgery and radio/chemotherapy is required.

Intestinal lymphomas

Incidence

Rare cause of intestinal malignancy.

Clinical features

Symptoms include:

- Abdominal pain.
- Intestinal obstruction.
- Diarrhoea.
- Anorexia.
- Anaemia (iron deficiency due to blood loss).

The symptoms are similar to those of any tumour in the small intestine or colon. A palpable mass may occasionally be present.

Diagnosis and investigation

Consider:

- Small bowel enema or follow-through will detect most lesions but is unlikely to distinguish it from other tumours.
- A CT of the abdomen will visualize the lesion and show enlargement of local lymph nodes, which is commonly seen in small bowel lymphomas. Biopsy will confirm the diagnosis.

Aetiology and pathogenesis

More frequently found in the ileum. Majority are of the non-Hodgkins B cell type arising from mucosa-associated lymphoid tissues (MALT). They tend to be of annular or polypoid masses in the terminal ileum. T cell lymphomas are seen in patients with coeliac disease and are characteristically ulcerated plaques or strictures in the proximal small bowel.

Complications

Extensive involvement will result in malabsorption.

Prognosis

Small tumours with surgical resection have a good prognosis of 75% at 5 years depending on the grade of lymphoma. T cell lymphomas have a poorer outcome, with an overall survival of 25% at 5 years.

Treatment

Surgery followed by radiotherapy and/or chemotherapy.

NEOPLASTIC PROBLEMS

Adenocarcinoma of small intestine

Incidence

Rare, but accounts for 50% of all tumours found in small intestine.

Clinical features

Commonly anaemia, abdominal pain, weight loss, and diarrhoea.

Diagnosis and investigtation

Consider:

- Barium follow-through/enema usually demonstrates a stricture.
- A CT of the abdomen demonstrates local invasion and any local lymph node involvement can also be detected.

Aetiology and pathogenesis

Coeliac and Crohn's disease have a higher incidence of adenocarcinoma of small bowel. The exact mechanism is unknown.

Treatment

Surgical resection of the affected area. Radiotherapy and chemotherapy are of limited value.

Carcinoid tumours

Incidence

Accounts for up to 10% of small intestinal tumours.

Clinical features

Most are asymptomatic. Approximately 10% are found incidentally on appendicectomy due to acute appendicitis. Occasionally, patients can present with an acute abdomen secondary to obstruction by the tumour.

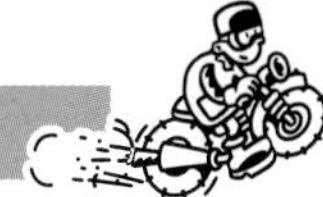

Carcinoid syndrome

This is seen in 5% of patients with carcinoid tumours when liver metastases are present. Characteristic features are:

- Facial flushing.
- Abdominal pain.
- Chronic diarrhoea (Fig. 20.5).

Right-sided cardiac lesions (i.e. tricuspid regurgitation or pulmonary stenosis) are found in half of the patients with carcinoid syndrome.

Diagnosis and investigation

Primary tumours are only diagnosed on histological specimens.

Liver ultrasound or CT scan confirms the presence of liver metastases. These deposits usually take up radiolabelled metaiodobenzylguanidine (MIBG) or octreotide if the diagnosis is uncertain.

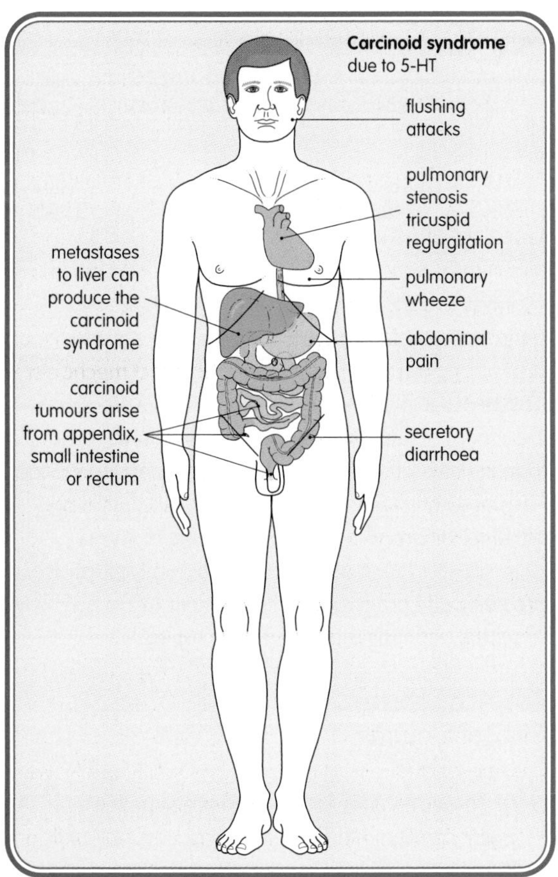

Fig. 20.5 Clinical features of carcinoid syndrome.

Urinary 5-hydoxyindole acetic acid (5-HIAA), the major metabolite of 5-hydoxytryptamine (5-HT), is increased in the urine.

Aetiology and pathogenesis

Originates from APUD (amine precursor uptake and decarboxylation) cells and the most common primary sites include the appendix, terminal ileum, and rectum.

The tumours secrete a number of vasoactive peptides, including serotonin (5-HT), bradykinin, and histamines, which cause the facial flushing, GI symptoms, and cardiac lesions.

Primary carcinoid tumours may secrete hormone (usually 5-HT, but also bradykinin and histamine), but its serum concentration is reduced by metabolism on first pass through the liver via the portal circulation from the gut. Once the tumour metastasizes to the liver, this 'protection' is bypassed and massive amounts of hormone reach the systemic circulation, where it produces symptoms of the carcinoid syndrome.

Prognosis

Most patients survive up to 5–10 years after diagnosis.

Treatment

Octreotide, a somatostatin analogue, is the standard treatment. It inhibits gut hormone release, so stops the flushing and diarrhoea. Inhibition of tumour growth can occur in some patients. Some tumours secrete different hormones, e.g. adrenocorticotropic hormone producing different clinical syndromes (e.g. Cushing's), and treatment will need to be tailored to the symptoms.

Peutz–Jeghers syndrome

Clinical features

Mucocutaneous pigmentation of the face, hands, and feet with multiple polyps along the intestines, giving rise to bleeding and occasionally intussusception.

Diagnosis and investigation

Barium enema or barium follow-through are carried out to demonstrate the extent of polyposis with confirmation by biopsy taken at colonoscopy or enteroscopy.

Aetiology and pathogenesis

Inherited as an autosomal dominant trait. The polyps are hamartomas and can occur anywhere along the GI tract, but particularly in the small bowel.

Complications

There is a small but a definite risk of malignant change of hamartomas.

Treatment

Polypectomies should be carried out along the bowel to look for dysplastic features but bowel resection should be avoided if possible.

INFECTIONS

Bacterial overgrowth

Clinical features

Mainly that of malabsorption, i.e. diarrhoea, steatorrhoea, and vitamin deficiency, especially B_{12}.

Diagnosis and investigation

Investigations to consider should include:

- Hydrogen breath test—oral lactulose or glucose is ingested and metabolized by the bacteria to hydrogen, which can be detected in expiration (Fig. 17.8). However, interpretation can be difficult because there are bacteria present in the oral cavity and rapid transit time will allow bacteria in the large intestine to break down lactulose.
- ^{14}C glycocholic acid breath test—^{14}C-labelled bile salt is ingested and bacteria deconjugates the bile salts releasing $^{14}CO_2$, which can be detected in exhaled breath. Rapid transit time will also cause a rise in radioactivity due to substrate reaching bacteria in the large intestines.
- Small intestinal aspiration—direct aspiration followed by aerobic and anaerobic cultures can be an alternative method for diagnosing bacterial overgrowth.

Aetiology and pathogenesis

Gastric acid normally kills most bacteria and intestinal motility keeps the jejunum free of bacteria. The terminal ileum usually contains faecal type of bacteria, i.e. *E. coli* and anaerobes.

Bacterial overgrowth occurs as a result of structural abnormality, i.e. Polya gastrectomy, small intestinal diverticulosis, strictures, or where stasis occurs allowing bacteria to grow. The condition can be seen in elderly people and in scleroderma (due to hypomotility).

Deconjugation of bile salts by the bacteria can result in fat malabsorption (steatorrhoea) and deficiency of the fat soluble vitamins A, D, E, and K. The bacteria can also metabolize vitamin B_{12} and interfere with its binding to intrinsic factor, hence causing B_{12} deficiency.

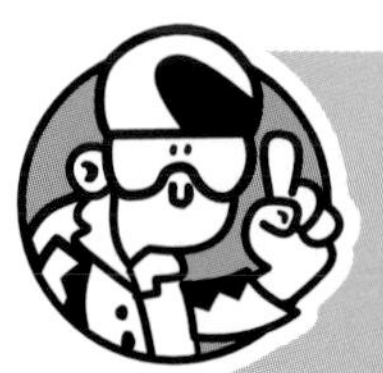

Patients with vitamin B_{12} deficiency due to bacterial overgrowth often have a high serum folate, due to its absorption following production by the bacteria.

Complications

Result from malabsorption of vitamin B_{12} and fat-soluble vitamins causing macrocytic anaemia, peripheral neuropathy, osteomalacia, etc.

Treatment

Treatment of underlying cause, e.g. strictures, blind loop in Polya gastrectomy, etc., may be required in the form of surgical resection. Multiple diverticulosis and other conditions may not be amenable to surgery.

Antibiotics, such as tetracycline or metronidazole, are used and prolonged or intermittent use is normally required. Vitamins may need to be replaced.

Tropical sprue

Clinical features

These consist of:

- Diarrhoea—Chronic diarrhoea predisposes to malabsorption, vitamin deficiencies, and malnutrition.
- Weight loss.
- Anorexia.

Diagnosis is reserved for people resident in epidemic areas such as Asia, South America, and parts of the Caribbean. Often, there is a preceding enteric infection.

Diagnosis

Investigations to aid diagnosis include:

- Stool culture is necessary to exclude other causes of infective diarrhoea (e.g. giardiasis).
- Jejunal biopsy shows partial villous atrophy but it is often less severe than that of coeliac disease.

Aetiology and pathogenesis

Likely to be an infective cause, but the exact aetiology is unknown. A number of pathogens have been implicated but conclusive evidence is unavailable. Different agents could be responsible for the presentation in different parts of the world.

Complications

Folate deficiency is common. Complications are a result of vitamin deficiency seen in any malabsorptive state.

Treatment

Improvement of symptoms on leaving the endemic area is common.

Most patients will require antibiotics, e.g. tetracycline, for up to 6 months. Folate and other vitamin supplements are also required.

Whipple's disease

Incidence

Rare. Particularly affects middle-aged males.

Clinical features

These include:

- Steatorrhoea.
- Abdominal pain.
- Fever.
- Weight loss.

Peripheral lymphadenopathy, migratory arthritis and pigmentation may also be seen.

Involvement of the brain causes a chronic encephalitis and may be the dominant feature.

Diagnosis and investigation

Small intestinal biopsy typically show villous atrophy and periodic acid–Schiff (PAS) positive macrophages, which represent the remains of dead bacteria.

Aetiology and pathogenesis

The bacteria responsible have been identified as *Tropheryma whippeli* and are presumed to be of a low infectivity. Exact mechanism of the disease is uncertain, but may involve a variety of immunodeficiency.

Treatment

Prolonged antibiotics, such as penicillin, tetracycline, or chloramphenicol,are effective and improvement can be dramatic. Supplements of relevant vitamins and minerals may be required for patients with severe malabsorption.

Tuberculosis

Incidence

Rare in the UK but should be suspected in areas where it is more common (e.g. Asia), and in patients infected with HIV presenting with relevant features.

Clinical features

These are similar to those of Crohn's disease, i.e. weight loss, abdominal pain, anorexia, anaemia, etc. (Fig. 20.6). Intestinal obstruction may occur. Right iliac fossa mass may be present. Can also present with tuberculous ascites mimicking malignant disease.

Diagnosis and investigation

Consider:

- Abdominal ultrasound—may show mesenteric thickening and lymph node involvement.
- Laparotomy for histological confirmation followed by bacteriological confirmation is the gold standard, but tuberculosis (TB) cultures can take up to 6 weeks.
- Chest X-ray—may show presence of pulmonary TB and so aid in the diagnosis of small intestine TB.

Aetiology and pathogenesis

Due to reactivation of the primary disease caused by *M. tuberculosis*. Bovine TB is very rare and is due to ingestion of unpasteurized milk. The ileocaecal area is the most commonly affected. Typical caseating granulomas are seen histologically.

Treatment

As for pulmonary TB, i.e. triple therapy of isoniazid, rifampicin, and pyrazinamide. Treatment should be extended up to 6–9 months.

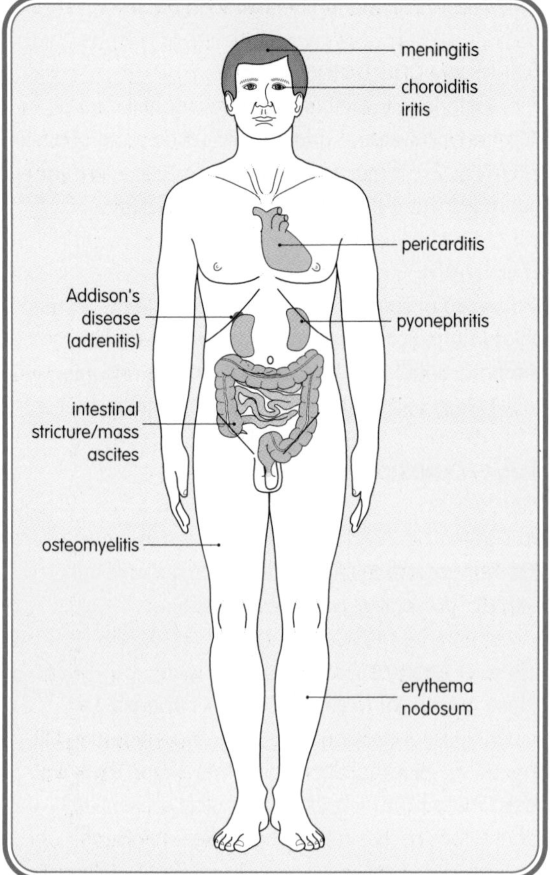

Fig. 20.6 Body map of features seen in extra-pulmonary tuberculosis.

Yersinia infection

Clinical features

In adults, it causes an enterocolitis characterized by fever, diarrhoea, and abdominal pain. It can also give rise to terminal ileitis, which often clinically mistaken for appendicitis.

Reiter's syndrome (conjunctivitis, arthritis, and non-specific urethritis) can sometimes occur after infection with Yersinia. Erythema nodosum and seronegative arthritis are not uncommon and are probably immune-related.

In children, the infection is more likely to cause mesenteric adenitis, giving rise to abdominal pain.

Diagnosis

Not routinely confirmed, but occasionally made on tissue diagnosis or lymph node biopsy (e.g. after appendicectomy).

Aetiology and pathogenesis

Caused by Yersinia enterocolitica (enterocolitis) and Yersinia pseudotuberculosis (terminal ileitis).

Treatment

Usually a self-limiting disease, and no specific treatment needed. In severe cases, tetracycline may be given.

Giardiasis

Incidence

Common in the tropics and is an important cause of travellers' diarrhoea.

Clinical features

Typical symptoms include:

- Watery diarrhoea.
- Nausea.
- Anorexia.
- Abdominal pain.
- Malabsorption.

Asymptomatic carriers are also seen.

Diagnosis and investigtation

Stool examination is important, but cysts can be seen only in fresh stool samples as they often die when stored.

Negative stool examination does not exclude the diagnosis because excretion of the parasite can be intermittent.

Duodenal aspirate/biopsy allows direct visualization of the parasite. Serology-specific IgG and IgM antibodies can be measured.

Aetiology and pathogenesis

Giardia lamblia is a protozoan that is found worldwide and epidemics have been reported in parts of Europe and North America.

Spread is by faecal–oral route and mainly via contaminated water supplies.

The organism colonizes within the small intestinal wall and can produce an asymptomatic infection. However, in most cases, villous atrophy occurs causing diarrhoea and malabsorption.

The exact mechanism of how *Giardia* causes villous atrophy is unknown, but immune-mediated response may be responsible. Bacterial overgrowth may account for some of the malabsorption seen.

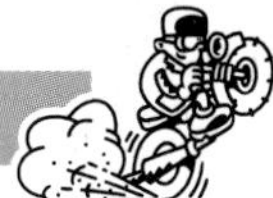

Complications

These are due to malabsorption of vitamins and malnutrition seen in small bowel disease.

Treatment

Metronidazole is the drug of choice given for 7–10 days with or without vitamin supplements.

Cholera

Clinical features

Incubation takes from a few hours to 6 days.

Diarrhoea is often profuse and watery (also painless). Classically likened to 'rice water' stool due to presence of mucus.

Circulatory collapse due to profound dehydration occurs in severe cases. Renal failure may ensue.

Diagnosis and investigation

Diagnosis is mainly made on clinical grounds.

Stool examination is helpful. Motile organism can be seen in freshly passed stool, but this is not specific for cholera, as a similar appearance can occur in Campylobacter infections. Stool cultures will normally confirm the diagnosis.

Aetiology and pathogenesis

Caused by the Gram-negative bacillus *Vibrio cholerae*. Infection is by faecal–oral route via contaminated water supplies and food sources. Exotoxins produced by the bacteria bind irreversibly to epithelial receptors along the small intestine which activate adenylate cyclase and, hence increase intracellular cAMP concentrations (Fig. 20.7). This, in turn, causes the stimulation of salt and water secretion into the intestinal lumen, resulting in a devastating loss of fluid and electrolytes. Reabsorption of fluid in the small intestine is also inhibited, contributing to the fluid loss.

Treatment

Fluid and electrolyte replacement either intravenously or orally is the mainstay of treatment.

Antibiotics such as tetracycline will shorten the duration of the illness but drug resistance is an increasing problem.

Strongyloidiasis

Clinical features

These include:

- Local skin erythema and itching where the larvae have gained entry.
- Respiratory symptoms, such as cough and rarely pneumonitis, approximately 7–10 days after initial penetration.
- Abdominal discomfort, intermittent diarrhoea, and constipation are seen approximately 3 weeks later when intestinal colonization occurs. Heavy infection

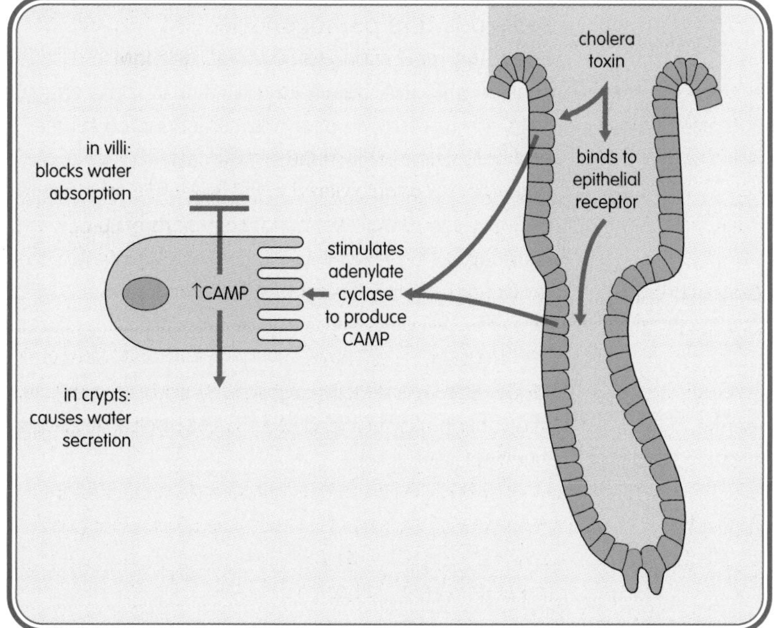

Fig. 20.7 Mechanisms of diarrhoea in cholera infection.

may produce more marked symptoms including steatorrhoea and intestinal malabsorption.

Diagnosis and investigation

Eosinophilia is commonly seen on full blood count. Larvae can be detected in fresh stool sample or duodenal aspirate.

Aetiology and pathogenesis

Due to infection with *Strongyloides stercoralis,* found especially in South America and Asia. Infection can persist for decades and new cases are still diagnosed on war veterans who were infected while abroad.

Adult worms reside in the crypts of the small intestine, causing inflammatory response and, hence, mucosal damage. The worms are excreted in the stool and autoinfection is common.

Complications

Disseminated strongyloidiasis is rare and often a fatal condition seen in people who have become immunocompromised for one reason or another.

Treatment

Thiabendazole or albendazole are effective treatments.

Hookworm infection

Incidence

Seen worldwide, and is said to affect a quarter of the world's population.

Clinical features

These include:

- Local skin irritation where the worm gains entry.
- Mild respiratory symptoms may be seen approximately 2 weeks later.
- Iron deficiency anaemia.

The most common cause of iron deficiency anaemia worldwide is hookworm infection.

Diagnosis and investigation

Full blood count shows a microcytic anaemia. Eosinophilia may be seen early in the infection. Ova can be seen in a fresh stool sample.

Aetiology and pathogenesis

Ancylostoma duodenale is responsible for the cases found in Europe and Middle East, whereas *Necator americanus* causes the disease in South East Asia, Far East, and sub-Saharan Africa.

The adult worm attaches to the small intestinal mucosa by its buccal capsule and feeds off blood from the mucosa.

Treatment

Mebendazole is the treatment of choice.

Roundworm infection

Incidence

Seen worldwide, but particularly common in poor rural areas.

Clinical features

Often asymptomatic. Nausea, vomiting, abdominal discomfort, diarrhoea, and intestinal obstruction occur with heavy infections.

Invasion of appendix or biliary tree will cause appendicitis and biliary obstruction, respectively.

Larvae in lung will cause pulmonary eosinophilia.

Diagnosis and investigation

Eggs can be seen on microscopic preparations from fresh stool samples.

Adult worm may appear from mouth or anus.

Aetiology and pathogenesis

Due to *Ascaris lumbricoides*, which can grow to a considerable size, causing malnutrition in some cases. Eggs are ingested via a faecally contaminated source and hatch into larvae in the small intestine. They can travel via the portal system to the liver and lungs, where they develop further. Pulmonary larvae may be coughed up to be swallowed back into the intestine to grow into mature worms up to 20 cm in length.

Treatment

Mebendazole is effective against the parasite. Surgical intervention may be needed for acute appendicitis and intestinal obstruction.

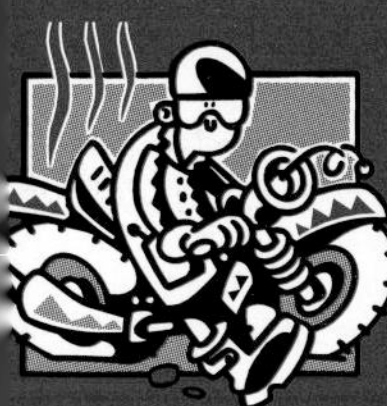

21. Colon

ANATOMY, PHYSIOLOGY, AND FUNCTION OF THE COLON AND RECTUM

The colon starts at the ileocaecal valve and joins the rectum at the rectosigmoid junction (Fig. 21.1).

The muscle wall consists of an inner circular layer and an outer longitudinal layer which is incomplete and comes together to form taenia coli.

The anal canal has:

- An internal sphincter (involuntary control).
- An external sphincter (voluntary control).

The main role of the colon is absorption of water and electrolytes, which takes place mainly in the ascending colon.

Entry of faeces into the rectum produces relaxation of the internal sphincter and the urge to defecate. Defecation is brought about by voluntary relaxation of the external anal sphincter and an increase in intra-abdominal pressure.

FUNCTIONAL DISORDERS

Irritable bowel syndrome

Incidence

A common condition, accounting for up to 40% of patients attending gastroenterology clinics. The majority of people affected are women.

Clinical features

These include:

- Abdominal pain that classically occurs in the left iliac fossa and is relieved by defecation and passage of wind.
- Alternating constipation and diarrhoea is common with passage of pellet-like stools or frequent small-volume bowel motions of a loose consistency. The patient may also complain of a sensation of incomplete emptying of the rectum.
- Abdominal distension and bloating is very suggestive of irritable bowel syndrome in the absence of bowel obstruction.
- Features of depression may also be present.

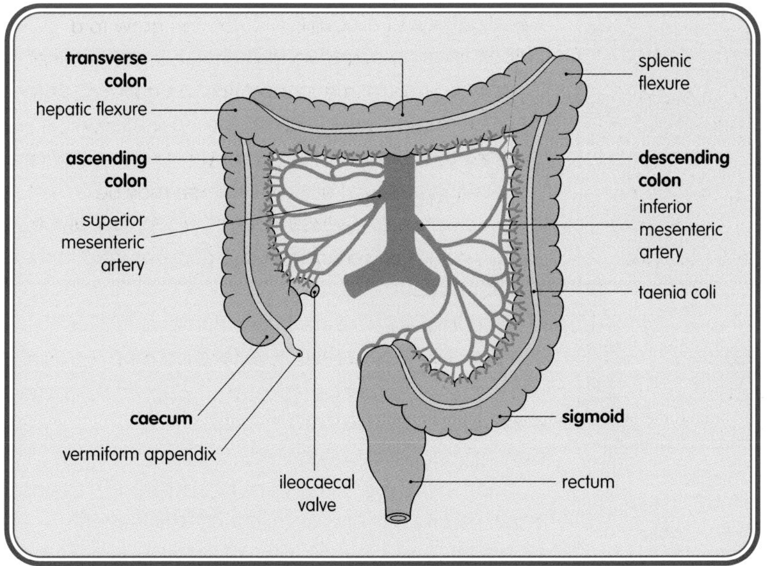

Fig. 21.1 Anatomy of the large intestine.

Diagnosis and investigation

Diagnosis is predominantly made on clinical grounds. Investigation such as routine full blood count and biochemistry will be normal.

Further investigations such as sigmoidoscopy and barium enema are usually only necessary to exclude any underlying pathology, especially in patients presenting over about 40 years of age.

Aetiology and pathogenesis

Precise aetiology is unclear, but it appears to be closely linked to psychological stress and patients often describe worsening of symptoms with high stress levels. The condition more commonly affects young females.

Intraluminal pressure readings are normal during symptom-free periods and pain is associated with increased force of contraction in the small intestine and colon during an attack, which may reflect an exaggerated response of the intestine to pyschological stress. Depression may be an important contributory factor.

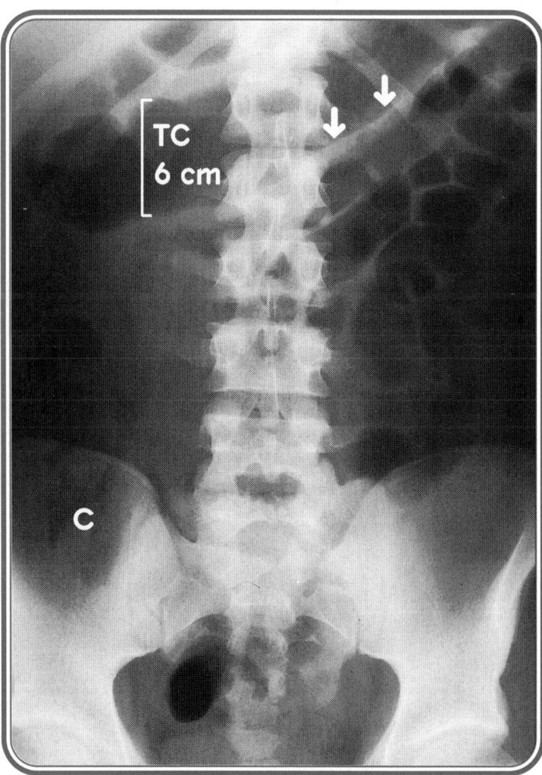

Fig. 21.2 Plain abdominal X-ray showing megacolon. Note the transverse colon (TC) 6cm and thumbprinting in the caecum (C), indicating severe mucosal oedema, which can also be seen between bowel layers (arrows).

Raised intraluminal pressure is associated with reduced intestinal bulk and development of diverticulosis, but increased fibre intake does not always improve symptoms and may make the condition worse.

Complications

There is an increased incidence of diverticular disease in later life probably due to long-standing increased intraluminal pressure.

Treatment

Reassurance is the key in the management of these patients, and it must be emphasized that the disorder is a functional one rather than one with a pathological cause. It is essential to relate your explanation to the patient's symptoms. High-fibre diets may benefit those with constipation as a dominant feature.

Antispasmodics, e.g. mebeverine, can be given for pain relief. Opioid drugs such as those containing codeine should be avoided, as they impede bowel transit and exacerbate the condition.

Megacolon

Clinical features

Constipation is characteristic, with a long, protracted history possibly with faecal impaction and soiling at a young age. Reduced rectal sensation is usual and anal tone may be increased on rectal examination.

Diagnosis and investigation

Investigations to consider:

- Barium enema or plain abdominal X-ray shows a dilated proximal colon (Fig. 21.2). A narrowed distal colon may be seen in Hirschsprung's disease.
- Deep mucosal rectal biopsy is necessary, especially in young patients, to confirm or exclude Hirschsprung's disease in which a segment of the rectum has absent or reduced ganglion cells in the submucosa.
- Manometry shows failure of internal sphincter relaxation in response to rectal distension.

Aetiology and pathogenesis

Can be congenital or acquired.

Congenital type is known as Hirschsprung's disease, which usually presents in childhood with chronic constipation and faecal soiling. Rectal biopsy shows an absence of ganglion cells in the submucosal plexus. Adults presenting with the condition may have segmental disease, hence initial biopsy may be normal and a deeper biopsy or a full thickness biopsy is required.

The most common cause of aquired megacolon is chronic constipation with or without laxative abuse. Causes of chronic constipation are many (Fig. 21.3). Chronic ingestion of laxatives results in depletion of ganglion cells.

Complications

Can result in subacute or acute bowel obstruction.

Treatment

Hirschsprung's disease is primarily treated by surgical resection of the affected colon.

Acquired megacolon is more difficult to treat because patients may have been taking laxatives for some time. Frequent enemas or manual evacuations may be needed. In severe cases surgical intervention is required.

Pseudo-obstruction

Clinical features

Similar to those of bowel obstruction, i.e. vomiting, distension, non-passage of flatus, etc., but unlike true obstruction, bowel sound is absent.

Aetiology and pathogenesis

Bowel paralysis is common after laparotomy due to manual handling and will return to normal within 2–3 days. Systemic conditions can also give rise to an adynamic bowel, e.g: drugs, electrolyte disturbance, septicaemia. It is commonly seen in intensive care patients.

Causes of chronic constipation
Low residue diet
Drugs, e.g. opioids, iron, anti-depressants
Metabolic conditions: hypothyroidism, hypercalcaemia
Neuropsychiatric conditions: Parkinson's, depression, stroke (immobility)
Obstruction and pseudo-obstruction
Painful anorectal conditions, e.g. fissure
Carcinoma of the colon

Fig. 21.3 Causes of chronic constipation.

Treatment

Correction of the underlying abnormality will usually result in the return of normal peristalsis.

INFLAMMATORY BOWEL DISEASE

Ulcerative colitis

Incidence

Average incidence is 5–8 out of 100 000 people in Europe and the USA.

Peak age of onset between 20–40 years of age. Women are affected more often than men.

Clinical features

Diarrhoea is the most prominent feature, usually associated with presence of blood and mucus. Patients may pass up to 20 loose motions per 24 hours during an acute attack.

Non-specific features such as malaise and anorexia are common, and extraintestinal manifestations also occur (Fig. 21.4).

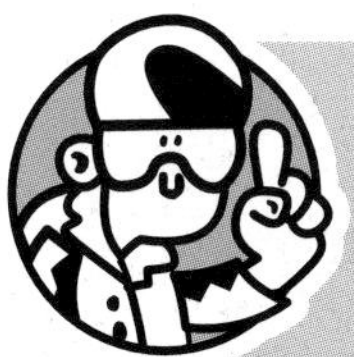

Abdominal pain in ulcerative colitis is an ominous feature and may indicate development of toxic megacolon or perforation.

Diagnosis and investigation

You should consider the following investigations:

- Full blood count, C reactive protein, blood cultures, and stool cultures, as for Crohn's disease.
- Raised biliary enzymes indicate the presence of primary sclerosing cholangitis.
- A plain abdominal X-ray is essential to exclude colonic dilatation.
- A barium enema shows ulceration, and the extent of

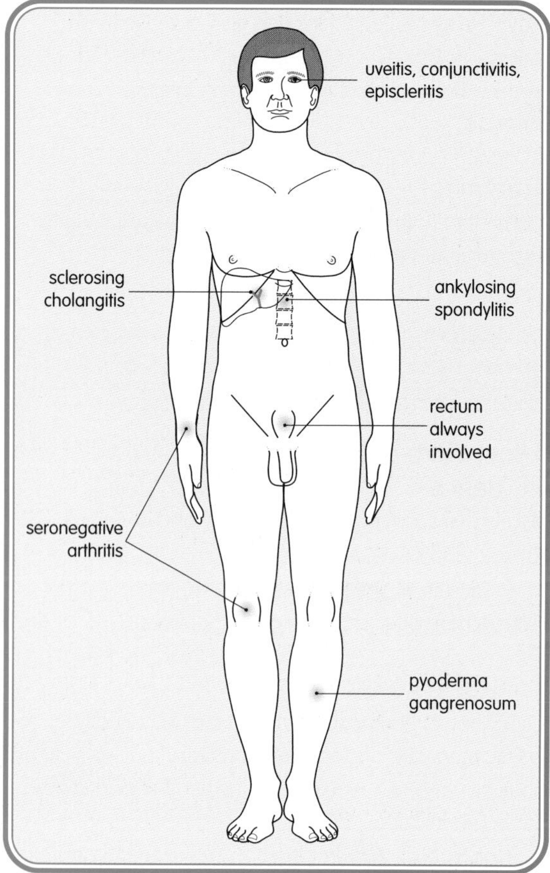

Fig. 21.4 Body map of extraintestinal features of ulcerative colitis.

colonic involvement may be seen in active disease. In long-standing chronic cases, characteristic 'lead-pipe' colon (Fig. 21.5) can be demonstrated.

- Colonoscopy is the preferred investigation because it offers the advantage of biopsy to differentiate from Crohn's disease and other forms of colitis. Mucosa is inflamed and friable and bleeds easily.

Aetiology and pathogenesis

Unknown aetiology but there is an association with HLA-B27 and ankylosing spondylitis which is suggestive of a genetic basis but no conclusive evidence is yet available.

Histological features are similar to those seen in infectious diarrhoea but no agent has been shown to be responsible.

Perinuclear antineutrophil cytoplasmic antibodies (pANCA) can be found in 60% of patients with ulcerative colitis, which suggests an underlying immunological cause, but it is difficult to ascertain whether the changes in autoantibodies are a cause or a result of the disease.

Patients with ulcerative colitis are more likely to be non-smokers or ex-smokers compared to the general population but the significance of this observation is unclear. Conversely, Crohn's disease is associated with smoking.

Ulcerative colitis affects the rectum and may extend along the whole length of the colon. Small bowel involvement is not seen in contrast to Crohn's disease, except in patients those with extensive disease affecting the terminal ileum ('backwash ileitis') (Fig. 21.5).

Macroscopically, the mucosa looks inflamed and bleeds easily and in severe disease, extensive ulceration is seen with neighbouring mucosa appearing like polyps ('pseudopolyps'). Fulminant colitis results in loss of the mucosal layer and involvement of the muscle layer, producing toxic dilatation.

Microscopically, the inflammation is limited to the mucosa and submucosa with inflammatory cells accumulating in the lamina propria and colonic gland to form crypt abscesses. Goblet cell depletion is also seen. Long-standing colitis results in fibrosis of mucosa and submucosa, hence loss of haustral pattern and a shortened and featureless colon ('lead pipe colon', Fig. 21.6).

Complications

Toxic megacolon is seen on plain abdominal X-ray. Dilatation of 5 cm or greater is associated with a risk of perforation and peritonitis. The patient is usually unwell with fever, abdominal tenderness, and tachycardia (Figs 21.2 and 21.7).

The risk of developing adenocarcinoma after 10 years of colitis is approximately 5% higher than the general population.

Cholangiocarcinoma arises with increasing frequency in patients with ulcerative colitis when primary sclerosing cholangitis is present.

Amyloidosis is probably related to high levels of circulating acute-phase protein during exacerbations.

Prognosis

The course of the disease is variable, but characteristically it is a chronic relapsing disease. Patients with proctitis alone have a good overall prognosis, with only 10% progressing to more extensive

Ulcerative colitis versus Crohn's disease		
	Ulcerative colitis	**Crohn's disease**
Clinical features	Bloody diarrhoea	Abdominal pain and weight loss
Macroscopic appearance	Usually confined to colon Ulceration superficial and continuous	Most often terminal ileum but can affect anywhere in GI tract Patchy transmural ulceration and skip lesions are common
Microscopic appearance	Crypt abscesses	Granulomas are common

Fig. 21.5 Contrasting features between ulcerative colitis and Crohn's disease.

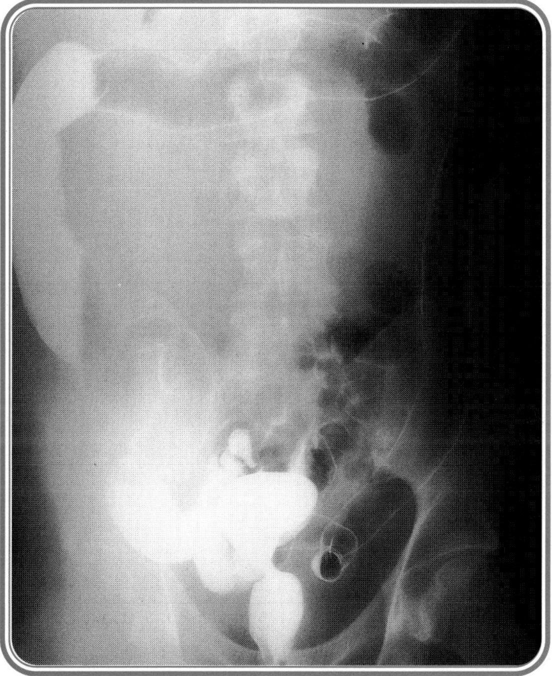

Fig. 21.6 Barium enema showing 'lead pipe' appearance in chronic ulcerative colitis.

Features of severe ulcerative colitis
Stool frequency >8 times/day with blood
Abdominal pain and tenderness
Fever >37.5°C
Tachycardia >100 bpm
C-reactive protein >20 mg/l
ESR >35 mm/h
Haemoglobin <10 g/L
Albumin < 30 g/L

Fig. 21.7 Features indicating severity in ulcerative colitis.

disease. Severe fulminant disease is associated with up to 25% mortality.

Treatment

Treatment options include:

- Corticosteroids given during an acute attack to gain remission. Topical treatment can be given for localized disease (proctitis) in the form of an enema. Long-term use of steroids should be avoided.
- 5-aminosalicylic acid (5-ASA) compounds are effective in reducing acute inflammation and maintaining remission in ulcerative colitis. Sulphasalazine is attached to sulphapyridine, which is broken down by bacteria to active 5-ASA. Olsalazine and mesalazine may be less toxic because they do not have a sulphur compound conjugated. These can be given in enema form for localized proctitis.
- Immunosuppression with azathioprine can be used for patients who are not responding to steroids.
- Surgical resection, usually in form of colectomy, is imperative for patients with complications such as toxic megacolon or perforation, and may be required in patients not responding to medical treatment.

Crohn's colitis

Clinical features

Crohn's disease can affect any part of the intestine including the colon and is occasionally confined to the colon alone (Crohn's colitis).

It can be difficult to differentiate Crohn's colitis from ulcerative colitis and the two conditions can overlap (referred to as indeterminate colitis).

The clinical picture is of abdominal pain and diarrhoea. Pain is more common than in ulcerative colitis and bleeding is far less common.

Investigation and diagnosis

These are basically the same as for ulcerative colitis. Differentiation from ulcerative colitis can be difficult.

The presence of granulomas and deep inflammation is suggestive of Crohn's colitis, whereas paucity of mucin and crypt abscesses are more in favour of ulcerative colitis.

Aetiology and pathogenesis

Up to 15% of patients will have clinical features of ulcerative colitis, but the biopsy will reveal the presence of granulomas which is pathognomic of Crohn's disease, therefore making the diagnosis difficult.

Recent genetic studies have shown that a presence of certain genes occurring simultaneously predisposes an individual to developing inflammatory bowel disease. It is now thought that ulcerative colitis and Crohn's disease may represent opposite ends of a spectrum, such that intermediate colitis exists, which may manifest clinically as Crohn's colitis.

Treatment

Standard treatment remains the same. However, it is important to distinguish between Crohn's and ulcerative colitis because there are important implications in their treatment. For example surgery is generally considered to be curative in ulcerative colitis, whereas this is clearly not the case for Crohn's disease.

Collagenous colitis

Clinical features

Occurs more commonly in women and presents as intermittent chronic watery diarrhoea. Abdominal pain may also be present. Patients are asymptomatic during remission.

Diagnosis and investigation

Stool culture, inflammatory markers, and colonoscopy are usually normal.

Diagnosis is based on histology which demonstrates the presence of a thickened subepithelial collagen layer (Fig. 21.8). There may also be intraepithelial lymphocytic infiltration, but this is more commonly seen in microscopic colitis (see below).

Aetiology and pathogenesis

There is an association with long-term use of non-steroidal anti-inflammatory drugs (NSAIDs) but an underlying immunological cause has been suggested, as this condition is more commonly seen in people with seronegative arthritis, Raynaud's phenomenon and coeliac disease.

Treatment

NSAIDs should be stopped. Antidiarrhoeal drugs are ineffective. Sulphalazine and cholestyramine have been tried with variable success rates. In persistent cases, short-term steroids can be used.

Microscopic colitis

Clinical features

Similar to collagenous colitis, i.e. intermittent diarrhoea, abdominal pain, etc. Again, the condition is more commonly found in women.

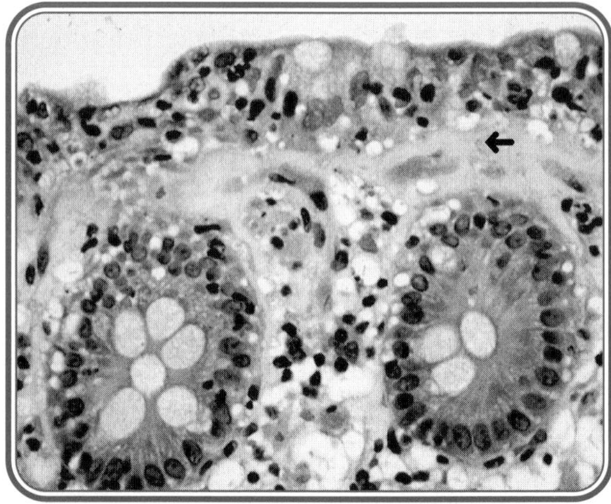

Fig. 21.8 Photomicrograph of collagenous colitis. Note the thickened amorphous layer just below the surface epithelial cells (arrow).

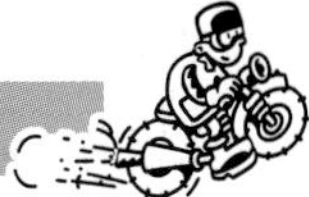

Diagnosis and investigation

These are as for collagenous colitis, except the biopsy shows intraepithelial lymphocytic infiltration without thickening of the collagen layer.

Aetiology and pathogenesis

An immune aetiology has also been suggested because there is an association with:

- Increased frequency of patients who have HLA-A1 haplotype.
- Decreased frequency of HLA-A3.

In addition, a minority of patients have subsequently been found to have coeliac disease.

Treatment

As for collagenous colitis. Cholestyramine may also be helpful.

NEOPLASTIC DISORDERS

Colonic polyps

Clinical features

Usually these polyps are an incidental finding as part of an investigation for abdominal pain, rectal bleeding, altered bowel habit, etc. In addition:

- Obstruction and intussusception can occur, especially in infants.
- Iron deficiency anaemia may be present if the polyp ulcerates or bleeds.
- Diarrhoea is seen with the villous type and can be severe enough to cause hypokalaemia.

Diagnosis and investigation

Investigations include:

- Barium enema—may demonstrate either solitary or multiple polyps.
- Endoscopy—is used to confirm and remove polyps for histological examination (see Fig. 17.19).

Aetiology and pathogenesis

The majority of polyps are adenomas (tubular, tubulovillous, or villous).

The malignant potential of any polyp is related to:

- Increasing polyp size.
- Polyp type, i.e. tubulovillous rather than metaplastic (Fig. 21.9).

Polyps can be solitary or multiple. Genetic and environmental factors have been implicated because they are more commonly seen in the Western world (10% of population), but no definite cause has been found. Almost all colonic carcinomas originate from a polyp and 90% of patients with colonic carcinoma will have polyps elsewhere in the colon. Five per cent of polyps removed at sigmoidoscopies are found to have invasive carcinoma.

Familial polyposis coli is an inherited autosomal dominant condition involving a gene located on the long arm of chromosome 5. There are polyps throughout the GI tract, especially in the colon, and patients commonly present in their teens. Hypertrophy and osteomas of the mandibles and long bones are commonly associated with this syndrome.

The other main type of polyps are the hamartomas such as Peutz–Jeghers syndrome (see Chapter 20). More commonly in children are juvenile polyps which histologically are shown to be mucus-retention cysts and mainly confined to the colon.

People who have Cronkhite–Canada syndrome have polyps similar to those of Peutz–Jeghers syndrome but in addition have ectodermal abnormalities such as nail dystrophy and skin pigmentation.

Complications

These include:

- Malignant change with increasing size.
- Bleeding, obstruction, and intussusception.

Prognosis

There is a 50% chance of recurrence after removal of an adenomatous polyp .

Treatment

This involves:

- Endoscopic removal of polyps—any lesions found on endoscopy or barium studies should ideally be removed to prevent malignant transformation (see Fig. 17.19).
- Surgical resection for patients with familial polyposis coli for whom individual polyps cannot be removed.
- Surveillance of patients who are at risk, i.e. polyposis coli and their first degree relatives.
- People who have had an adenoma should have regular colonoscopy to remove recurrence or detect new polyps.

Colorectal carcinoma

Incidence

The second most common carcinoma in the UK affects approximately 20 out of 100 000 people. Peak age at diagnosis is between 60 and 65 years. Disease is rare in Africa and Asia and it is thought to be environmental rather than genetic factors.

Aetiology and pathogenesis

Western diets of high animal fat and low fibre have been linked to colorectal carcinoma, possibly due to stagnation of intestinal content which increases contact time between potential carcinogens and the bowel wall.

Familial polyposis coli and inflammatory bowel disease are risk factors for the development of colonic tumours. The relationship between inflammatory bowel disease and carcinomas is not clear cut but it does not appear to be directly associated with chronicity of inflammation. It is possible that the risk for development of colonic carcinoma is an inherited one because the age of onset is more important than the severity of the disease.

Colonic carcinoma is now thought to be a result of a multiple genetic alteration that occurs in a progressive, stepwise manner. Oncogenes that normally regulate cell division and differentiation may undergo mutation due to external stimuli, producing hyperplasia, followed by metaplasia, and eventually dysplasia and tumour. Most commonly associated with colonic carcinoma are the c-KRAS and c-MYC oncogenes. The APC gene on the long arm of chromosome 5 is responsible for familial polyposis coli, which may have a role in development of colonic carcinoma (Fig. 21.9).

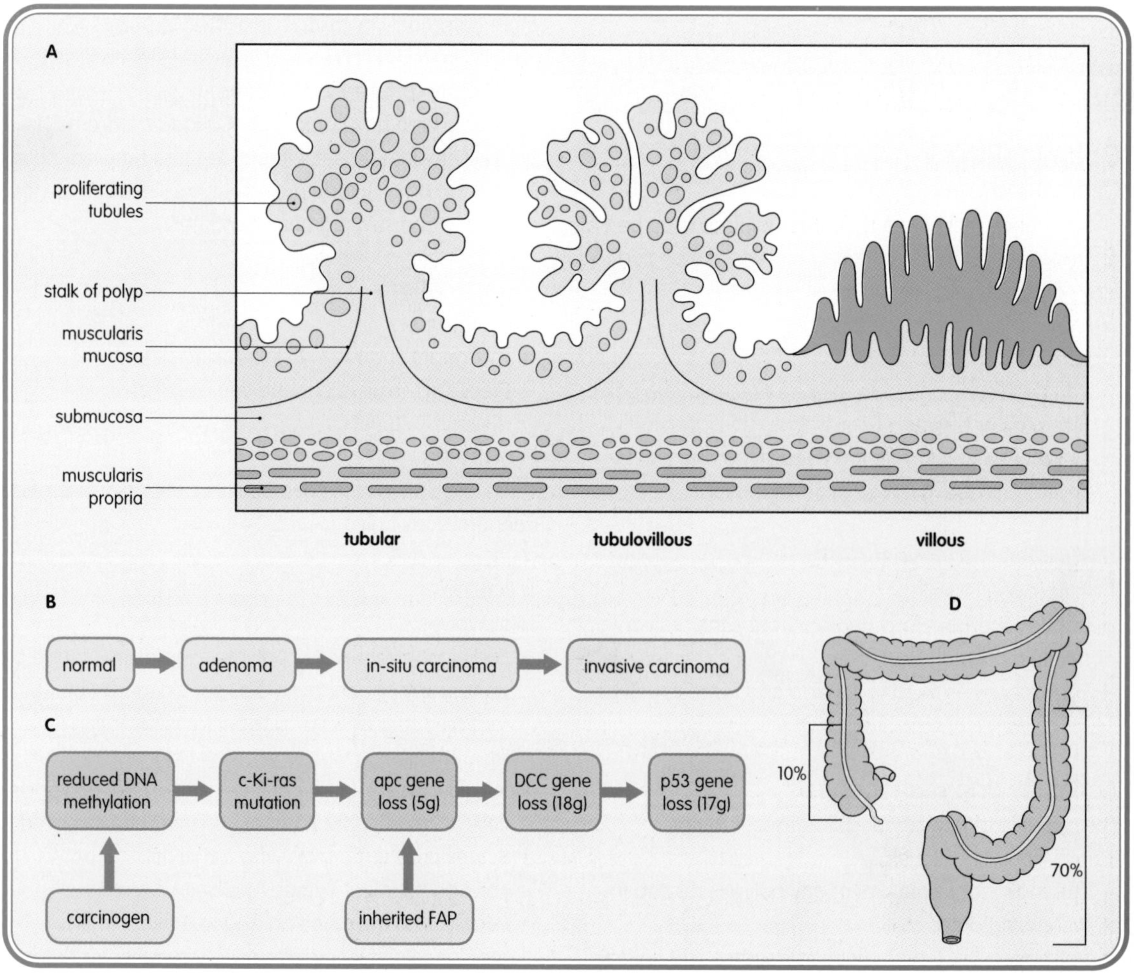

A

proliferating tubules
stalk of polyp
muscularis mucosa
submucosa
muscularis propria
tubular
tubulovillous
villous

B

normal → adenoma → in-situ carcinoma → invasive carcinoma

C

reduced DNA methylation → c-Ki-ras mutation → apc gene loss (5g) → DCC gene loss (18g) → p53 gene loss (17g)
carcinogen (→ reduced DNA methylation)
inherited FAP (→ apc gene loss (5g))

D

10%
70%

Fig. 21.9 (A) Types of colonic polyps. (B) A summary of the polyp cancer sequence in the colon. (C) Molecular changes involved. (D) Two-thirds of colon cancers occur within 60 cm of the anal verge and within reach of a flexible sigmoidoscope.

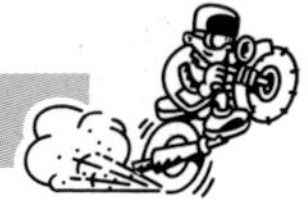

Dukes' classification of colonic cancer is shown in Fig. 21.10.

Hereditary colonic carcinomas have been described, and the gene responsible is located on chromosome 2. These patients have tumours at an early age, i.e. peak incidence at 40 years, and typically have a right-sided lesion (Lynch syndrome type I). Some of these patients also have an increased incidence of other carcinomas such as endometrial, brain, and lung, as well as other GI carcinomas (Lynch syndrome type II).

Approximately two-thirds of tumours arise from the rectosigmoid colon and these tumours typically start off as a flat lesion and later become bulky, polypoid, and ulcerate. Similar types of lesions are found in the caecum and ascending colon. Lesions in the descending colon tend to be annular and produce the typical 'apple core' lesion on barium enema.

The tumours produce a variable amount of mucin, and histologically signet ring cells can be seen where the nucleus is pushed to one side due to cytoplasmic mucus.

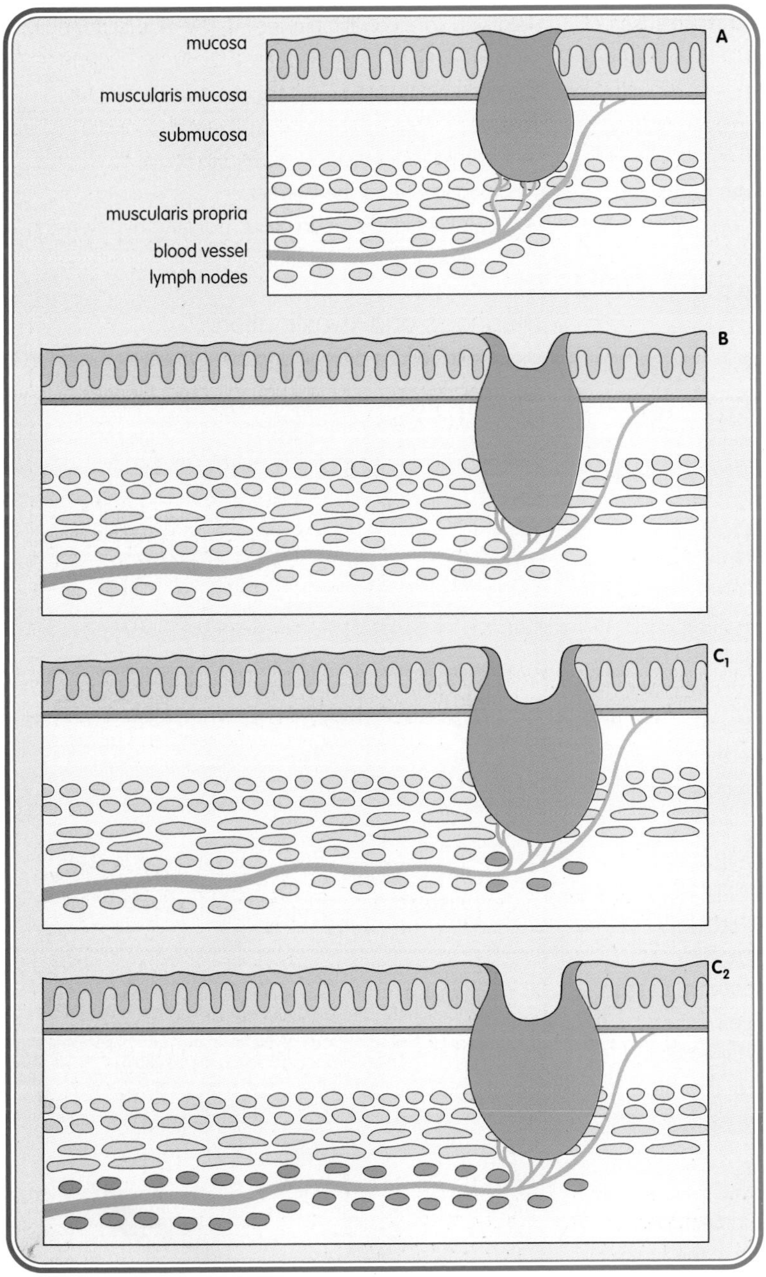

mucosa
muscularis mucosa
submucosa
muscularis propria
blood vessel
lymph nodes
A
B
C_1
C_2

Fig. 21.10 Dukes' classification of colonic cancer. (A), the tumour is confined to the bowel wall; (B) it extends through the muscle coat but does not involve lymph nodes; (C) all layers are affected, with the proximal lymph node affect in C_1 and both the proximal and the highest resected nodes positive in C_2.

Clinical features

The main features are:

- Anaemia, weight loss, abdominal pain, or loose bowel motions are the most common features. A mass may be palpable in the right iliac fossa, especially with caecal lesions. Rectal bleeding or obstruction is more common with left-sided lesions, e.g. rectosigmoid.
- Altered bowel habits are seen in >50% of all patients.
- Perforation and abscess formation is not uncommon, and jaundice due to liver metastases can occur in advanced cases.

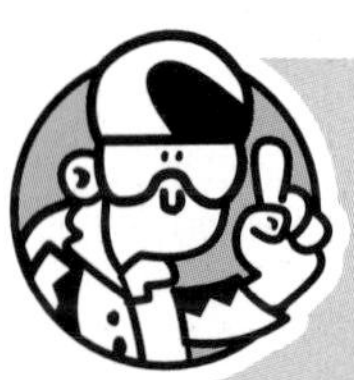

Rectal examination is an essential part of the examination as often a tumour can be palpated.

Diagnosis and investigation

Investigations of use include:

- Full blood count—may detect iron deficiency anaemia, which is common.
- Faecal occult blood—is often positive but can be seen in any cause of underlying GI bleed, e.g. duodenal ulceration.
- Barium enema—is still the investigation of choice in most centres. Poor bowel preparation can make interpretation difficult.
- Rigid sigmoidoscopy—is easily performed on an outpatient basis, but only identifies rectosigmoid tumours.
- Flexible sigmoidoscopy—can detect up to 70% of tumours and is a better investigation in combination with barium enema to examine the remainder of the colon. Colonoscopy is reserved for patients unsuitable for barium enema or in doubtful cases. Adequate bowel preparation is essential.
- Abdominal ultrasound—is sensitive for detecting metastases in the liver before surgical resection.

Treatment

The mainstays of management are:

- Surgical resection with end-to-end anastomosis or end colostomy depending on the site of the tumour.
- Chemotherapy with or without radiotherapy—given to patients with Dukes' B and C which can improve survival (Fig. 21.10). Chemotherapy can sometimes be given to patients with liver metastases, but the results are disappointing.

Prognosis

See Fig. 21.11. Overall survival is 30% at 5 years.

Angiodysplasia

Incidence

Relatively rare condition affecting the elderly population.

Clinical features

To note:

- Chronic iron deficiency anaemia is due to chronic blood loss from the GI tract.
- Acute GI bleeding can occur, causing hypotension and shock in some patients.

Diagnosis and investigation

Diagnosis can be difficult and often involves repeated gastroscopy and colonoscopy to detect the lesion:

- Red cell radioisotope-labelled scanning can be helpful to identify the site of blood loss.

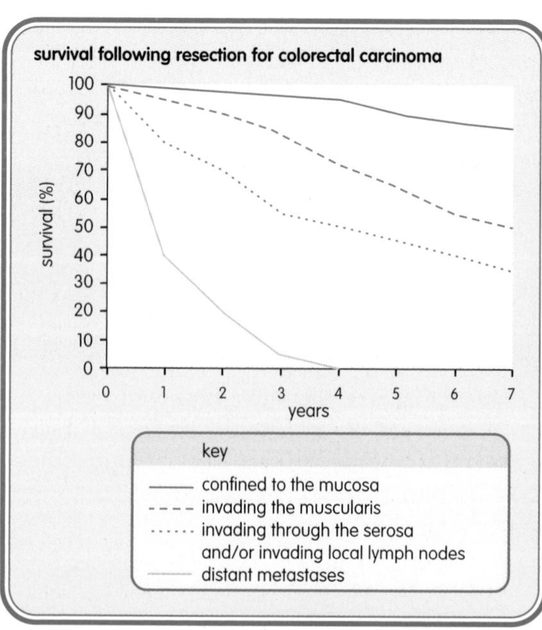

Fig. 21.11 Survival following resection for colorectal carcinoma according to Duke's staging. Note that survival is commensurate with that of the normal population if the tumour is confined to the mucosa.

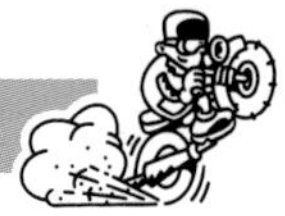

- Selective angiography may demonstrate abnormal blood vessels or the site of active bleeding.

Aetiology and pathogenesis

The underlying aetiology is unknown but the condition is most likely to be acquired because it affects mainly the elderly population. There is an association with aortic stenosis, and approximately half the patients will have some form of cardiac disease. It can occur in anywhere along the GI tract, but more commonly in proximal colon, caecum, and terminal ileum.

Treatment

Diathermy during colonoscopy can be successful for small lesions. Larger proximal lesions will need surgical resection. Hormonal treatment with progesterone derivatives can result in regression of the lesions.

ANORECTAL CONDITIONS

Haemorrhoids

Clinical features

The main symptoms are:

- Rectal bleeding occurring at the end of defecation.
- Perianal irritation and itching are also seen.

Diagnosis and investigation

Proctoscopy reveals blood vessels classically seen at the 3, 7, and 11 o'clock positions.

Aetiology and pathogenesis

Haemorrhoids result from enlargement of the venous plexuses at the lower end of anal mucosa.

Raised intra-abdominal pressure inhibits venous return and hence venous engorgement. Common contributing factors are constipation, pregnancy, excessive straining to pass urine or stool, etc.

A minor degree of rectal prolapse is common. Oestrogen-related venous dilatation may also contribute to development of haemorrhoids in pregnancy.

Rectal bleeding occurs as a result of trauma by passage of hard stools. Symptoms are usually intermittent and exacerbated by constipation.

Mucus secreted by glandular epithelium can block skin pores, which causes secondary infection by bacteria and *Candida*, followed by local skin irritation. Haemorrhoids can be classified into internal and external. They may be painful if they thrombose (Fig. 21.12).

Complications

Thrombosis of the haemorrhoids is painful and irreducible. However, it is a self-limiting condition and eventually atrophy and fibrosis of the thrombosed haemorrhoids occurs, leaving visible anal tags.

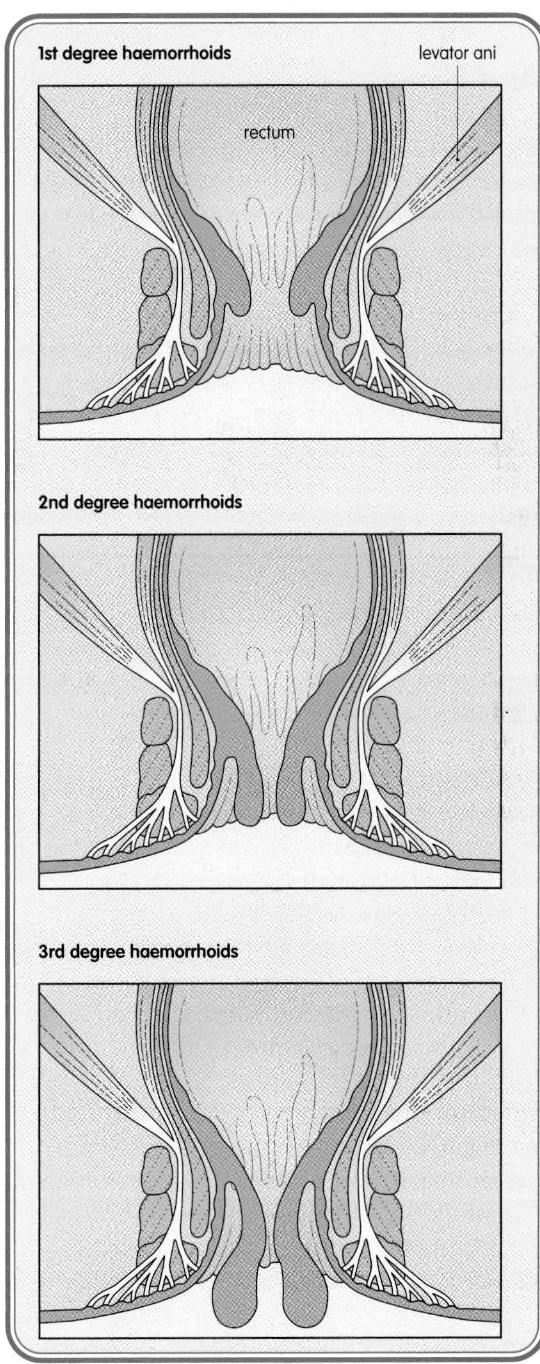

Fig. 21.12 Anatomical representation of haemorrhoid classification.

Treatment

In mild cases, a high-fibre diet is all that is required to improve the underlying constipation.

- Injection of sclerosing agent or elastic band ligation may be needed in more troublesome cases.
- Surgical resection is reserved for irreducible prolapsed and problematic cases.

Anal fissures

Clinical features

Rectal pain during defecation associated with rectal bleeding is the classic presentation. Pain, in turn, will cause anal spasm and aggravate the constipation that caused the condition originally.

Diagnosis

Often made on clinical grounds. Rectal examination is extremely painful and rarely possible. If rectal examination is required, then local or general anaesthesia may be used.

A small skin tag or sentinel pile may be seen at the anus and parting of the buttocks may reveal the fissure itself.

Aetiology and pathogenesis

Usually the result of passage of a large constipated stool causing a tear in the anal mucosa. Over 90% of cases are in the midline of the posterior margin.

Treatment

Treatment depends on the type of fissure:

- Acute fissures are treated with local anaesthesia and prevention of further constipation with either a bulking agent or osmotic laxative.
- Chronic fissuring may require surgical intervention in the form of anal stretch or more recently lateral internal sphincterotomy, which has a better result with regard to incontinence in later age.

Pruritus ani

A common complaint. The majority of cases are secondary to poor hygiene and some degree of faecal incontinence, especially in elderly people. Associated conditions such as haemorrhoids, threadworm infestation, or fungal infection should be excluded.

In the absence of any underlying cause, treatment should include good personal hygiene and keeping the area dry. Use of topical steroids should be avoided.

Rectal prolapse

Incidence

Common among elderly people and young children.

Clinical features

Tenesmus is a feeling of incomplete defaecation which can be due to prolapse. Rectal bleeding can occur due to mucosal ulceration secondary to stool trauma. Incontinence of faeces may be seen.

Complete prolapse of the rectal wall can sometimes be seen through the anus (Fig. 21.13).

Diagnosis and investigation

Usually made on history and examination. However:

- Sigmoidoscopy may reveal a 'solitary' rectal ulcer approximately 8–10 cm above the anal verge, usually on the anterior rectal wall. These 'solitary' ulcers can also be multiple.
- Prolapse can often be seen when the patient is asked to voluntarily strain as if to pass a stool.
- Defaecating proctogram is a very useful, if undignified, examination if the prolapse is internal but producing significant symptoms.
- Endoscopic ultrasound can be useful to determine whether muscle damage has occurred (possibly due to obstetric trauma) as this can be repaired surgically.

Aetiology and pathogenesis

The condition results from excessive straining when opening bowels. In the initial stages, the prolapse only occurs after defaecation and returns spontaneously, but later the condition worsens and prolapse may appear on standing.

In early stages, prolapse of the mucosa or rectal wall may remain internal to the anal sphincter, hence the patient may experience discomfort but no obvious abnormality can be seen.

Treatment

Childhood prolapse rarely requires surgical treatment. Parents should be reassured because the prolapse will almost always be reduced either spontaneously or with gentle manipulation. A high-fibre diet should be given, and the child taught not to strain at defaecation.

Minor prolapses often do not require treatment because they reduce themselves and only appear after straining. General advice such as a high-fibre diet and avoidance of straining should be given. Patients with

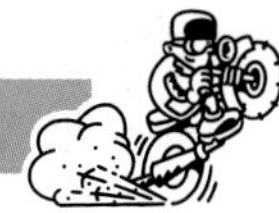

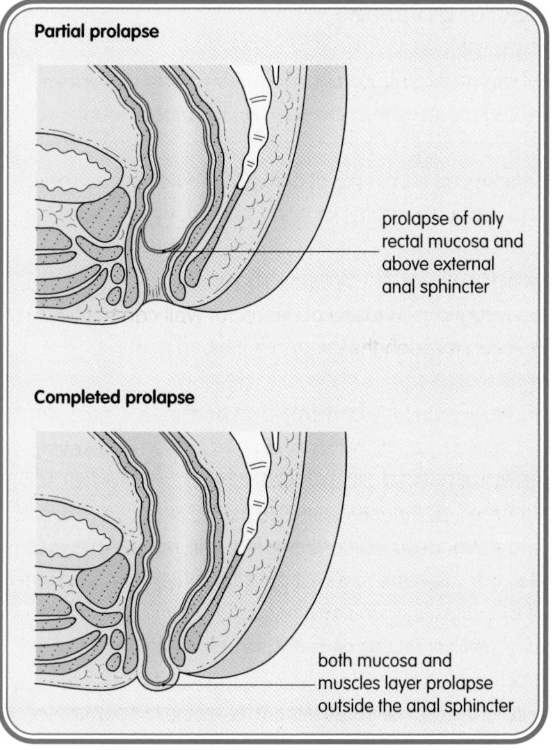

Fig. 21.13 Classification of rectal prolapse.

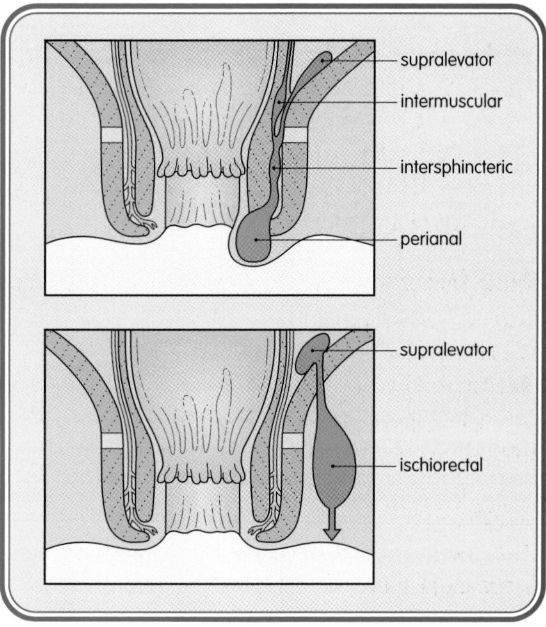

Fig. 21.14 Illustration showing how perianal infection can develop into abscess or fistula.

severe prolapse should be treated surgically by posterior fixation of the rectum to the sacral wall. Sphincter repair may also be necessary if incontinence is a problem due to a weakened sphincter.

Anorectal abscesses

Clinical features

Pain depends upon the site of the abscess:

- A fluctuant mass sitting just beneath the inflamed skin is typical of perianal and ischiorectal abscesses.
- A tender mass on rectal examination may be due to intersphincteric or pararectal abscesses.

Systemic features of infection such as fever and neutrophilia may occur.

Aetiology and pathogenesis

More often seen in patients with diabetes, Crohn's disease, or other causes of immunosuppression, but do occur in otherwise healthy individuals. The condition is due to infection of the anal glands which tends to spread along the anal duct through the external sphincter and its surrounding tissues (Fig. 21.14).

Treatment

Surgical drainage is required in all cases, except for those that are very minor for which antibiotics alone can be given. Antibiotics are routinely given after the drainage procedure.

Anal fistula

Clinical features

Intermittent discharge over the perianal area from the fistula. The fistula itself can be seen as a small area of granulation tissue around the anal margin. It is often dismissed as incomplete healing of anorectal abscess. Underlying Crohn's disease should be excluded or confirmed.

Diagnosis and investigation

Examination under anaesthesia is usually required to establish the site of the proximal opening by a probe.

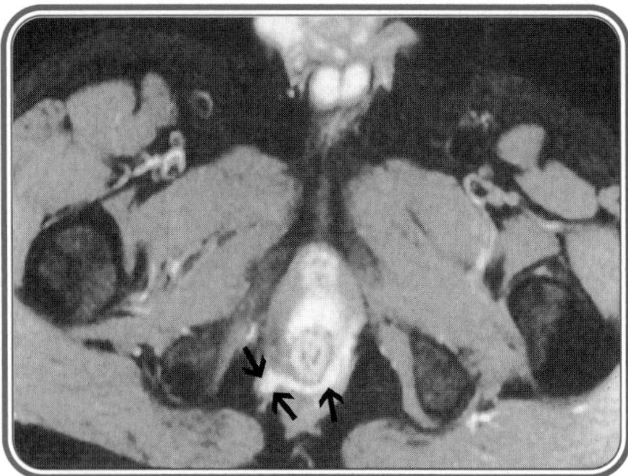

Fig. 21.15 Magnetic resonance scan demonstration of anal fistula tracking around the back of the anal canal and through the muscularis on the right side (arrows).

Occasionally, a dye is injected into the distal orifice to identify the opening (fistulogram).

Aetiology and pathogenesis

Anal fistula is a common complication of anorectal abscesses as the anal gland infection spreads to form an abscess and drains externally in the form of a fistula. An MR scan demonstration of anal fistula is shown in Fig. 21.15. Crohn's disease is also a cause of anal fistula, and they are often multiple.

Treatment

Once the proximal opening has been identified, the fistula can be laid open and healing by secondary intention occurs, providing the fistula does not involve the anal sphincter.

Fistulae that involve the sphincter will require a specialist anorectal surgeon for preservation and repair of the sphincter to provide continence.

Fistulae caused by Crohn's disease should be treated with conservative treatment as for active Crohn's disease. Surgical treatment usually involves an ileostomy.

INFECTIONS

Bacterial infection of the colon

Incidence

The most common cause of diarrhoea worldwide, especially affecting travellers outside their own country.

Clinical features

These include:

- Diarrhoea, abdominal pain, fever, and vomiting.
- Leucocytosis may be seen on full blood count.

Clinical and biochemical dehydration not uncommon, especially at extreme of ages, i.e. elderly and infants.

Diagnosis and investigation

Investigations of use include:

- Routine biochemistry and full blood count.
- Stool culture.
- Sigmoidoscopy and biopsy if diarrhoea is persistent.

Aetiology and pathogenesis

Common pathogens include species of *E. coli, Shigella,* and *Salmonella* which are spread via faecal–oral route and are often the result of poor food hygiene. Invasion of the colonic epithelium occurs and in some cases with certain strains of *E. coli*, an enterotoxin is produced.

Clostridium difficile infection is typically seen after broad spectrum antibiotic therapy, but especially clindamycin. Disturbance of normal colonic flora caused by antibiotics allow proliferation of *C. difficile* and toxin production. On sigmoidoscopy, plaques of inflammatory exudates can be seen giving the appearance of pseudomembranes (pseudomembranous colitis). Direct person to person spread can also occur.

Diagnosis can be made by isolation of the toxins in the stool.

Treatment

Rehydration is required either intravenously or orally. Once stool cultures have confirmed the diagnosis, appropriate antibiotics should be started. If the patient is severely ill, ciprofloxacin can be started once stool and blood cultures have been taken. If *C. difficile* is suspected or confirmed, then metronidazole or vancomycin is the drug of choice.

Antidiarrhoeal agents, e.g. loperamide should be avoided if possible because it impairs the clearance of the pathogen from the bowel.

Amoebiasis

Incidence

Occurs worldwide, but more commonly in tropics.

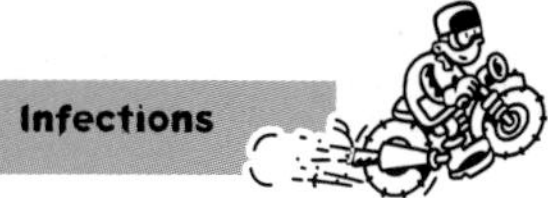

Clinical features
In acute infection these include:
- Abdominal pain.
- Diarrhoea (often bloody).
- Nausea and vomiting.

Fulminant colitis and toxic dilatation can rarely occur.

Diagnosis and investigation
Investigations:
- Fresh stool samples are required for identification of amoebic cysts.
- Specific antibody can be measured in the serum.
- Sigmoidoscopy demonstrates ulceration of the colonic mucosa but it is not diagnostic.

Aetiology and pathogenesis
The disease is caused by *Entamoeba histolytica* which is digested in its cyst form via contaminated food or water, or direct person-to-person spread. Multiplication of the organism takes place in the colon, where they invade the colonic epithelium, causing ulceration. Not all who are infected will have clinical disease and some become asymptomatic cyst carriers.

Complications
Uncommon. Perforation due to toxic dilatation can occur. Strictures can occur in chronic infection. Hepatic abscesses are not uncommon (see Chapter 22).

Treatment
Metronidazole is the drug of choice. Improve hygiene to reduce person-to-person spread.

Cryptosporidiosis
Clinical features
Symptoms include:
- Watery diarrhoea.
- Fever.
- Abdominal pain.

Toxic dilatation and sclerosing cholangitis can be seen in patients with AIDS.

Diagnosis and investigation
Parasite can be identified by modified Ziehl–Nielsen stain of faeces or intestinal biopsy.

Aetiology and pathogenesis
The parasite is found worldwide with its major reservoir in cattle, and is likely to be spread via contaminated water supplies.

Healthy individuals will have a self-limiting gastroenteritis and often the diagnosis is not confirmed. People who are immunocompromised tend to have a devastating illness with long and protracted chronic diarrhoea.

The organism also causes sclerosing cholangitis in the immunocompromised patient.

Treatment
No effective treatment is found as yet. Good hygiene prevents spread of the infection.

Schistosomiasis
See also Chapter 22 and Fig. 22.27.

Clinical features
The main features are:
- Fever.
- Urticaria.
- Nausea.
- Vomiting.
- Bloody diarrhoea.

Diagnosis and investigation
Consider the following investigations:
- Specific antibodies can be detected by serology.
- Eggs can be isolated from stool, urine, or rectal biopsy.
- Sigmoidoscopy reveals mucosal ulceration which is not diagnostic.

Aetiology and pathogenesis
Schistosoma mansoni predominantly affects the colon, causing erythema and ulceration of the mucosa. A localized granulomatous reaction may be mistaken for colonic cancer. Progressive fibrosis leads to stricture formation but obstruction is rare.

Schistosoma japonicum affects the small intestine and proximal colon and epithelial dysplasia is seen with chronic infection which is now accepted to be a premalignant condition.

Complications
Periportal fibrosis and portal hypertension. Ectopic

deposition of eggs elsewhere in the body, e.g. lung and brain.

Treatment
Praziquantel is currently the drug of choice.

Whipworm infection
Incidence
Found worldwide and prevelance can be as high as 90% in poor communities with poor hygiene.

Clinical features
Usually asymptomatic.

Heavy infestation causes bloody diarrhoea associated with weight loss, abdominal discomfort and anorexia. Involvement of appendix causes appendicitis.

Diagnosis and investigation
Stool examination for eggs.

Sigmoidoscopy—adult worms may be seen attached to the rectal mucosa.

Aetiology and pathogenesis
Caused by *Trichuris trichura*. Adult worms are more commonly found in the distal ileum and caecum. The whole colon may be affected in heavy infection.

The adult worm embeds itself in the colonic mucosa, causing damage and ulceration, leading to protein and blood loss in severe cases.

Treatment
Mebendazole is the treatment of choice.

Threadworm infection
Incidence
Occurs worldwide, but more prevalent in temperate climates. Outbreaks are seen in institutional establishments and areas of overcrowded living conditions.

Clinical features
Pruritus ani is intense and usually nocturnal due to egg laying by the female worm.

Submucosal abscess is rare and due to secondary bacterial infection of the colonic mucosa.

Diagnosis and investigation
Adult worms may be seen directly leaving the anus. Clear adhesive tape can be applied to the perianal region to allow the identification of eggs microscopically.

Aetiology and pathogenesis
Caused by *Enterobius vermicularis* and commonly affects children. Adult worms reside in the colon and female worms migrate to the perianal region to lay their eggs. Superficial damage to the colonic mucosa is common during heavy infestations.

Autoinfection via scratching and poor hygiene aggravates the problem. Rarely, migration to the peritoneum and visceral organs occurs.

Treatment
Mebendazole given as two single doses, 2 weeks apart is effective. Asymptomatic family members should also be treated.

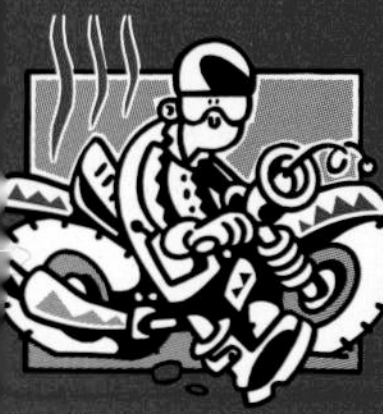

22. Liver

STRUCTURE AND FUNCTION OF THE LIVER

The predominant pathological mechanisms affecting the liver are:

- Necrosis.
- Inflammation.
- Fibrosis.

The site at which these disease processes occur may produce different clinical syndromes, and the functions of the liver (Fig. 22.1) may be affected differentially:

- Centrilobular processes affect synthetic and metabolic functions and hepatocellular necrosis produces an enzyme rise predominantly of alanine transaminase (ALT) and aspartate transaminase (AST) (Fig. 22.2).
- Centrifugal or periportal processes have less effect on synthetic function but disproportionate effects on portal pressure and bile duct excretory function. Disease here tends to cause disproportionate increase in the 'biliary' enzymes alkaline phosphatase and gamma glutamyl transferase (Fig. 22.2).
- Alcoholic liver disease tends to have effects throughout all parts of the lobule and most progressive diseases ultimately will also involve both portal tracts and centrilobular areas.

Functions of the liver	
Function	**Substrate examples**
Synthetic function	Albumin (half-life 20 days) Transferrin (half-life 3 days) Coagulation factors (all of them)
Storage	Glycogen, triglyceride, iron (ferritin), vitamin A
Metabolic homeostasis	Maintenance blood glucose (glycogenolysis and gluconeogenesis)
Metabolic activation and transformation	Vitamin D, lipoproteins
Metabolic deactivation and detoxification	Sex steroids, ammonia, drugs
Excretion	Bilirubin

Fig. 22.1 Functions of the liver.

HYPERBILIRUBINAEMIAS

Unconjugated hyperbilirubinaemia

Gilbert syndrome

Incidence and diagnosis

The most common congenital hyperbilirubinaemia affecting 2–5% of the population. It is:

- Usually detected incidentally on routine checks as a raised bilirubin.
- More commonly manifest in males.

The patient is often asymptomatic, and a positive family history of jaundice may be seen in 5–10% of cases. Serum bilirubin is usually less than 50 mmol/L (normal <17).

Diagnosis is made on the basis of an increase in unconjugated bilirubin following an overnight fast or during a mild illness.

Aetiology and pathogenesis

Aetiology of the syndrome involves a reduction in enzyme activity (glucuronosyl transferase or UGT-1), but many other factors can affect this, hence its variable presentation. UGT-1 is a cytoplasmic enzyme that conjugates bilirubin to allow it to be excreted in a soluble form. Recently, a mutation in the promotor region (TATA box) of the mRNA for this enzyme was described, which reduces the efficiency of transcription of this enzyme. It is possible that Gilbert syndrome represents an extreme end of a normal distribution.

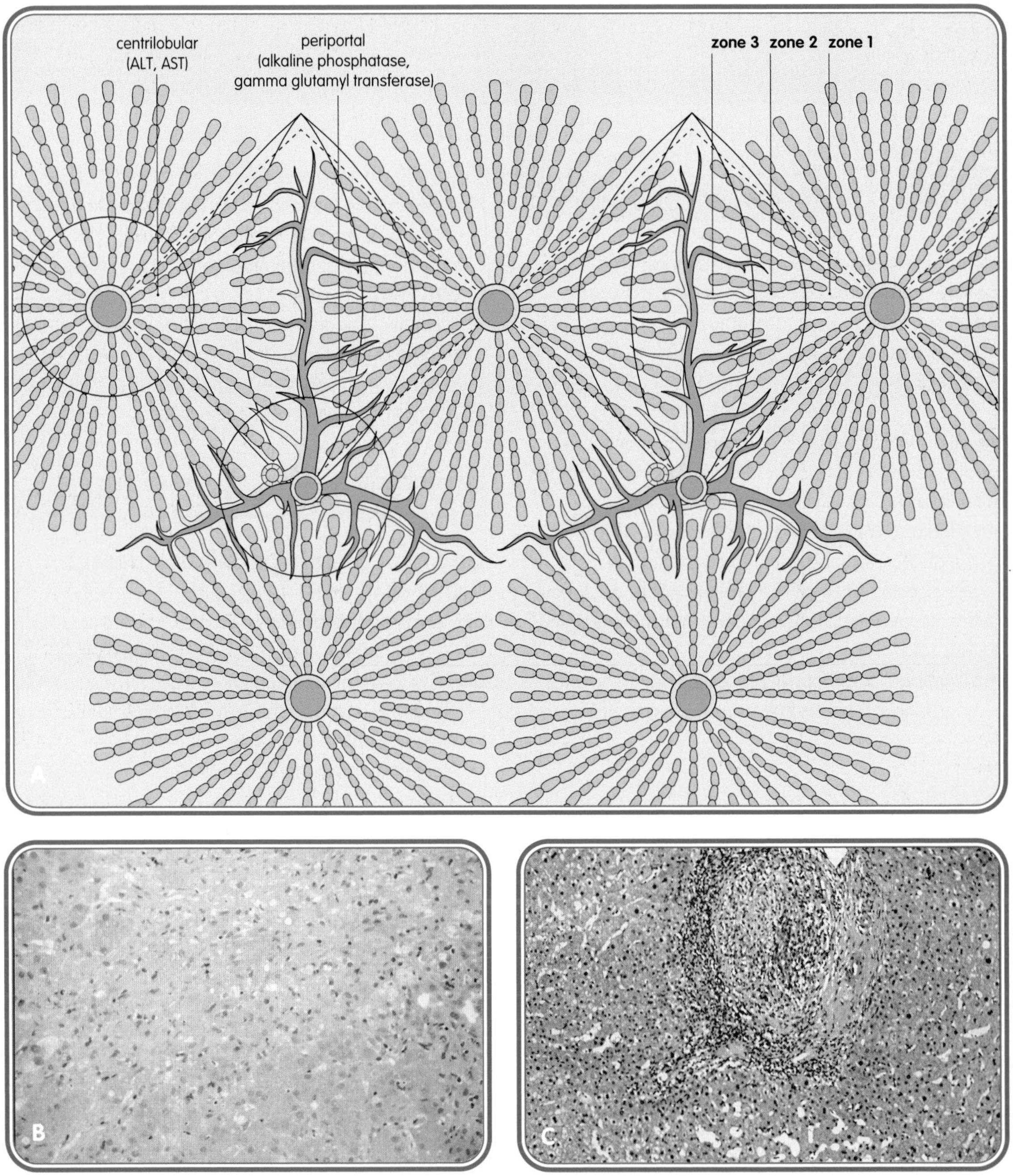

centrilobular (ALT, AST)
periportal (alkaline phosphatase, gamma glutamyl transferase)
zone 3 zone 2 zone 1
A

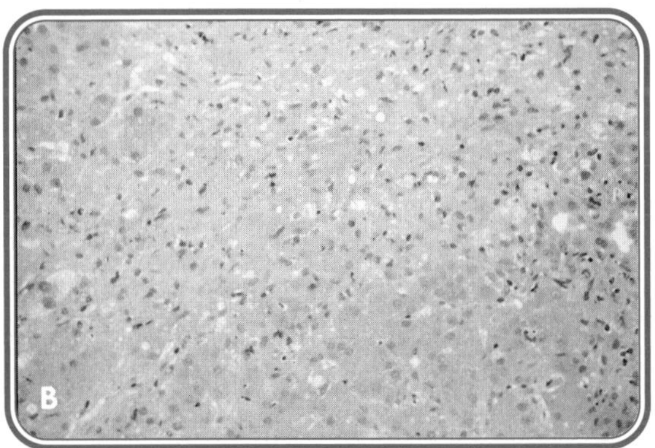

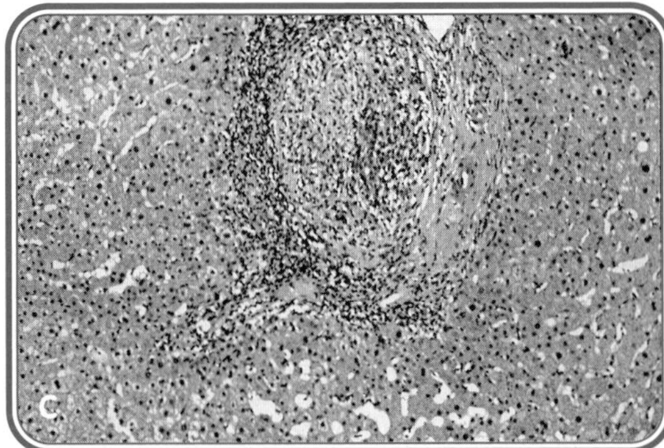

Fig. 22.2 (A) Hepatic lobular architecture showing functional zones and centrilobular or centripetal predilection for pathological processes. Different enzymes predominate in the different zones and their detection in serum may reflect liver damage in those zones. (B) Centrilobular necrosis with inflammation. (C) Inflammation centred on portal tract with early fibrosis.

Prognosis

This is excellent. It is important to reassure the patient that the condition is not serious and avoid any unnecessary investigations in the future. No treatment is required.

Crigler–Najjar syndrome

Two types have been described, both exceedingly rare conditions:

- Type I (autosomal recessive)—complete absence of glucuronosyl transferase.

- Type II (autosomal dominant)—decreased level of glucuronosyl transferase.

Type I deficiency: presents as neonatal jaundice due to unconjugated bilirubinaemia, fatal in first year of life. Serum bilirubin can rise to 600–800 mmol/L. Death is from kernicterus.

Type II deficiency: survival into adulthood is not uncommon. Serum bilirubin is usually less than 300 mmol/L. Kernicterus can be prevented by induction of the enzyme with phenobarbitone.

Liver biopsy is normal and transplantation is the only treatment.

Conjugated hyperbilirubinaemia

Dubin–Johnson syndrome

Incidence and diagnosis

This is a rare and benign disorder that usually presents in adolescence. Plasma bilirubin is conjugated.

A bromsulphthalein (BSP) clearance test in Dubin–Johnson syndrome has a second recirculation peak at 90 minutes. Liver biopsy is stained black due to centrilobular melanin deposits.

Aetiology and pathogenesis

The condition is believed to be due to the failure to excrete conjugated bilirubin and is inherited as an autosomal recessive pattern due to a defect in a transporter protein in the bile canaliculi.

Prognosis and treatment

No specific treatment is required and the prognosis is excellent.

Rotor syndrome

Also a benign and probably autosomal dominant condition of conjugated hyperbilirubinaemia. It can be distinguished from Dubin–Johnson syndrome by a normal liver biopsy. Prognosis is also excellent for this syndrome.

VIRAL HEPATITIS

Traditionally, viruses with a predilection to cause hepatitis have come to be classified alphabetically. Currently at least six different viruses are known to infect humans (A, B, C, D, E, and G). Other viruses such as cytomegalovirus (CMV), Epstein–Barr virus, yellow fever also infect the liver.

Hepatitis A

Incidence

Most common type of hepatitis worldwide, most often affects the young. Epidemics are associated with overcrowding and poor hygiene and sanitation. Transmission is by the faecal–oral route or ingestion of contaminated water or shellfish.

Clinical features

In the prodromal phase:

- Symptoms mimic viral gastroenteritis (nausea, vomiting, diarrhoea, headache, mild fever, malaise and abdominal discomfort).
- A distaste for cigarettes said to be characteristic in young adults.

The icteric phase occurs after 10–14 days (some patients remain anicteric) and resolves in 2–3 weeks:

- Mild symptoms such as malaise and fatigue may persist for months.
- Liver enlargement is common during the icteric phase; the spleen is palpable in approximately 10%.

Diagnosis and investigation

Diagnosis is usually made on clinical grounds. A definitive diagnosis can be made if there is a rising titre of anti-HAV IgM and/or demonstration of viral particles in stools by electron microscopy. Elevated anti-HAV IgG titre reflects previous exposure to hepatitis A and thus lifelong immunity. Transaminases are moderately elevated (500–1000 IU/L) but normalize rapidly (Fig. 22.3).

Aetiology and pathogenesis

Hepatitis A is a pico-RNA-virus excreted in the faeces of an infected person approximately 2 weeks before the onset of jaundice and up to 1 week thereafter. The disease is most infectious just before the onset of jaundice. The RNA virus is relatively heat resistant withstanding 60°C for up to 30 minutes, hence it thrives in areas of poor hygiene.

Complications

Rare, but myocarditis, arthritis, vasculitis, and very occasionally, fulminant hepatic failure have been described.

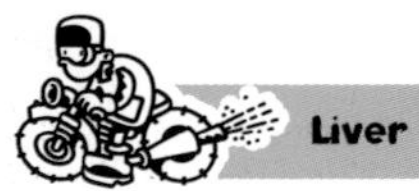

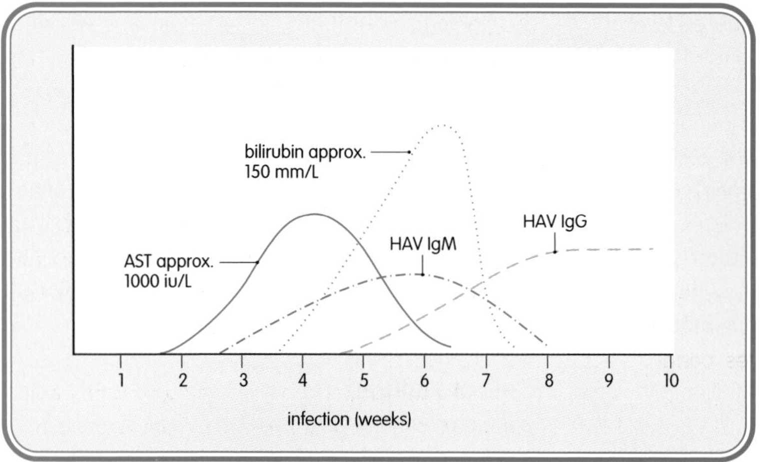

Fig. 22.3 Laboratory tests and their time course in hepatitis A infection.

Prognosis

Most patients recover completely without any sequalae; some have a self-limiting relapse of hepatitis. A few have a prolonged cholestatic jaundice (3–4 months) but in general the prognosis is excellent. Often the course is more prolonged in adults or immunocompromised patients.

Hepatitis A infection does not have a carrier status. Progression to chronic viral disease does not occur but in some individuals may precipitate autoimmune liver disease. Previous infection confers lifetime immunity.

Aims and indication for treatment

Unless the patient is very unwell, hospital admission is unnecessary. Treatment otherwise is supportive. Vaccination or hyperimmune globulin should be offered to people at high risk.

Treatment plans

Antiemetics can be given for nausea and vomiting, intravenous fluids for dehydration, and simple analgesia for headaches. It is important to maintain caloric intake.

Hepatitis B

Incidence

Symptomless infected carrier rate 0.1% in UK and USA, 20% in parts of Asia and Africa (worlwide prevalence of carriers estimated at 300–400 million).

Transmission:

- Contaminated blood products (incidence has fallen dramatically since the introduction of screening in UK, Europe, and USA in the late 1970s).
- Contaminated instrumentation (IVDU).
- Sexual intercourse with infected partner.
- Vertical transmission (most common mode worldwide).
- Viral particles have been isolated from insects such as mosquitoes.

Aetiology and pathogenesis

HBV is a DNA virus that replicates in the liver where the core antigen incorporates itself into the host genome and the host's DNA polymerase transcribes for the virus and may be the prime factor for the development of hepatocellular carcinoma.

Body fluid contact is essential for transmission. Infection in the birth canal during parturition is the most important mode worldwide, creating a large 'carrier state' reservoir of infection. In developed countries, promiscuous sexual practitioners and intravenous drug users form the largest reservoir of infection.

Hepatitis B syndromes may be acute, chronic, or the carrier state.

Clinical features

Features of acute hepatitis B include:

- Incubation time: 60–160 days (average 90 days).
- Non-specific prodromal symptoms: arthralgia, anorexia, abdominal discomfort.
- Jaundice, fever, and hepatomegaly are usual features.
- Urticarial or maculopapular rash may appear, together with a polyarthritis thought to be secondary to immune-mediated complexes.
- History of contact with contaminated source is usual

(especially travellers to the Orient, drug addicts, accidental injury to health workers, etc.).

Features of chronic hepatitis B include:

- Most chronic carriers are asymptomatic.
- Majority discovered incidentally, e.g. blood donor screening, occupational health checks, routine liver function tests, etc.
- Patients with chronic active hepatitis may present with features or complications of chronic liver disease or cirrhosis: jaundice, ascites, portal hypertension, hepatic failure.
- Chronic hepatitis predisposes to cirrhosis of the liver and an increased risk of hepatocellular carcinoma, especially in males.

Investigation and diagnosis

Transaminases may be very high in the acute stage (1000–5000 IU/L) falling rapidly after the first week; chronic hepatitis produces only a mild elevation of ALT or AST.

Serology (Fig. 22.4): surface antigen (HBsAg) is the first serological marker to appear (6 weeks to 3 months); 'e' antigen (HBeAg) follows, reflecting viral replication, high infectivity, and more severe disease. This usually disappears before HBsAg, but its persistence correlates with HBV DNA in blood. HBsAg and HBeAg may be present in either acute or chronic HBV infection.

Anti-HBe antibodies appear from approximately 8 weeks after infection and their presence reflects low infectivity. Such seroconversion may occur spontaneously after several decades or with interferon. Anti-HBs antibodies appear late (>3 months) and confer lifelong immunity.

Antibodies to core antigen (HBcAg, IgM) were measured in the past when there was a window period where HBsAg disappeared and anti-HBsAg was not detectable but this has largely superseded by detection of core DNA by polymerase chain reaction (PCR).

Complications

Fulminant hepatitis and death occurs in 1% of patients. Extrahepatic complications: arteritis and glomerulonephritis may be immune-complex mediated. Variation in the viral genome (mutants) are becoming more common; often associated with fulminant hepatitis

Prognosis

Up to 90% of acute infections resolve without sequelae:

- 5–10% of patients become chronic carriers (carrier rate is much higher following vertical transmission possibly due to immature immune response to the virus in the neonate).
- 5% develop chronic active hepatitis, which may progress to cirrhosis or hepatocellular carcinoma in cirrhotic patients, especially males (25% lifetime risk).

Aims of treatment

Acute infection: as in hepatitis A infection, symptomatic relief is all that is required with extra care taken when handling of body fluids. Fulminant hepatitis carries a grave prognosis, requires intensive care and possible liver transplantation. Chronic hepatitis can be treated

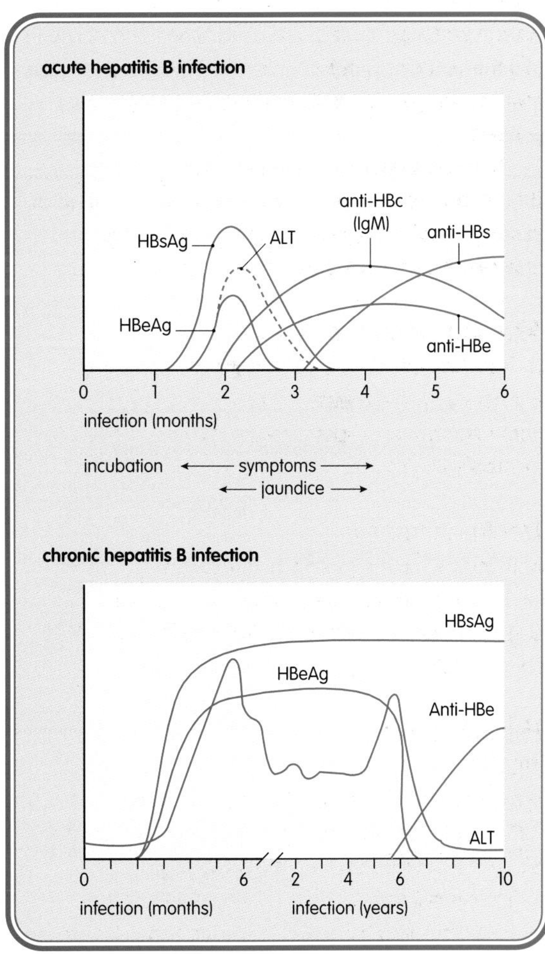

Fig. 22.4 Laboratory tests and their time course in hepatitis B infection. (Redrawn with permission from: Kumar PJ, Clarke ML. *Clinical Medicine* 3rd ed. London: Baillière Tindall; 1994.)

with alpha-interferon to seroconvert from HBeAb negative to HBeAb positive. The success rate is variable, especially in cases of vertical transmission.

Vaccination is successful in preventing transmission. When combined with immunoglobulin at birth, thus successfully prevents vertical transmission. Hyperimmune globulin or lamivudine, a nucleoside analogue, are used to prevent recurrence after transplantation.

Indication for treatment

Patients who are HBeAg positive and HBeAb negative have raised liver transaminases and evidence of chronic active hepatitis on liver biopsy and should be offered interferon treatment (Fig. 22.5).

Treatment plan

Subcutaneous injection of interferon alpha (5–10 mega units three times weekly) are used. Dose and duration of treatment are dependent on the patient's tolerance of side effects (a flu-like syndrome and headaches). All pregnant hepatitis B virus mothers should plan for vaccination of newborn at parturition. Vaccination should also be offered to other people at risk, such as intravenous drug users, health care personnel, and travellers to high risk areas.

Poor prognostic factors in hepatitis B and C

Hepatitis B	Hepatitis C
Possibly duration of infection; age >40 years	Age at acquisition: older fare worse
Any signs, e.g. spider naevi, ascites	Viral inoculation or load may have a role; genotype 1b seem to fare less well
Activity on liver biopsy, especially if cirrhotic	Bridging fibrosis or cirrhosis on liver biopsy
Males fare worse than females	Males fare worse than females
Concomitant disease	Possibly higher iron stores and alcohol intake cause synergistic damage
Development of hepatocellular carcinoma, especially in males	Development of hepatocellular carcinoma, especially in males

Fig. 22.5 Poor prognostic factors in hepatitis B and C .

Hepatitis C

Incidence

Previously known as non-A, non-B hepatitis and now thought to be responsible for up to 90% of such cases. The hepatitis C virus was identified in 1988 and routine screening of blood products has been available only since 1991.

Transmission:

- Contaminated blood products.
- Contaminated instrumentation (IVDU).
- Sexual, vertical, and breast milk transmission is uncommon (5%).

Clinical features

Features include:

- Clinical jaundice occurs in less than 20% of patients.
- Fatigue and malaise are common.
- Extrahepatic manifestations such as arthritis, cryoglobulinaemia, and aplastic anaemia are rare.

A minority of patients with cirrhosis may have its attendant potential complications of portal hypertension, hepatic failure, or hepatoma.

Diagnosis

Most commonly, patients are referred for investigation of abnormal liver enzymes found incidentally or are referred by the blood transfusion service when they are discovered to be antibody positive:

- Transaminases are usually only slightly elevated (ALT 50–150 IU/L).
- Bilirubin and synthetic function is usually normal.
- Ferritin may be elevated.
- Antibodies to hepatitis C are found in the serum using ELISA or radioimmunoassay kits.
- Viral RNA is detectable by reverse transcription polymerase chain reaction (RT-PCR).
- Liver histology shows a spectrum from fatty infiltration through lobular hepatitis to cirrhosis.

Aetiology and pathogenesis

Hepatitis C is a single-stranded RNA virus with several immunogenic subtypes, hence allowing epidemiological studies to establish modes of transmission.

Complications and prognosis

- 70% develop chronic indolent hepatitis of varying severity.
- 20% progress to cirrhosis.

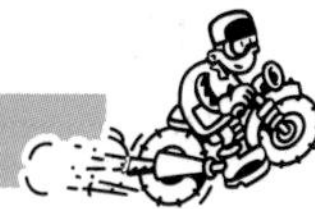

Advanced age at infection, male gender, and high viral load predict a more rapid progression. Fulminant hepatitis is a rare but fatal complication (Fig. 22.5).

Aims of treatment
To reduce the level of viral replication in the liver and thus liver damage and cirrhosis, interferon alpha is the drug of choice.

Indications for treatment
Most criteria are based on severity of inflammation on biopsy. Hepatitis C virus antibody positivity and RT-PCR positive are prerequisites. There is some evidence that selection by certain criteria improves response rate (e.g. young age or low body weight, females, low iron indices).

Treatment plan
Alpha-interferon 3–6 mega units for 3–6 months achieves a biochemical response (normalization of ALT) in approximately two-thirds patients and a clearance of virus detectable by RT-PCR in less than 50%. Treatment is continued for 6–12 months in PCR responders, but response is sustained in only about half of those treated. Currently there is no vaccine for hepatitis C. Recently the combination of interferon with ribavirin has been shown to approximately double the response rate associated with the use of interferon alone.

Hepatitis D
Incidence
Also known as the delta virus, it is an incomplete RNA particle which is unable to replicate by itself. It occurs as a co-infection with hepatitis B virus and is particularly seen in IV drug abusers but can affect any patient with hepatitis B.

Diagnosis
Co-infection is indistinguishable from acute hepatitis B infection, but occasionally superinfection produces an active flare-up of hepatitis with a rise of liver transaminases. Clinical jaundice may not be obvious.

Presence of IgM anti-delta virus with IgM anti-HBcAg confirms co-infection and IgM anti-delta is replaced by IgG anti-delta over 6–8 weeks. IgM anti-delta in presence of IgG anti-HBcAg indicates superinfection because IgM anti-HBcAg is replaced by IgG antibodies after the initial infection. Hepatitis D RNA can be measured in the serum and liver, and is seen in both acute and chronic infection.

Aetiology and pathogenesis
The incomplete RNA particle is enclosed within HBsAg, suggesting that it is unable to replicate by itself but is activated in the presence of hepatitis B infection.

Complications
Fulminant hepatitis is a serious complication and is more common after co-infection. Chronic infection with hepatitis D is usually the case in the form of cirrhosis.

Aims of treatment
Supportive for fulminant hepatitis. Reduction of viral replication with interferon to reduce the risk of developing cirrhosis.

Indications for treatment
Chronic active hepatitis as demonstrated on liver enzymes and biopsy.

Treatment plan
As for other chronic viral hepatitis with interferon alpha, where it can induce remission but as with hepatitis C infection, relapse is common on withdrawal of treatment.

Hepatitis E
In summary of hepatitis E:

- An RNA virus spread via the faecal–oral route.
- Predominantly seen in developing countries
- Mortality rises from 1% to 20% in pregnant women; the reason is still at present unclear.
- Hepatitis E RNA can be detected in serum or stool by PCR.
- Treatment as for hepatitis A is only symptomatic.
- No carrier state is associated and it does not progress on to chronic active hepatitis.
- Improved sanitation and hygiene are essential for prevention and control.

A summary of hepatitis viruses is shown in Fig. 22.6.

Hepatitis G
Hepatitis G (also called GB-C) has recently been identified and has some sequence homology with hepatitis C. It has been found in about 2% of blood donors who have been screened, but there is not a routine screening test available. It is thought not to cause acute or chronic hepatitis but its precise clinical relevance is still not clear.

Hepatitis viruses				
Type	**Spread**	**Incubation**	**Prevention**	**Treatment**
A	Faecal–oral	2–6 weeks	Immunoglobulin or vaccine	Not specific
B	Contaminated body fluid: vertical, blood, semen	2–6 months	Hepatitis B immunoglobulin or vaccine	Alpha-interferon Lamivudine
C	Contaminated blood	6–8 weeks	None available	Alpha-interferon Ribaviron
D	Contaminated blood Requires hepatitis B	Unknown	Prevention of hepatitis B	None
E	Faecal–oral	2–9 weeks	Improve hygiene	None

Fig. 22.6 Summary of hepatitis viruses.

Epstein–Barr virus (infectious mononucleosis)

Incidence and diagnosis

A common disease of the young, although it can occur at any age.

Fever, malaise, tonsillar, and glandular enlargement are typical mild jaundice associated with abnormal liver function tests is common.

Paul–Bunnell or Monospot test is positive and a rise in IgM antibodies to EBV is diagnostic of infectious mononucleosis. In addition, atypical lymphocytes are seen in the peripheral blood.

Aetiology and pathogenesis

Usually transmitted via saliva ('kissing disease') with an incubation time of 4–5 weeks.

Large mononuclear cells are seen to infiltrate the portal tracts but liver architecture is preserved.

Complications and prognosis

Hepatitis due to EBV carries an excellent prognosis, with a majority of patients retaining normal liver function.

Cytomegalovirus (CMV)

Predominantly in immunosuppressed patient: causes a hepatitis occasionally with fatal consequences.

- CMV may be detected in urine but isolation and growth is slow.
- A rising IgM titre to CMV is most reliable for the diagnosis of acute infection.
- Liver biopsy shows intracytoplasmic inclusion bodies and giant cells.

OTHER INFECTIONS INVOLVING THE LIVER

Toxoplasmosis

Rare in the UK. Clinical features in an adult are indistinguishable from infectious mononucleosis caused by Epstein–Barr virus (negative Monospot test).

A congenital form of the infection can occur if a mother is infected during pregnancy.

Clinical features

Lymphadenopathy associated with a febrile illness is the most common form of presentation.

Maculopapular rash, hepatosplenomegaly, and reactive lymphocytes may be seen together with a biochemical rise in serum transaminases with or without clinical hepatitis. Rarely, chorioretinitis and myocarditis occurs, but more commonly seen in immunocompromised.

Diagnosis

Rising IgM titres are diagnostic. The organism can also be isolated by injecting tissues, e.g. bone marrow or cerebrospinal fluid (CSF) from the patient, into the peritoneum of mice and peritoneal fluid examined 7–10 days later.

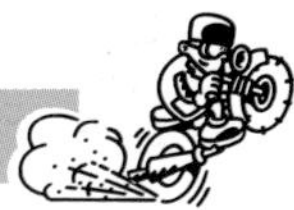

Aetiology and pathogenesis

Caused by *Toxoplasma gondii*, which is an intraplasmic protozoan that requires an animal host, such as cats or sheep, in addition to the intermediate human host. Infection is caused by ingestion of cysts via food contaminated by faeces of animal host.

Treatment

No treatment is required in mild cases because it is a self-limiting disease in people with normal immune systems.

Pyrimethamine and sulphadiazine can be given for severe cases and the patient should be treated for up to 1 month. Spiramycin can be given as an alternative to pyrimethamine during pregnancy (due to its teratogenic effects).

Good hygiene when animal handling is essential for prevention of the disease.

Leptospirosis

Also known as Weil's disease.

Clinical features

Acute systemic infection, i.e. fever, arthralgia, headache, anorexia.

Jaundice, hepatomegaly, renal failure, skin rash, and haemolytic anaemia in more severe cases.

Diagnosis and investigations

Blood, CSF, and urine cultures will isolate the organism. Specific rising titres of IgM antibody are diagnostic.

Aetiology and pathogenesis

Majority of cases are due to a Gram negative organism *Leptospira icterohaemorrhagiae* excreted by rats in their urine. Other Leptospira species are found in the urine of cattle, dogs, and pigs.

They gain access via abrasions in the skin or mucous membrane, and those particularly at risk are sewer workers, pot holers, and people who participate in watersports.

Complications

Renal and hepatic failure is seen in severe cases.

Prognosis

Mortality can be as high as 20%, especially in elderly people.

Treatment

Penicillin is an effective antibiotic. Alternatively, erythromycin and tetracycline can be used.

Brucellosis

Incidence

Extremely rare in UK. More commonly found in countries where raw unpasteurized milk is consumed. Must be considered in people with prolonged fever of an unknown cause.

Clinical features

The symptoms of an acute infection are often non-specific and insidious:

- Fever.
- Arthralgia.
- Weight loss.
- Headache.
- Night sweats.

Hepatomegaly and lymphadenopathy are commonly seen.

In chronic infection, the symptoms may persist for several months with bouts of fever and splenomegaly. Chronic derangements of liver biochemistry may be seen.

Diagnosis and investigations

Investigations to consider:

- Blood cultures are positive during acute infections in approximately half of patients. Rising titres are diagnostic.
- Liver biopsy may reveal presence of granulomas, but these are not specific for brucellosis.

Aetiology and pathogenesis

A zoonosis due to a coccobacillus largely spread by ingestion of unpasteurized milk. Three species are recognized: *Brucella abortus* (cattle), *Brucella melitensis* (goats and sheep) and *Brucella suis* (pigs).

The organism travels via the lymphatics and infect lymph nodes and reticuloendothelial systems. Hypersensitivity may account for the formation of granulomas.

Treatment

A prolonged course of tetracycline and rifampicin is given. Alternatively, co-trimoxazole can be used.

METABOLIC AND GENETIC LIVER DISEASE

In general, the following conditions often progress to chronic liver disease, but are considered separately here.

Haemochromatosis

Incidence

An autosomal recessive disorder due to excess iron accumulation affecting approximately 0.5% of the Caucasian population, with a heterozygote frequency of up to 10%.

Clinical features

Features are dependent on sex, dietary intake, age, and associated toxins (e.g. alcohol) (Fig. 22.7). Men tend to present earlier due to the protective mechanism of menstrual blood loss in women.

Patients may present between the fourth and fifth decade with the classic triad of

- Skin pigmentation (melanin deposition).
- Diabetes ('bronze diabetes').
- Hepatomegaly if the iron deposition is severe.

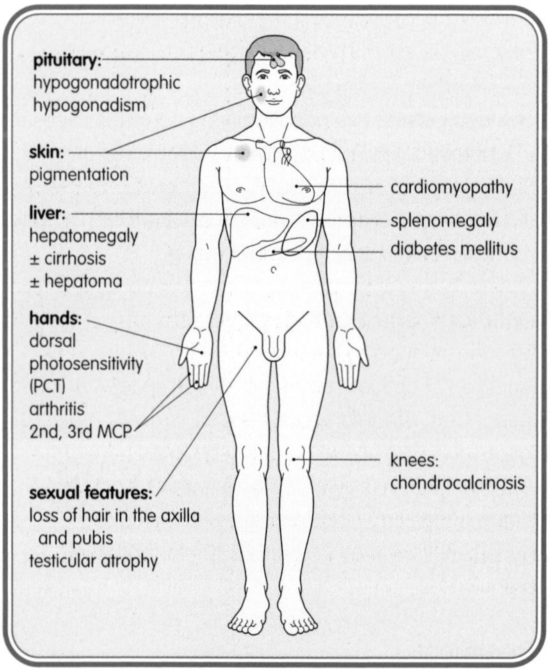

pituitary: hypogonadotrophic hypogonadism
skin: pigmentation
liver: hepatomegaly ± cirrhosis ± hepatoma
hands: dorsal photosensitivity (PCT) arthritis 2nd, 3rd MCP
sexual features: loss of hair in the axilla and pubis testicular atrophy
cardiomyopathy
splenomegaly
diabetes mellitus
knees: chondrocalcinosis

Fig. 22.7 Body map for haemochromatosis. (MCP, metacarpophalangeal joint; PCT, porphyria cutanea tarda.)

Other common presentations include gonadal atrophy and loss of libido secondary to pituitary dysfunction, cardiac failure, arthritis in small joints of the hand and chondrocalcinosis in the knees.

Diagnosis and investigation

Investigations include:

- Serum iron—usually elevated with a low total iron binding capacity.
- Transferrin saturation: grossly elevated (often 100%; normal <50%) but levels can also be moderately raised in heterozygotes.
- Serum ferritin: usually grossly elevated (>1000 μg/L; normal <300 males, <200 females). Ferritin can also be elevated in rheumatoid or other inflammatory diseases or in alcoholic liver disease, as it is an acute-phase protein. This occasionally causes confusion (see later).
- Liver biopsy—definitive test for diagnosis and at the same time assesses the extent of liver damage. Increased parenchymal iron deposition is also seen in alcoholic cirrhosis. Iron is demonstrated by Perl's potassium cyanide stain producing a Prussian Blue appearance if haemosiderin iron is present. Iron deposition is graded I–IV depending on degree and distribution. Grades III and IV are usually diagnostic of haemochromatosis. A hepatic iron index of <1.9 (mg iron per mg dry weight liver divided by the patient's age in years) is also diagnostic and is useful for differentiating genetic haemochromatosis from iron loading in alcoholic liver disease.

Aetiology and pathogenesis

Normally, iron absorption is regulated in the proximal small intestine according to the body's requirements for iron. In haemochromatosis, the regulatory mechanism is faulty, leading to inappropriate levels of absorption even when iron stores are massive.

The condition is characterized by increased deposition in the liver parenchymal cells in which extensive pigmentation and fibrosis develops and eventually cirrhosis occurs.

Increased iron content also occurs in endocrine glands, the heart, and skin.

Iron accumulation is gradual throughout life and there is a threshold below which tissue damage may not occur (e.g. 5 mg/g in the liver), hence the late presentation.

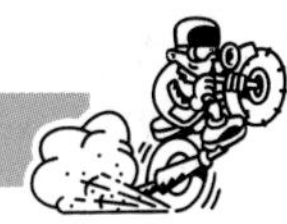

There is an association with HLA-A3, B14, and B7 groups. Recently, a mutation (C282Y) in a gene (HFE) close to HLA on chromosome 6 has been identified as a probable cause.

Complications

If untreated, cirrhosis is a common end-point followed by liver failure, which may be accompanied by portal hypertension.

Up to one third of male patients who have cirrhosis may develop hepatocellular carcinoma (Fig. 22.8).

Treating patients reverses the tissue damage and improves the survival rate. However, the risk of malignant change may persist if cirrhosis is already present.

Screening of first degree relatives in the form of ferritin levels is now routine to make a diagnosis before the development of irreversible liver damage.

Aims and indications for treatment

To reduce serum ferritin to within normal levels and limit the progression of liver damage in all patients who have a positive diagnosis of haemochromatosis.

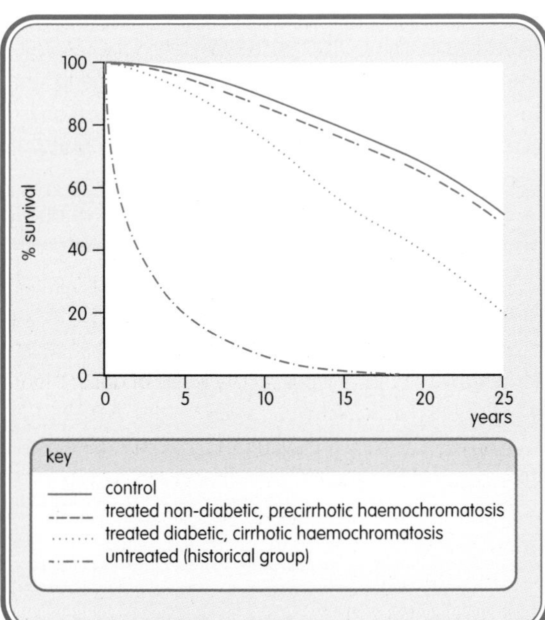

Fig. 22.8 Survival with iron overload depends on the development of complications. Even so, depletion of iron stores prolongs survival. Life expectancy is normal if treatment is started before the onset of end-organ damage.

Treatment plan

This should consist of:

- Venesection—a unit of blood (450 ml) contains 250 mg iron. Weekly venesection is required for 6–12 months to remove the 20–40 g excess iron present. Regular removal of 2–3 units of blood per year thereafter maintains ferritin levels within normal limits.
- Chelating agents, e.g. desferrioxamine, can be used for patients who cannot tolerate venesection. Ascorbic acid should be avoided by these patients.

Wilson's disease (hepatolenticular degeneration)

Incidence

A rare inborn error of copper metabolism affecting approximately 3 out of 100 000 people.

Clinical features

These include:

- Signs of chronic liver disease with neurological manifestation of basal ganglia damage, i.e. tremor, dysarthria, choreo-athetosis, and eventually dementia.
- Kayser–Fleischer copper brown ring in Descemet's membrane in the cornea (often requires slit lamp to see).
- Renal tubular damage giving rise to renal tubular acidosis and renal failure if severe.
- Haemolytic anaemia and osteoporosis in rare cases (Fig. 22.9).

Diagnosis and investigation

Serum copper and caeruloplasmin are usually low or normal. Urinary copper is grossly elevated in 24 hour collection (>10 times the normal range).

A definitive diagnosis depends on a liver biopsy and the amount of copper deposition, although elevated copper levels are found in chronic cholestasis.

Aetiology and pathogenesis

The condition is due to an autosomal recessive gene located on chromosome 13. There are at least 30 mutations described resulting in a faulty transporter protein (ATP7B) which excretes copper from the liver via the Golgi complex.

Complications

These may include:

- Cirrhosis, and liver failure will follow if left untreated.

- Neurological manifestations can be severe and disabling.
- Renal failure from renal tubular acidosis.

Prognosis

Early diagnosis and treatment can lessen the risk of mortality and morbidity considerably, but once neurological features are established, these are often irreversible.

Aims and indications for treatment

All patients with Wilson's disease are treated in order to reduce copper deposition and to avoid life-threatening complications.

Treatment plan

Lifelong oral intake of penicillamine is an effective treatment, but serious side effects can occur, limiting its usage. Urine copper levels should be monitored. All first degree relatives should be screened for early treatment.

Penicillamine and trientene (triethylamine) are copper chelating agents that have been shown to be effective. They increase urinary copper excretion, but do not completely decopper the liver, instead causing the copper to be associated with metallothionein protein. Zinc treatment is also effective in reducing copper absorption and increasing metallothionein synthesis.

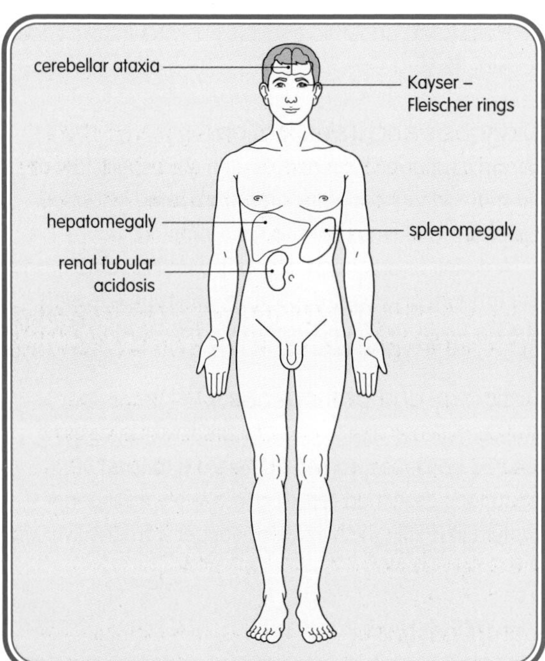

Fig. 22.9 Body map for Wilson's disease.

Alpha-1-antitrypsin deficiency

Incidence

Inherited as a rare autosomal recessive disorder. Alpha-1-antitrypsin is a protease inhibitor produced in the liver that mediates various inflammatory processes.

Clinical features

These include:

- Late-onset liver cirrhosis (>50 years).
- Early-onset of pulmonary basal emphysema (5% of homozygotes by 40 years).

Diagnosis and investigations

Investigation of use:

- Low serum alpha-1-antitrypsin level (alpha-1 AT).
- Liver biopsy—changes of cirrhosis with PAS positive staining globules within hepatocytes.
- Genotype—depending on the amino acid mutation various severity of the disease can occur, i.e. ZZ have the worse prognosis (Fig. 22.10).

Aetiology and pathogenesis

The gene responsible is located on chromsome 14. The variant of alpha-1 AT is characterized by position on a electrophoretic strip, i.e. M (medium), S (slow), and Z (very slow).

- Normal genotype is MM. S and Z variants are due to a single polypeptide mutation, resulting in reduced

Alpha-1-antitrypsin deficiency	
PiMM	Normal phenotype
PiMZ	Heterozygous for alpha-1-antitrypsin deficiency (variable type)
PiSZ	Heterozygous for alpha-1-antitrypsin deficiency
PiZZ	Homozygous for alpha-1-antitrypsin deficiency (severe type)

Fig. 22.10 Variants in alpha-1-antitrypsin deficiency. (Pi, protease inhibitor.)

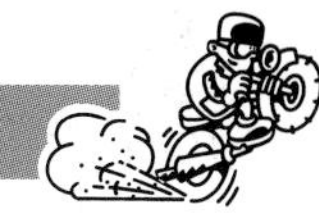

synthesis and secretion of normal alpha-1 AT. S produces approximately 60% of activity produced by M, and Z only 15%.

- Clinical phenotypes can be homozygous (e.g. ZZ) or compound heterozygous (e.g. MZ, MS, SZ).

Complications

Liver and respiratory failure due to cirrhosis and basal emphysema, respectively, usually occurs.

Prognosis

Up to 15% of patients with ZZ genotype will develop cirrhosis by the fifth decade and 5% will develop emphysema by the fourth decade.

Treatment plan

There are no specific treatments available. Treatments for chronic liver disease apply. Patients with hepatic failure should be considered for liver transplantation. Smoking should be strongly discouraged.

Cystic fibrosis

Incidence

More patients are now surviving into adolescence and adulthood, and the incidence of liver complications has risen. Up to 10% of patients may have established cirrhosis by their mid-20s.

Clinical features

Newborn infants may present with obstructive jaundice in the first few weeks of life due to the accumulation of viscous secretions in a similar fashion to meconium ileus. Recovery is usual within 6 months, but some will die of hepatic failure in infancy.

In those who survive, symptomatic liver disease can be seen up to 15% of adolescents.

Aetiology and pathogenesis

Thought to be due to obstruction of the biliary tree by mucus plugs, but the lesions can be patchy and can be missed on liver biopsy. Liver cirrhosis occurs in most cases in those with hepatic involvement.

Portal hypertension and splenomegaly may occur as a consequence of liver cirrhosis.

Prognosis

It is now recognized that the underlying liver disease is a significant prognostic factor for overall survival in cystic fibrosis. Patients with marked liver impairment have a worse outcome which may influence the timing of transplantation.

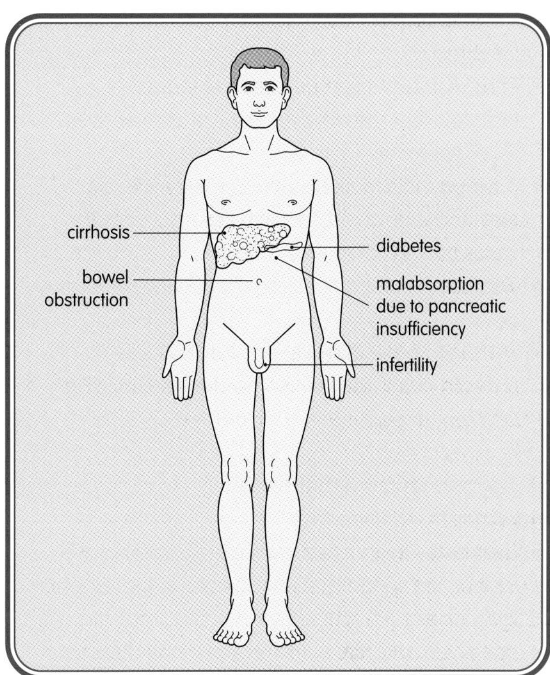

Fig. 22.11 Body map of extrarespiratory manifestations of cystic fibrosis.

Treatment

Treatment of cirrhosis is the same regardless of the underlying aetiology. Patients who are suitable maybe considered for heart–lung–liver transplant which will significantly improve their outcome (Fig. 22.11).

CHRONIC LIVER DISEASE

This section deals predominantly with chronic liver disease with an autoimmune basis. Other causes of chronic liver disease are discussed under each relevant section.

Primary biliary cirrhosis (PBC)

Incidence

Predominantly affects women with a female to male ratio of 10:1, presenting commonly between fourth and sixth decades.

Clinical features

These are:

- Pruritus, which often precedes jaundice; hepatosplenomegaly and signs of chronic liver disease are late features.
- Asymptomatic patients often present with an elevated level of alkaline phosphatase or with associated autoimmune disease.
- Xanthomas and other deposits of cholesterol may be seen.
- Metabolic bone disease may develop due to reduced absorption of fat soluble vitamin D (Fig. 22.12).

Diagnosis and investigation

Investigations to undertake:

- Liver tests—high levels of alkaline phosphatase initially, with derangement of other enzymes when cirrhosis occurs. Albumin and prothrombin time are preserved until late in the course of the disease. A rising bilirubin heralds progression to the last stage of disease and is a useful prognostic indicator.
- Autoantibodies—antimitochondrial antibodies (M_2 subtype) are detected in over 95% of cases. Lower titres of smooth muscle antibody and antinuclear factor are often also present. IgM is generally raised.
- Serum cholesterol raised secondary to cholestasis.
- Liver biopsy—there is a characteristic picture of lymphocytic infiltration around the portal tract, together with plasma cells and occasionally granulomas, resulting in bile duct fibrosis, progressing to cirrhosis (see p. 170).

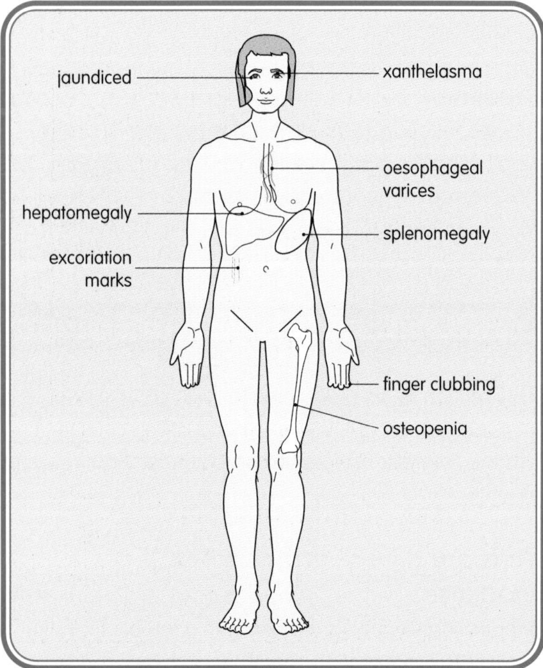

Fig. 22.12 Body map of primary biliary cirrhosis.

Aetiology and pathogenesis

The aetiology is unknown, but PBC is considered to be an autoimmune disease and is associated with other autoimmune phenomena such as hypothyroidism and sicca syndrome (xerostomia and xerophthalmia). Antimitochondrial antibodies (AMA) especially to M_2 antigen, are found in the majority of cases, but their presence in high titres does not correlate to the clinical or pathological picture, hence it may play no part in the pathogenesis of the disease but it is a very specific marker.

The antigen appears to be the E2 component of the pyruvate dehydrogenase enzyme complex on the inner mitochondrial membrane. Sensitized T cells may account for the damage seen because patients with PBC have impaired cell-mediated responses and the reduction in T suppressor cells may allow cytotoxic T cells to cause ductule damage.

High levels of IgM may be due to a defect in B cells to convert from secretion of IgM to IgG.

Complications

Complications include:

- Cirrhosis and hepatic failure eventually developing in most cases.
- Other autoimmune disorders, e.g. rheumatoid arthritis, scleroderma, autoimmune thyroid disease etc., occur more often than in the normal population.
- Membranous glomerulonephritis and renal tubular acidosis can also be associated features.

Prognosis

Median survival from time of symptoms is 8–12 years, but asymptomatic patients at presentation may not seem to progress for many years. Death is from progressive liver failure or its complications, including hepatoma (Fig. 22.13).

Aims and indications for treatment

Mainly symptomatic, as response to medical treatment is often disappointing. Steroids and penicillamine have no beneficial effects and are contraindicated due to their side effects.

Treatment plan

Treatment should include the following:

- Ursodeoxycholic acid has been shown to benefit some patients with an improvement in biochemical and histology profiles. Cyclosporin, azathioprine, and colchicine have also been shown to have some effect but are not used routinely due to their side effects.
- Pruritus is difficult to treat: cholestyramine reduces bile salt absorption in the enterohepatic cycle and may be helpful.
- Fat-soluble vitamins (i.e. A, D, and K) are given to correct deficiencies.
- Liver transplant is indicated in severe disease.

Treatment of hyperlipidaemia is not usually required.

Primary sclerosing cholangitis (PSC)

Incidence

A rare condition in which over 60% of cases are associated with inflammatory bowel disease (patients may have no bowel symptoms and the diagnosis is made subsequently on histology or barium enema). Approximately 10% patients with ulcerative colitis may have overt or subtle evidence of PSC. More commonly presents in males (3:1).

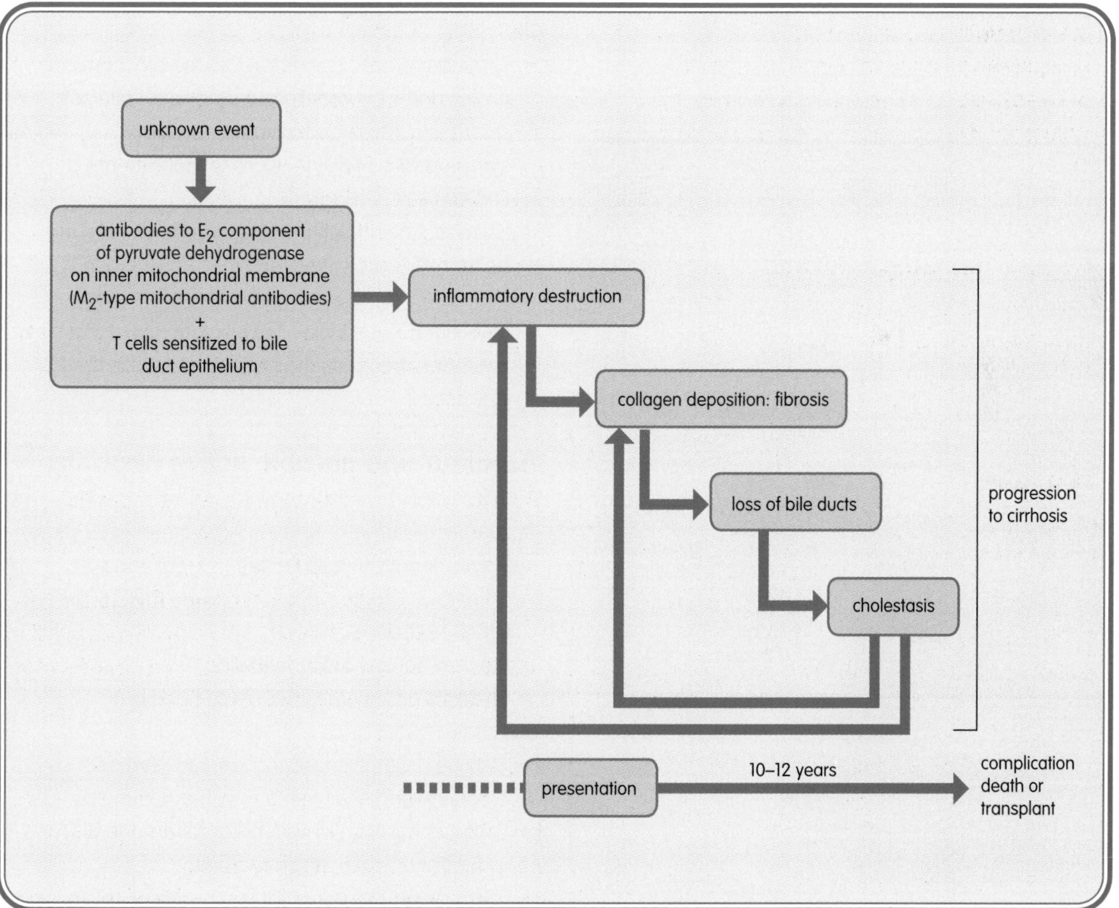

Fig. 22.13 Pathogenic mechanisms and progression in primary biliary cirrhosis.

Clinical features

These include:

- Symptoms associated with inflammatory bowel disease, particularly ulcerative colitis.
- Abdominal pain and jaundice with or without pruritis.
- Cirrhosis and its complication in late stages.
- Asymptomatic.

Diagnosis and investigation

Investigations to consider include:

- Liver function test—high alkaline phosphatase with or without hyperbilirubinaemia.
- Liver biopsy—a progressive fibrous obliterating cholangitis is seen. Polymorph infiltration of bile ducts is characteristic.
- ERCP—characteristic 'bead-like' appearance can be seen due to multiple strictures throughout bile ducts (Fig. 22.14).

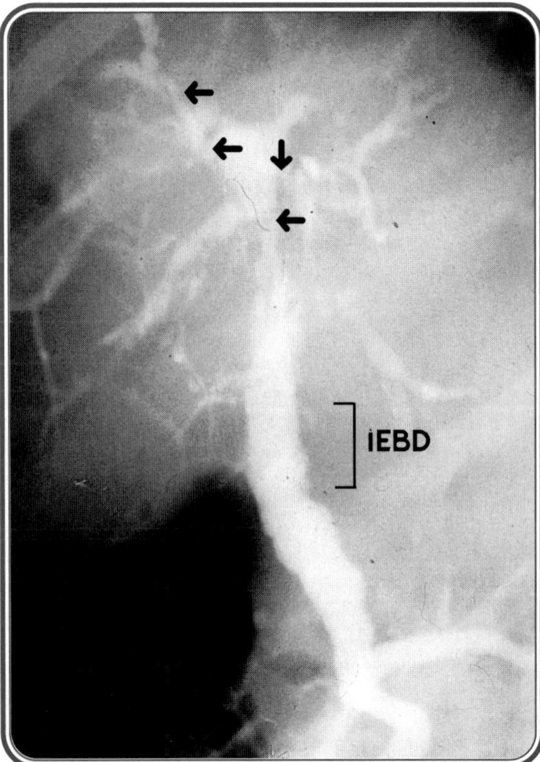

Fig. 22.14 ERCP showing typical beading, irregular ducts in PSC, and intrahepatic strictures (arrows).. (IEBD, irregular extrahepatic bile duct)

Aetiology and pathogenesis

Possible underlying autoimmune phenomenon, but exact mechanism is unknown. Certain HLA types are associated with a worse outcome.

Some patients with AIDS appear to have a similar sclerosing cholangitis which may be due to underlying infective cause, possibly *Cryptosporidium* infection.

Complications

Are those of cirrhosis and liver failure in addition to those associated with inflammatory bowel disease.

Up to 30% patients may develop cholangiocarcinoma in the long term.

Prognosis

Often runs a benign course with an exception in a few cases where hepatic failure can be rapid.

Indications for treatment

These are:

- Ursodeoxycholic acid improves the biochemical profile and may ameliorate secondary bile salt damage. Otherwise treatment is mainly symptomatic. Steroids and azathioprine are of limited use.
- Isolated strictures, if present, can be stented or balloon-dilated.
- Liver transplantation is indicated in late stage disease. A Roux loop biliary-enteric anastomosis is necessary because the patient's own bile duct is diseased.

Autoimmune chronic active hepatitis

Incidence

Occurs more commonly in young women (<25 years) and occasionally in middle age (50–60) years.

Clinical features

These may consist of the following:

- Presents as an acute hepatitis in one quarter of cases.
- May be asymptomatic for years and present as chronic liver disease with or without jaundice.
- Features associated with an autoimmune disease, e.g. arthritis, rash, fever, malaise.
- Cirrhosis and its potential for complications in long-standing cases.

Diagnosis and investigation

Tests to consider include:

- Liver function test—elevated bilirubin and ALT; increased globulins, particularly IgG; derangement of clotting factors and hypoalbuminaemia.
- Full blood count—normocytic normochromic anaemia, thrombocytopaenia, leucopaenia (changes also consistent with systemic lupus erythematosus).
- Liver biopsy—piecemeal necrosis of chronic active hepatitis.
- Autoantibodies—positive antismooth muscle antibodies (present in 60%) (Fig. 22.15).

Aetiology and pathogenesis

Unknown cause. Thought to be immune-mediated because there are abnormalities in T suppressor cells which may result from autoantibody production against hepatocyte antigens. An elevated IgG indicates defects in humoral response.

Association with other autoimmune disease (e.g. pernicious anaemia, systemic lupus erythematosus, thyroid disease, etc.) suggests cell-mediated response to own tissues. Lupus erythematosus cells (LE) are found in a number of liver biopsies, hence the old term 'lupoid hepatitis'.

A number of drugs, e.g. methyldopa, ketoconazole, isoniazid, may cause a chronic hepatitis similar to the autoimmune variety and in some cases are related to acetylation of the drug by the liver, i.e. 'slow' acetylators are at an increased risk of developing chronic active hepatitis (CAH) compared with 'fast' acetylators.

Complications

Cirrhosis and liver failure. Patients are also more likely to develop other organ-specific autoimmune diseases.

Prognosis

Remission and exacerbation for several years followed by cirrhosis is characteristic. Half will die within 5 years if no treatment is given compared with 90% survival rate with treatment.

Aims and indications for treatment

Early diagnosis and treatment are the key in order to lessen the risk of mortality and morbidity.

Treatment plan

Corticosteroids to induce remission and subsequent addition of azathioprine as a steroid-sparing agent are the mainstay of treatment.

Sarcoidosis and liver

Sarcoidosis is a chronic disease characterized by the presence of non-caseating granulomas which predominantly affect the lung, lymph nodes, and the skin, but the liver is also rarely affected.

The underlying aetiology is unknown and the majority of cases present as bilateral hilar lymphadenopathy.

It is a rare cause of hepatosplenomegaly, by producing portal hypertension either as a direct consequence of the granulomas compressing the portal venules or periportal scarring causing an obstruction.

Interpretation of autoantibody tests in liver disease

Antibody	Inference	ALT, AST elevation	Alk Phos, GGT elevation	Raised immunoglobulins	Diagnostic test
AMA	PBC	Slight	Moderate	Mainly IgM, some IgG	AMA-M2 subtype, liver biopsy
SMA, ANF, LKM	AICAH	Moderate	Slight	Mainly IgG	Liver biopsy
pANCA	PSC	Slight	Moderate	Some IgG	ERCP

Fig. 22.15 Comparison of antibody profiles in autoimmune liver disease. (AICAH, autoimmune chronic active hepatitis; ALT, alanine transaminase; Alk Phos, alkaline phosphatase; AMA, antimitochondrial antibody; ANF, antinuclear antibody; AST, aspartate transaminase; GGT, gamma-glutamyl transferase; LKM, liver kidney microsomal antibody; pANCA, antineutrophil cytoplasmic antibody; PBC, primary biliary cirrhosis; PSC, primary sclerosing cholangitis; SMA, smooth muscle antibody.)

In cases of difficulty in diagnosing systemic sarcoidosis, a liver biopsy may be diagnostic especially in the presence of abnormal liver enzymes. Serum angiotensin-converting enzyme (ACE) is elevated and a Kveim skin test (which is no longer available) is positive.

Hepatic complications are those of portal hypertension with or without decompensated liver disease.

Treatment is with systemic steroids to induce remission of the disease.

Alcoholic liver disease

Incidence and diagnosis

Approximately 1% of the population are alcoholic, i.e. psychologically or physically dependent:

- 20–30% of these develop alcoholic liver disease.
- Approximately 25% of liver cirrhosis is due to alcohol.

Current recommendations for safe alcohol consumption: 21 (male) and 14 (female) units per week.

- A unit of alcohol (approximately 10 g) represents a measure of spirit, a glass of wine, or half a pint of beer (see Fig. 14.3).
- An intake of 20 units (or more) per day is associated with a high risk of hepatocellular damage.

Clinical features

Diagnosis is made mainly on the history, and the extent of liver damage can be determined by liver biochemistry and liver biopsy.

Symptoms can often be vague, including nausea, vomiting, abdominal pain, and diarrhoea, and may be attributable to the effects of alcohol *per se*. More extensive hepatocellular damage may manifest from jaundice to hepatic failure.

Extrahepatic manifestations include:

- Wernicke's and Korsakoff's syndromes.
- Proximal myopathy.
- Peripheral neuropathy.
- Gastritis and erosions.
- Porphyria cutanea tarda.
- Neglect.
- Psychosocial difficulties.

Pathogenesis

Three main types of liver damage are described:

- Fatty change.
- Alcoholic hepatitis.
- Fibrosis.

Fatty change

Ethanol is metabolized in the liver, which results in hepatic fatty acid synthesis and reduced fatty acid oxidation leading to accumulation and fatty destruction of the hepatic cells (Fig. 22.16). Similar changes can also be seen in obesity, diabetes, starvation, and pregnancy.

There is thought to be no permanent hepatocellular damage, hence fatty change returns to normal with abstinence from alcohol.

Alcoholic hepatitis

Infiltration with polymorphonuclear leucocytes and hyaline material (Mallory bodies) is typical. Fatty change often coexists with alcoholic hepatitis. Mallory bodies may also be seen in this form of chronic active hepatitis; they are not specific to alcoholic damage.

Fibrosis

Characterized by fibrosis with nodular regeneration which implies previous or continuing liver damage. A micronodular pattern progresses to macronodular in later stages.

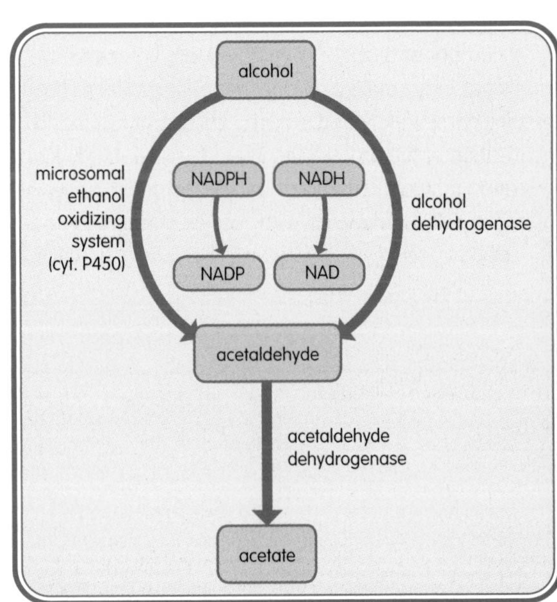

Fig. 22.16 Biochemical pathways for metabolism of alcohol. Alcohol under normal circumstances is converted to acetaldehyde by the action of alcohol dehydrogenase. In heavy drinkers, induction of the cytochrome P450 enzyme system occurs, hence increasing the metabolism of alcohol. Free radicals are a by-product of NADP and NAD production causing hepatocellular damage.

Diagnosis and investigations

A background of chronic liver disease and a history of heavy alcohol consumption is highly indicative of alcoholic liver disease.

Other investigations may aid diagnosis:

- Full blood count—often reveals a macrocytosis (a sensitive indicator of heavy alcohol consumption). Iron deficiency anaemia may be seen in cases of chronic gastrointestinal bleed due to varices or gastric or oesophageal erosion. Leucocytosis is common.
- Liver biochemistry: gamma glutamyl transferase is another indicator of heavy alcohol intake. In the presence of hepatitis, raised AST, ALT, bilirubin, and alkaline phosphatase will be seen. AST is usually only moderately raised at levels below 300 IU/L; ALT is usually less than half that value and it has been suggested that the AST:ALT ratio is a useful indicator of alcoholic liver disease when in excess of 2. Low albumin may suggest underlying cirrhosis. Associated hyperlipidaemia with haemolytic anaemia can occasionally be seen (Zieve syndrome).
- Clotting screen—prolonged prothrombin time is typical of alcoholic hepatitis due to reduced production of clotting factors by the liver.
- Ultrasound will demonstrate fatty change and if there is macronodular cirrhosis may demonstrate an irregular margin with irregular intrahepatic foci mimicking metastatic disease.
- Liver biopsy is the gold standard of diagnosis. Difficulty may arise due to deranged clotting and a transjugular liver biopsy may be necessary. Features of fatty change and cirrhosis will be seen. End-stage cirrhosis seen on histology will not distinguish its underlying aetiology.

Complications

Liver failure and cirrhosis.

Prognosis

Dependent on abstinence. Patients without established cirrhosis have a 5-year survival of 60% if they continue drink alcohol, which rises to 90% if they discontinue. Cirrhotic patients have an even poorer prognosis with 5-year survival rate of 35%.

Treatment

Abstinence from alcohol is vital. Acute alcohol withdrawal, i.e. hallucinations, tremor, and fits (delirium tremens), should be treated with a sedative such as diazepam or chlordiazepoxide. Multivitamins, especially vitamin B complex, should be given in addition to high protein and calorie supplements except in cases of hepatic encephalopathy.

Treatment of cirrhosis is described separately.

CIRRHOSIS

Cirrhosis is the end-stage of all progressive liver disease.

Clinical features

Cirrhosis *per se* is usually asymptomatic. Symptoms arise due to either the underlying disease or when complications of cirrhosis ensue.

Abdominal examination may reveal:

- Hepatomegaly or splenomegaly (if portal hypertension is present).
- Ascites.
- Dilated umbilical veins (caput medusae; Fig. 22.17).

Stigmata of chronic liver disease in the skin include anaemia, jaundice, palmar erythema, Dupuytren's contracture, finger clubbing, leuconychia, pruritus, spider naevi, and xanthomas.

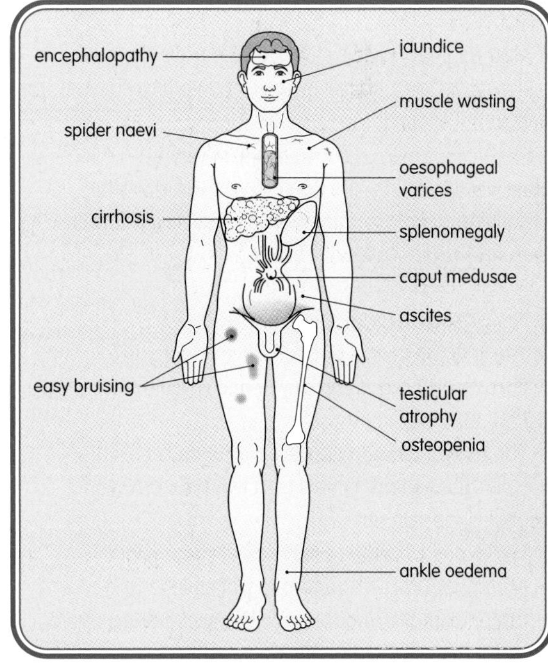

Fig. 22.17 Body map showing features of cirrhosis.

There may be endocrine features, such as loss of hair, testicular atrophy, parotid enlargement, gynaecomastia, amenorrhoea, and a loss of libido (see Fig. 22.17).

Neurological features include drowsiness, confusion, flapping of hands, constructional apraxia, and fetor hepaticus (portosystemic encephalopathy).

Fluid retention may be apparent in the abdomen (ascites) or as ankle oedema.

Investigations

Investigations to consider include the following:

- Biochemistry can be surprisingly normal but some abnormality will often be present with slightly raised transaminases and alkaline phosphatases. In severe cases, all liver enzymes will be abnormal. Low sodium and albumin are also seen.
- Full blood count may reveal anaemia due to GI bleeding secondary to variceal bleeding. Macrocytosis can be a direct effect of alcohol in addition to vitamin deficiency.
- Coagulopathy is a very sensitive indicator of liver dysfunction and is reflected in the prolonged prothrombin time.
- Alpha-fetoprotein is raised in hepatocellular carcinoma.
- Ultrasound demonstrates fatty change, size, and fibrosis as well as hepatocellular carcinoma.
- Endoscopy identifies and allows treatment for varices.
- Liver biopsy may be indicated for patients in whom the underlying aetiology is unknown or to assess the severity of cirrhosis.

Other investigations are useful in establishing the underlying aetiology, e.g. hepatitis serology, ferritin, caeruloplasmin, autoantibodies.

Aetiology and pathogenesis

Cirrhosis of the liver is a result of cell necrosis followed by fibrosis and regeneration, hence nodule formation (Fig. 22.18).

The most common cause worldwide is chronic hepatitis B infection, whereas in the Western world, alcohol is the culprit.

Two types of cirrhosis have been described:

- Macronodular—regenerating nodules are generally larger and of a variable size. They are often due a result of chronic hepatitis B or C infection.
- Micronodular—contains nodules that are <3 mm in size, uniformly affects the liver, and is more often seen with ongoing alcohol abuse. However, a mixed picture can be seen and the underlying cause does not necessarily reflect the histological change.

Complications

Portal hypertension

Portal vascular resistance is increased due to collagen deposition and fibrosis seen in liver cirrhosis and, hence formation of varices in the gastro-oesophageal junction (p. 173). In addition, sodium retention and vasoactive substances such as nitric oxide (due to accumulation of toxic metabolites) will increase plasma volume and splanchnic vasodilatation, respectively, and thus maintain portal hypertension.

Bleeding from the varices will result in haematemesis and melaena and can be precipitated by trauma (e.g. food bolus) or rising portal venous pressure (i.e. worsening liver cirrhosis).

Ascites

This is a result of fluid in the peritoneal cavity, and its pathogenesis involves several physiological processes.

A

Causes of cirrhosis
Alcohol excess
Chronic viral hepatitis, especially B and C
Genetic diseases, e.g. haemochromatosis, alpha-1-antitrypsin deficiency
Chronic liver diseases, e.g. primary biliary cirrhosis, chronic active hepatitis
Cryptogenic where no aetiology is apparent but the patient presents with complications

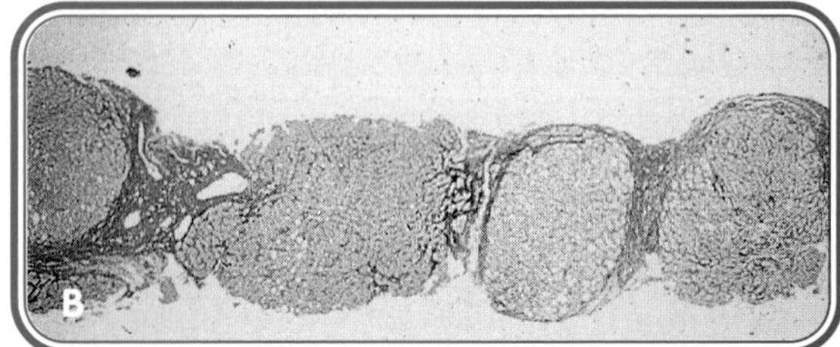

Fig. 22.18 (A) Common causes of cirrhosis. (B) Low power photomicrograph of needle liver biopsy showing fibrous nodular formation and established cirrhosis.

Sodium and water retention occur due to renin–angiotensin release secondary to arterial vasodilatation, caused by vasoactive substances such as nitric oxide. Portal hypertension *per se* causes fluid to accumulate in the peritoneal cavity due to increased hydrostatic pressure, hence further reduces intravascular volume and stimulates sodium and water retention via aldosterone.

Ascites may be aggravated by low albumin and thus a lowered oncotic pressure of the plasma as a result of reduced production by the liver.

Spontaneous bacterial infection of ascites is a serious complication that carries a significant risk of mortality (50%). Common pathogens include *E. coli, Klebsiella,* and other gut bacteria. Clinical deterioration, fever, and neutrophilia should raise the possibility of infected ascites. Aspiration of ascitic fluid should be performed for Gram stain and culture. Treatment with broad spectrum antibiotics such as cefotaxime should be used.

Hepatic encephalopathy

Toxic metabolites that are usually detoxified by the liver accumulate in the bloodstream and pass through the blood–brain barrier to cause encephalopathy. Ammonia produced by the breakdown of proteins by intestinal bacteria appears to play a role in hepatic encephalopathy.

Clinically, the patient is confused, disorientated, has slurred speech, and in severe cases, convulsion and coma. Coarse flapping of hyperextended hands, hepatic fetor (sweet-smelling breath due to ketones), and constructional apraxia (unable to draw a five-pointed star) can also be seen.

Acute onset usually has a precipitating factor which can potentially be reversible (e.g. bleeding or infection).

Hepatorenal syndrome

Characterized by cirrhosis, jaundice, and renal failure.

It is thought to be due to a depletion in intravascular volume, activation of the renin–angiotensin system, and vasoconstriction of the renal afferent arterioles, hence reduced glomerular filtration.

Other mediators have also been implicated that are related to prostaglandin synthesis and the syndrome can be precipitated by the use of non-steroidal anti-inflammatory drugs (NSAIDs). More commonly, the condition is a result of diuretic use or excessive paracentesis causing intravascular volume depletion.

The renal abnormality is thought to be functional because transplanted kidneys from a donor patient with heptorenal syndrome to a recipient will result in a normal functioning kidney. However, extreme cases will cause tubular necrosis and renal damage.

The patient should be treated for prerenal failure and the condition carries a very high mortality.

Hepatocellular carcinoma

Development of cirrhosis is itself a risk factor for hepatocellular carcinoma (see under Liver tumours).

Prognosis

Grading of prognosis is made on the Child's criteria (Fig. 22.19). In general, there is a 50% survival in 5 years).

Treatment

Generally consists of managing the complications that arise.

Modified Child classification			
Child's class	**A**	**B**	**C**
Serum bilirubin mmol/L	Normal	Up to twice normal	More than twice normal
Serum albumin g/L	Normal	30–35	Less than 30 g/L
Ascites	None	Minimal and responds to diuretics	Moderate or marked
Encephalopathy	None	None or mild irritability	Grades II, III, IV
Coagulopathy	None	Prothrombin time ≤4 s prolonged	PT ≥5 s prolonged

Fig. 22.19 Modified Child classification of cirrhosis based on functional capacity of the liver. Class C carries a poor prognosis.

For treatment of bleeding varices, see p.174.

If ascites is present, spontaneous bacterial infection must be excluded and if found, appropriate therapy should be started.

A reduction in dietary sodium will allow the reabsorption of ascitic fluid back into the circulation.

Diuretic therapy is used to increase renal excretion of sodium and hence excess water. Spironolactone is the diuretic of choice because it is a specific aldosterone antagonist and hepatic dysfunction results in secondary hyperaldosteronism because of failure to break down aldosterone in the liver. Further diuresis may be required and the use of loop diuretic such as frusemide is effective, but the patient is at risk of hyponatraemia, dehydration, and hypokalaemia. Paracentesis is often carried out for symptomatic relief (up to 20 L can be drained).

Hypovolaemia is problematic because ascites reaccumulates at the expense of circulating volume. This can be avoided by administration of salt-poor albumin or plasma expanders such as gelofusin.

Various shunts can be inserted for persistent ascites such that they drain peritoneal fluid into the internal jugular vein but infection and blockage of the shunts limits their use.

For hepatic encephalopathy an underlying preciptating cause should be found and appropriate treatment instigated, i.e. correction of electrolyte imbalance, treatment of sepsis, etc. Laxatives and enemas should be given to reduce ammonia load.

A low protein diet should be given in order to reduce nitrogenous waste which exacerbates encephalopathy.

Oesophageal and gastric varices

Incidence

Major complication of cirrhosis, whatever the underlying aetiology. Up to 70% of cirrhotic patients will develop varices and up to 40% of these will bleed.

Portal vein thrombosis causes non-cirrhotic portal hypertension.

Clinical features

Acute GI bleed in the form of melaena or haematemesis due to rupture of varices may be the presenting feature. Other features may include:

- Stigmata of chronic liver disease: palmar erythema, spider naevi, proximal myopathy or muscle wasting, pigmentation or jaundice, hypogonadism.
- Splenomegaly is usually present due to underlying portal hypertension.
- Features of liver failure, e.g. encephalopathy, ascites, jaundice, etc.

Diagnosis and investigations

These include:

- Full blood count, biochemistry, clotting etc., as for anyone with an acute GI bleed. A low platelet count may indicate hypersplenism due to portal hypertension. Prolonged prothrombin time is an indicator of diminished hepatic synthetic function.
- Endoscopy is essential to confirm the diagnosis and differentiate variceal haemorrhage from other causes.
- Liver biopsy may be required if aetiology of liver disease is in doubt once the acute episode has been treated.
- Ultrasound and Doppler studies may be useful to diagnose hepatic or portal vein thrombosis.

Aetiology and pathogenesis

Due to presence of portal hypertension which can be:

- Presinusoidal.
- Sinusoidal.
- Postsinusoidal.

When portal pressures rises above 10–12 mmHg (normal = 5–8 mmHg), collateral communication with the systemic venous system occurs instead of blood flowing into hepatic vein. Portosystemic anastomosis occurs at gastro-oesophageal junction, ileocaecal junction, rectum, and anterior abdominal wall via the umbilical vein (Fig. 22.20).

Presinusoidal

Blockage of the portal vein before its entry to the liver, e.g. portal vein thrombosis possibly due to congenital venous abnormality or umbilical sepsis. Pancreatic disease is the most common cause in adults. Other causes include schistosomiasis. Doppler studies usually identify the blockage.

Sinusoidal

The majority of cases are due to cirrhosis, where portal vascular resistance is increased due to distorted architecture and perivenular fibrosis. This can also occur in congenital hepatic fibrosis and non-cirrhotic

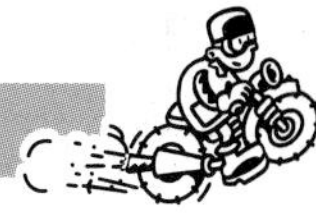

portal hypertension, where the histology shows mild portal tract fibrosis without cirrhosis.

Postsinusoidal

Budd–Chiari syndrome where there is occlusion of the hepatic veins as they exit the liver. The patient usually has a hypercoagulable state, underlying myeloproliferative disorder, or extrinsic occlusion by tumour or mass.

Portal hypertension develops if the condition becomes chronic. Other causes include constrictive pericarditis and right-sided cardiac failure.

Complication

Risk of developing encephalopathy is high with an acute variceal bleed.

Prognosis

Overall risk of recurrence after an acute episode is 80% over 2 years. Each variceal bleed carries a mortality risk of 15–40%.

Aims of treatment

To resuscitate in the acute episode and stop bleeding from the varices. Once this is successfully carried out, then preventive measures should be started.

Treatment

Resuscitation aims to replace depleted intravascular volume with plasma expanders, crystalloids, or blood if available (as with all major GI bleeds).

Urgent endoscopy is required, during which sclerosant is injected in or around the varices to cause inflammatory obliteration (see Fig. 17.18). Alternatively, elastic band ligation of the varices at endoscopy produces thrombotic obliteration (Fig. 22.21). Repeat sclerotherapy or banding is usually needed to prevent further bleeds.

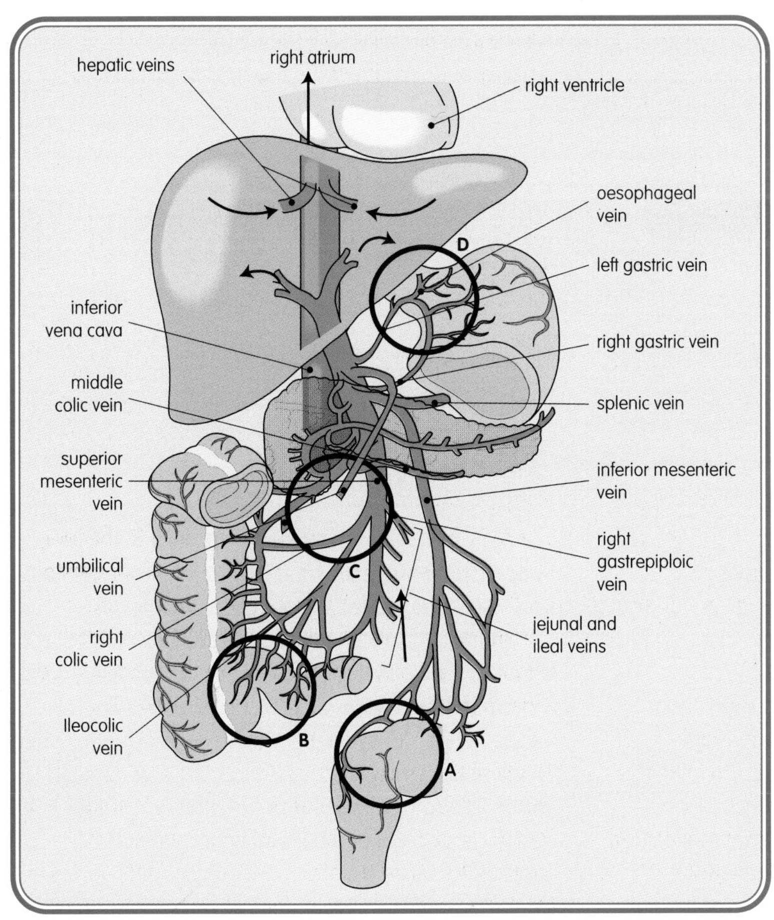

Fig. 22.20 Portal vasculature and sites of portal systemic anastomoses. Sites of portosystemic anastomoses are indicated by black circles. (A) Rectal varices or haemorrhoids. (B) Ileocaecal varices. (C) Umbilical varices (caput medusae). (D) Gastro-oesophageal varices. Varices at the gastro-oesophageal junction bleed most commonly only because they traverse the greatest pressure gradient between the negative pressure in the thorax and the positive pressure abdominal cavity.

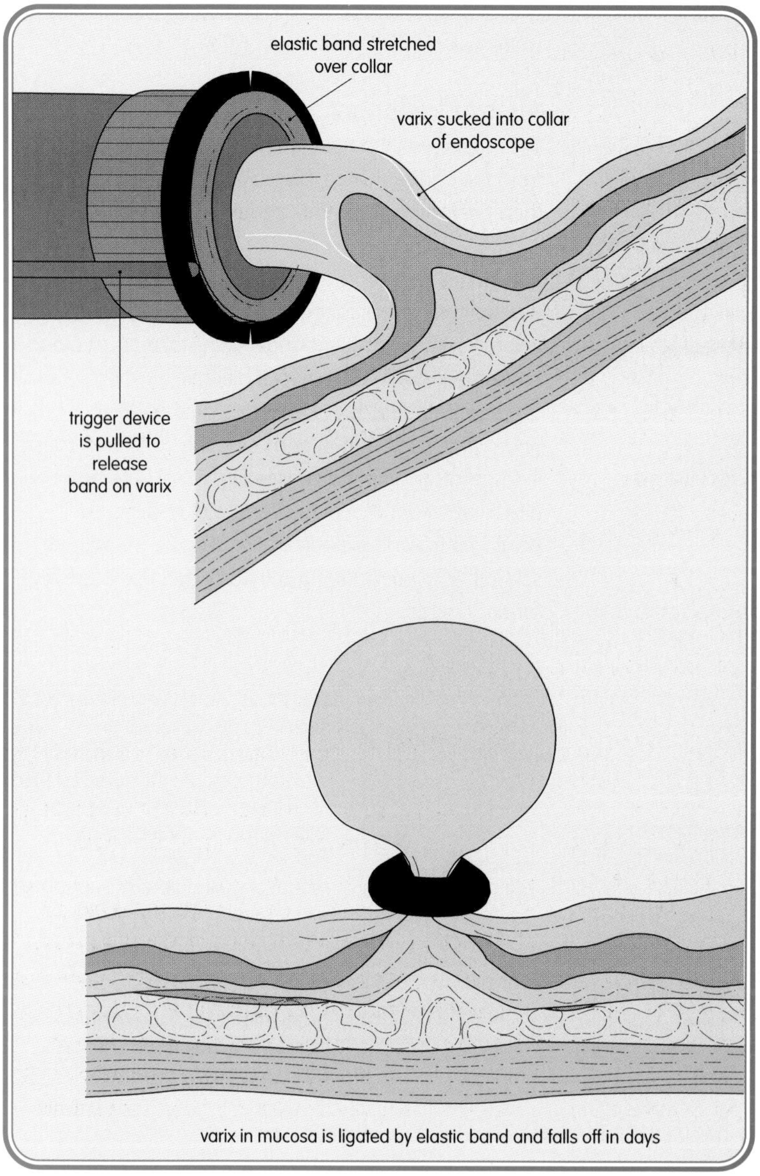

elastic band stretched over collar

varix sucked into collar of endoscope

trigger device is pulled to release band on varix

varix in mucosa is ligated by elastic band and falls off in days

Fig. 22.21 Strategy to control variceal haemorrhage by elastic band ligation.

Vasoconstrictor agents, such as octreotide (somatostatin analogue), can be used as an adjuvant therapy. The aim is to cause splanchnic vasoconstriction and, hence restrict portal blood flow.

Balloon tamponade is now mainly reserved for patients for whom sclerotherapy is temporarily unavailable or the procedure has failed. An inflatable tube is passed into the stomach and the balloon inflated with air. Traction on the balloon is maintained for 12 hours until the varices have collapsed. An alternative design of tube also has an oesophageal balloon. Prolonged inflation of the balloon is associated with mucosal ulceration and rupture of oesophagus. It also increases the risk of aspiration pneumonia.

Transjugular intrahepatic portocaval shunt (TIPS) is a shunt formed between the systemic and portal venous system to treat varices (Fig. 22.22). A guide wire is passed under X-ray control via the internal jugular vein to the hepatic vein and passes into the liver. Contact is made through the liver substance with the portal venous circulation and a metal endoprosthesis is inserted to create the shunt. Encephalopathy occurs in up to 30% patients. Recurrence of varices can occur if the stent thromboses.

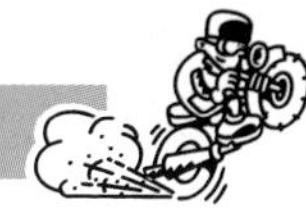

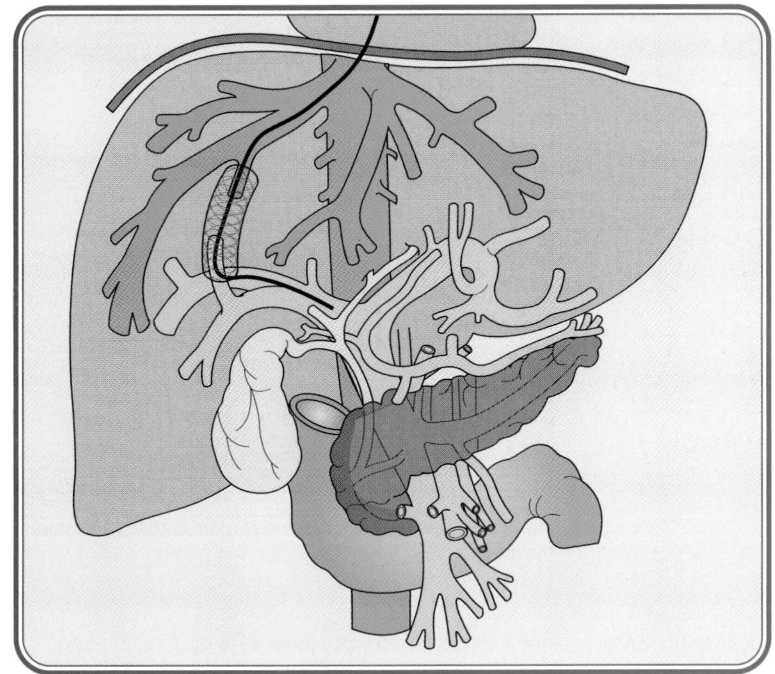

Fig. 22.22 Schematic representation of TIPS procedure.

Surgery is rarely performed nowadays. Oesophageal transection can be done as an emergency with ligation of the vessels. Portosystemic shunts (mesocaval or splenorenal) can also be undertaken surgically but have a high incidence of encephalopathy. Narrow gauge stents can improve the results but have no advantage over TIPS.

A beta-blocker, e.g. propranolol, can be given to reduce portal pressure by reducing cardiac output and allowing vasoconstriction of splanchnic arteries by inhibiting the effects of β_2 receptor-mediated vasodilatation. This is the drug of choice in maintenance therapy to prevent secondary haemorrhage following obliteration of varices.

TUMOURS OF THE LIVER

The most common tumours are metastatic spread from another primary site, e.g. GI tract, breast, thyroid, and bronchus. Primary tumours of the liver are usually malignant.

Hepatocellular carcinoma

Incidence

One of the most common malignant diseases worldwide but rare in the Western world.

Clinical features

Include:

- Usually non-specific, i.e. weight loss, malaise, fever, right upper quadrant pain, and in late stages, ascites (may be bloodstained).
- Cirrhotic patients who develop the above clinical features should have malignant change excluded.
- An enlarged irregular tender liver is more likely to be found in secondary metastasis or pre-existing cirrhosis than primary hepatocellular carcinoma.
- Metastasis to lung and bone may produce pleural effusions and pathological fractures, respectively.

Diagnosis and investigations

Investigations to consider:

- Liver function test—normal or mild abnormality of enzyme is usual in established inactive cirrhosis. A rise in ALT or AST may be indicative of tumour necrosis.
- Alpha-feto protein raised.
- Liver ultrasound will identify majority of liver tumours.
- Liver biopsy required for tissue diagnosis and normally done under ultrasound guidance.

Aetiology and pathogenesis

In areas where hepatitis B and hepatitis C are prevalent, over 90% of patients with hepatocellular carcinoma have positive serology and an equal number have pre-existing cirrhosis. The aetiology is presumed to be the integration of the virus into the host genome.

Most patients with cirrhosis, whatever the underlying cause, are at risk of developing hepatocellular carcinoma, but especially patients with hepatitis B and genetic haemochromatosis. Hepatoma development is more common in males than females with cirrhosis.

Prognosis

Very poor. <5% survival at 6 months.

Treatment

Little response to radiotherapy or chemotherapy. Isolated lesions may be surgically resected.

Other tumours of the liver

Adenomas

Rare. Associated with the oral contraceptive pill. Can present as an incidental finding or due to intrahepatic bleeding. Treatment by resection required only if complications develop.

Haemangiomas

Most common benign tumour of the liver and usually found incidentally on ultrasound. No treatment is required. If diagnosis is in doubt, then angiography is required.

Focal nodular hyperplasia (FNH)

This condition as its name suggests causes nodules in the liver, but hepatic function is normal. It is more common than hepatic adenoma but has no malignant potential. Its importance is that it can be mistaken for cirrhosis either on radiological scanning or even on histology from a needle biopsy. It is usually asymptomatic and found incidentally, but is believed to be related to the oral contraceptive pill. In these circumstances, it is thought that about 50% become symptomatic, usually with pain in the right upper quadrant. Symptomatic cases are treated by surgical resection.

DRUGS AND THE LIVER

Many drugs are metabolized by liver enzymes and some are excreted in bile. Some drugs are fat-soluble and their bioavailability can be affected by bile salt micellar concentration in the intestine. Plasma proteins, especially albumin synthesized in the liver, affect the kinetics of many drugs. Hence liver dysfunction and disease can impair absorption, transport, metabolism, and excretion of several drugs (Fig. 22.23). Care must be taken when using most drugs in the presence of liver disease. Conversely, several drugs can cause liver damage.

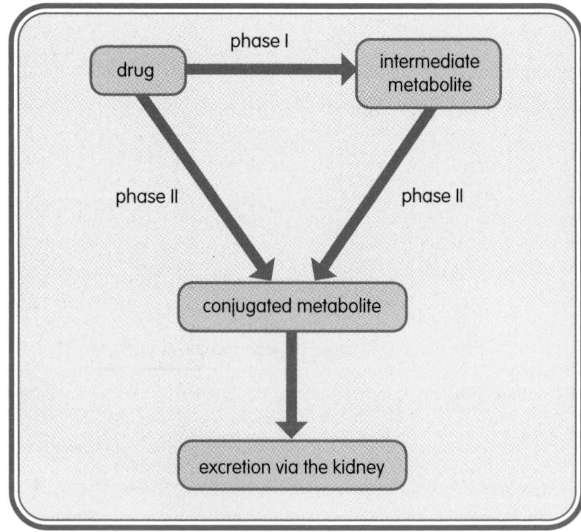

Fig. 22.23 Biochemical pathways of drug metabolism in the liver.

Drug toxicity to the liver

Incidence

Up to 10% of jaundice is caused by drugs via different mechanisms.

Aetiology and pathogenesis

Drug toxicity can be:

- Dose or duration related (e.g. azathioprine, methotrexate).
- Idiosyncratic (e.g. flucloxacillin, clavulanic acid).
- Due to overdose toxicity (e.g. paracetamol).

Three types of pathology are described (Fig. 22.24):

- Acute hepatitis typically occurs 2–3 weeks after starting the drug and normally resolves after cessation. In the case of halothane, repeated exposure sensitizes the patient and can cause fulminant hepatitis suggesting an immunological cause. Clinically, this can mimic severe viral hepatitis.
- Cholestasis—bile stasis causes a functional obstruction, hence biochemically it produces jaundice with pale stools and dark urine usually after

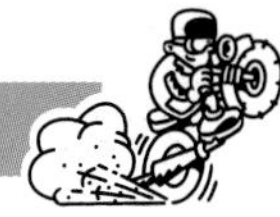

Drugs affecting liver function	
Pattern of liver damage	**Drugs**
Hepatitis	Anti-tuberculous: rifampicin, isoniazid Anti-fungal: ketoconazole Anti-hypertensive: atenolol, verapamil Anaesthetics: halothane
Cholestasis	Anti-psychotics: chlorpromazine Antibiotics: erythromycin, clavulanic acid, flucloxacillin Immunosuppressives: cyclosporin A Contraceptives and anabolic steroids
Necrosis	Paracetamol, carbon tetrachloride

Fig. 22.24 Drugs known to cause disturbance in liver function.

4–6 weeks. The cause of bile stasis is unclear but inflammatory infiltration of bile ducts and interference with excretory transport proteins has been implicated. Anabolic steroids and oral contraceptives can cause profound cholestasis.

- Necrosis—mainly dose-dependent. Toxic metabolites are normally detoxified by the liver, e.g. conjugation by glutathione, and once the level of glutathione falls, toxic metabolites accumulate and liver necrosis follows. Concurrent ingestion of enzyme-inducing drugs, e.g. alcohol, severely ill patients, or starvation will render these individuals more susceptible to toxicity.

Clinical features

These can range from mild elevation of liver enzymes to acute fulminant hepatic failure:

- Jaundice is usually secondary to an acute hepatitis or cholestasis but rarely it can be due to haemolysis.
- In the majority of cases derangement of liver enzymes is found on routine examination before clinical jaundice develops.
- Nausea and vomiting or abdominal pain may occur.
- Pruritus, steatorrhoea, and dark urine if cholestasis occurs.

Diagnosis and investigation

Find out about the history of drug ingestion.

Liver enzymes can show an acute hepatitic picture (raised ALT or AST) or a cholestatic/obstructive picture (raised alkaline phosphatase and gamma glutamyl transpeptidase). Jaundice may be present in either type.

Complications and prognosis

Fulminant hepatitis secondary to halothane-induced hepatitis has a mortality rate of up to 20%, but this is rare. Hepatic failure following acute liver necrosis most often and predictably follows paracetamol overdose.

Treatment

Withdrawal of the offending drug is usually all that is required, although in some cases, such as chlorpromazine-induced cholestatic hepatitis, it may take up to 12 months or longer before the liver biochemistry returns to normal.

Paracetamol toxicity

The analgesic paracetamol is commonly used for self-poisoning but this is a potentially treatable condition. Sadly, delayed presentation can often be fatal. As this is such a common clinical scenario, it is worth describing in detail.

Clinical features

Note that:

- Nausea and vomiting usually occur within the first 24 hours.
- Liver failure can be seen between 72 and 96 hours if left untreated. Acute renal failure can occur with or without liver failure.

Diagnosis and investigation

Paracetamol levels are plotted on a chart (Prescott nomogram) and correlated to time postingestion to establish the need for treatment, but the timing may be difficult because the history from the patient is often unreliable. It is safer to treat than to wait or rely on levels. Useful investigations include:

- Clotting screen—the prothrombin time is the most sensitive indication of hepatic damage.
- Liver biochemistry usually shows raised ALT and AST sometimes to very high levels (10 000), but these do not correlate well with toxicity or give any prognostic information.
- Electrolytes are usually normal. Raised creatinine indicates significant renal damage and a level >300 μmol/L predicts a serious outcome.
- Arterial gases—a low pH (<7.3) has a significantly poorer prognosis in patients presenting late (i.e. >24 hours) (Fig. 22.25).

Aetiology and pathogenesis

Paracetamol is converted to a toxic metabolite, N-acetyl-p-benzoquinonimine, which under normal circumstances is inactivated by conjugation with glutathione. In overdose, glutathione is depleted, hence there is a build up of toxic metabolite, thus hepatocellular necrosis (Fig. 22.26).

Patients with underlying liver impairment, e.g. chronic alcoholics or cirrhosis, or those concurrently taking an enzyme-inducing drug, e.g. phenytoin, are at greater risk of hepatocellular damage, hence threshold for treatment should be lowered.

Complications

Fulminant hepatic failure is a serious and often fatal complication which is more often seen in those presenting later than 16 hours post-ingestion.

Treatment

N-acetylcysteine infusion is the treatment of choice, which replenishes hepatic glutathione by providing the sulphydryl group it requires. The decision of whether treatment is required is based on serum paracetamol levels taken 4 hours or more post-ingestion and the likelihood of severe hepatic damage is predicted. Oral methionine can be given as an alternative, but its absorption is unreliable, especially if the patient is vomiting.

Serum paracetamol levels are unreliable in patients

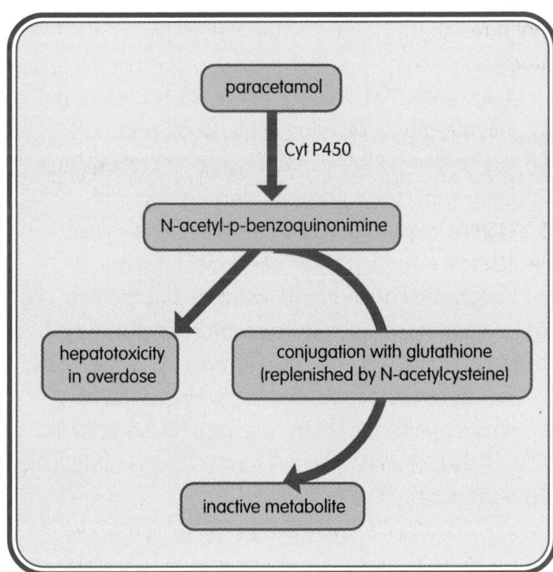

Fig. 22.26 Biochemical mechanism of paracetamol toxicity and prevention.

Poor prognostic factors for liver failure

	Paracetamol	Non-paracetamol
Aetiology		Non-ABC hepatitis
		Drugs
Age		<10, >40 years
Encephalopathy	Present on day 2	Present
Serum creatinine	>300 μmol/L	>300 μmol/L
Prolonged prothrombin time	>100 s	>50 s
pH	<7.3	

Fig. 22.25 Factors associated with a poor prognosis in liver failure.

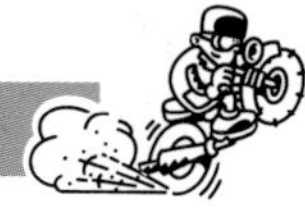

who present later than 16 hours post-ingestion, hence if there is any doubt, treatment should be started and stopped when subsequent liver biochemistry and clotting are found to be normal.

Patients presenting within 1 hour of ingestion should be given activated charcoal, as this will reduce the absorption of the drug from the GI tract.

Patients at risk of severe liver damage or with fulminant hepatic failure should be referred to a specialist unit for expert care and possible liver transplantation.

Prognosis

Patients who recover from hepatocellular damage do not have any residual liver impairment and can be treated as normal.

LIVER ABSCESSES

Pyogenic abscess

Incidence

An uncommon complication of intra-abdominal sepsis, e.g. diverticulitis, appendicitis, perforated bowel, etc., but it can occur sporadically without any overt sign of other sources of infection.

Clinical features

These include:

- Non-specific symptoms such as swinging fever, anorexia, weight loss, abdominal pain, malaise.
- Jaundice, tender hepatomegaly, and septicaemic shock in some cases.
- A reactive pleural effusion in the right lower lobe may be seen.

Diagnosis and investigation

Consider:

- Full blood count—normocytic normochromic anaemia, increased neutrophils.
- Liver tests—raised alkaline phosphatase, raised bilirubin (if bile ducts are obstructed).
- Blood cultures—positive only in approximately one third of cases.
- Liver ultrasound—cystic lesions (single or multiple) are seen and ultrasound-guided biopsy of the lesion with culture will yield organism and its sensitivity.
- Chest X-ray—a raised right hemidiaphragm with or without pleural effusion may be seen.
- Further imaging, e.g. CT scan of abdomen, may be required to identify primary source of infection.

Aetiology and pathogenesis

E. coli is the most common pathogen isolated. Others include *Strep. faecalis* (enterococcus), *Strep. milleri, Proteus sp., Staph. aureus,* and anaerobes.

Abdominal infection spread to the liver via the portovenous system is likely to be the most common cause, but direct spread from biliary infection or perinephric abscess can also occur.

Complications and prognosis

Few or no complications will occur if the abscess is single and adequately treated. Rupture of the abscess can occur, producing a peritonitis from which there is a significant increase in the risk of mortality.

Multiple abscesses have a poorer outcome than unilocular, with a mortality rate of over 50% in some cases depending on the underlying cause.

Treatment

Treatment options include:

- Aspiration of the abscess under ultrasound control should be done as a therapeutic intervention as well as a diagnostic procedure.
- Surgical intervention may also be required if aspiration is unsuccessful or if multiple abscesses are unsuitable for aspiration.
- Broad-spectrum antibiotics are given immediately to cover likely organisms, including anaerobes, until sensitivity is known.

Amoebic abscess

Incidence

Occurs worldwide and it is endemic in the tropics and subtropics.

Clinical features

The main symptoms are:

- Diarrhoea as part of amoebic dysentry (but not always).
- Non-specific, e.g. malaise, anorexia, fever, abdominal pain.
- Tender hepatomegaly with or without right pleural effusion.

Rarely, clinical jaundice is seen.

Diagnosis and investigation

Investigations include:

- Liver tests—raised alkaline phosphatase.
- Blood cultures—usually negative.
- Amoeba serology—does not indicate current disease as it remains positive after the disease has resolved.
- Liver ultrasound—single or multiple cysts are seen: aspiration of the cyst yields an 'anchovy sauce'-like substance.

Aetiology and pathogenesis

Caused by *Entamoeba histolytica* initially causing a diarrhoea illness and spread via the portovenous system into the liver. The initial bowel infection may not be clinically apparent. Inflammation of the portal tracts and development of single or multiple abscesses follows.

Complications

Rupture of the cyst causing peritonitis and secondary infection.

Prognosis

Good overall prognosis if treated adequately.

Treatment

Metronidazole is the antibiotic of choice, given for 2 weeks. Cysts should be aspirated for diagnostic and therapeutic purposes.

Surgical drainage may be necessary in resistant cases or multiple large abscesses.

PARASITIC INFECTION OF THE LIVER

Hydatid disease

Incidence

Occurs worldwide, but more common where sheep and cattle farming are the main source of living. Rare in the UK, except for parts of Wales where there are large communities of sheep farmers.

Clinical features

These are:

- Asymptomatic.
- Right upper quadrant discomfort due to cystic enlargement and jaundice if obstruction of bile duct occurs.
- Rupture in the abdominal cavity may cause fever, abdominal pain, and peritonitis.
- Hepatomegaly due to cystic formation.

Diagnosis and investigation

Investigations include:

- Full blood count—peripheral eosinophilia is typically seen.
- Haemagglutination test—positive for hydatid disease.
- Liver function test—normal unless obstruction of bile duct occurs causing jaundice.
- Liver ultrasound—cystic lesion with or without daughter cysts.
- Plain abdominal X-ray—not routinely done but calcification of the cyst may be seen incidentally.

Aetiology and pathogenesis

Caused by ingestion of *Echinococcus granulosus*, which is a dog tapeworm, and its embryo via contaminated fruit and vegetables or direct ingestion due to poor hygiene (Fig. 22.27).

Within the duodenum, the embryo hatch, enter the portovenous system and systemic spread to lung, kidney, and brain can occur in as well as the liver.

Complications

Cyst rupture and secondary infection are the main complications. Rupture in the bronchus and renal tract may cause haemoptysis and haematuria, respectively. Brain cyst may present as epilepsy due to its space-occupying effects.

Prognosis

If adequately treated, complete recovery is expected.

Treatment

Sterilization of the non-communicating cyst, e.g. by injection of formalin or oral albendazole (can also reduce the size of cysts), followed by surgical resection of the intact cyst. Fine needle aspiration is not routinely done due to risk of anaphylactic reaction to cyst contents.

Asymptomatic calcified cysts are usually left without treatment.

Prevention is by reducing carriage in domestic animal and improving hygiene.

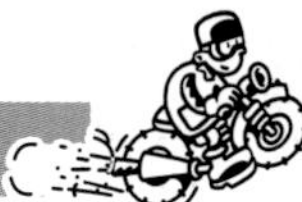

Schistosomiasis

Incidence

Prevalent worldwide affecting over 200 million people mainly in the tropics.

Clinical features

The main features are:

- Acute inflammatory response at the site of penetration through skin by the cercariae ('swimmer's itch').
- Fever, myalgia, malaise, GI upset, i.e. vomiting and diarrhoea in the acute phase.
- Chronic infection produces hepatomegaly with or without portal hypertension.

Diagnosis and investigation

Investigations of use:

- Full blood count—eosinophilia.
- Liver function test—raised alkaline phosphatase.
- Immunological test—positive result does not indicate current infection as antibodies remain after the disease has resolved.
- Detection of ova in stool, liver, or rectal biopsy.

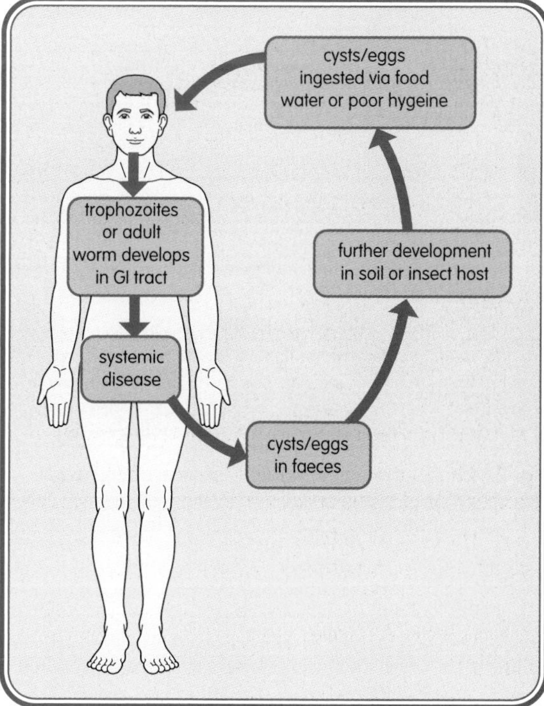

Fig. 22.27 Body map with parasitic life cycle.

Aetiology and pathogenesis

Predominantly caused by *Schistosoma mansoni* (Africa and South America) and *Schistosoma japonicum* (China and SE Asia). Mode of infection is via swimming or bathing in contaminated water with its intermediate host as the snail.

The infective form of the parasite, cercariae, penetrates the skin and migrates via the portovenous system into the liver where the parasite matures and eventually migrates along the portal and mesentric vein to produce a large amount of eggs, which leave the body by penetrating the intestinal wall to be excreted back into the river to complete its life cycle.

Granulomatous reaction to the trematode occurs in the liver producing a periportal fibrosis and hepatomegaly.

Complications

Portal hypertension and oesophageal varices occur in advanced cases, but cirrhosis is not usually seen.

S. japonicum produces a large number of eggs and systemic deposition of ova in lungs or brain can occur, producing epilepsy in the latter case. It also causes extensive chronic colitis and can cause premalignant changes in some cases.

Prognosis

Despite adequate treatment, fibrosis and risk of portal hypertension remains.

Aims and indications for treatment

The aim is to cause the trematode to vacate the portal and mesenteric vein and migrate to the liver or lung, where they are destroyed by the host's cell-mediated response. There may be difficulty in curative treatment, as the reinfection rate is high and it therefore may not be appropriate to attempt a cure.

Treatment

Praziquantel is an effective agent for all Schistosoma species. Abdominal pain and diarrhoea are common shortly after start of treatment.

Fascioliasis

Incidence

A zoonosis that infects sheep, cattle, and goats. Transmitted to humans via contaminated vegetables. Occurs worldwide, including UK.

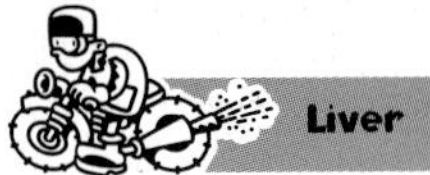

Clinical features

These include:

- Fever, malaise, hepatomegaly, abdominal discomfort, weight loss.
- Urticarial reaction due to migration of parasite.
- Jaundice and cholangitis due to its presence in the biliary tract.

Diagnosis and investigation

Investigations to consider:

- Full blood count—eosinophilia
- Liver function test—features of obstructive jaundice.
- Serological test— specific complement fixation test are now available.
- Ova are detected in stool in up to one third of cases, hence duodenal aspirate is required.

Treatment

Bithionol or praziquantel are effective treatments.

POLYCYSTIC LIVER SYNDROMES

Polycystic liver disease covers many different disorders that have in common cystic lesions of the liver. Classification is difficult.

Incidence

The most important entity is adult polycystic liver disease in which multiple cysts that do not usually communicate with the biliary tree develop in the liver. This condition is inherited as an autosomal dominant trait and its incidence is approximately 1/5000 births. A related but less common condition is inherited as a recessive trait and often involves communication with the biliary tree.

Caroli's disease is a variant comprising cystic dilatation of the biliary tree.

Congenital hepatic fibrosis is often included under the umbrella classification as microcysts are common.

Polycystic liver disease is frequently associated with cyst formation elsewhere. Cysts are found in the kidney in 60% of cases and other viscera, especially the pancreas, in 5% of cases.

Clinical features

The clinical importance of these cysts (Fig. 22.28) is that they are often found incidentally during investigation for other problems and occasionally cause diagnostic confusion. Sometimes cysts present with pain, usually due to haemorrhage. Cysts related to the biliary tree or kidney can become infected.

Unless they are symptomatic in these ways, cysts of the liver or kidney do not usually present any problems. Cysts that communicate with the biliary tree are thought to have some malignant potential.

Treatment

As most cysts are asymptomatic, usually no treatment is indicated. Cysts causing haemorrhage or pain may require drainage, surgical fenestration or resection. Cysts in the biliary tree occasionally require endoscopic drainage or resection .

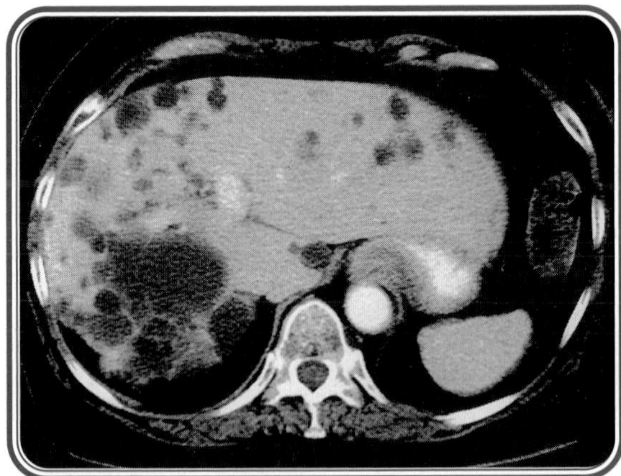

Fig. 22.28 Computed tomography scan of abdomen showing multiple cysts of different sizes in the liver.

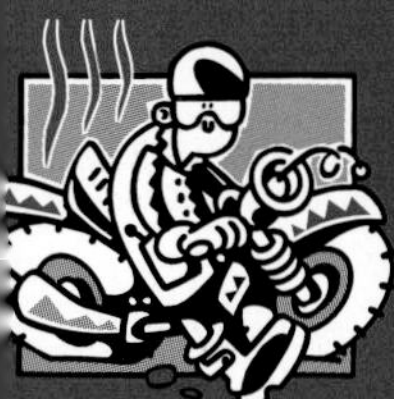

23. Biliary Tract

ANATOMY, PHYSIOLOGY, AND FUNCTION OF THE HEPATOBILIARY SYSTEM

Bile canaliculi between hepatocytes form ductules that coalesce into bile ducts in the portal tracts. These eventually form the right and left hepatic ducts which leave the respective lobes of the liver and join together to form the common hepatic duct at the porta hepatis. The cystic duct from the gallbladder inserts into the lower end of the common hepatic duct to form the common bile duct, which courses through the head of pancreas to emerge in the second part of the duodenum together with the pancreatic duct (Fig. 23.1).

Bile consists of:

- Water.
- Bile acids—these are synthesized from cholesterol, and act as a detergent for lipid stabilizers to form micelles with their hydrophilic and hydrophobic ends to enable absorption and digestion of fats.
- Cholesterol.
- Bilirubin—this is predominantly a by-product of the breakdown of red blood cells in Kupffer cells. Bilirubin is unconjugated and water insoluble. Conjugation occurs in the liver to allow excretion in the small intestine with bile. In the terminal ileum, bacterial enzymes deconjugate the molecule and a small proportion of free bilirubin (water insoluble) is reduced to urobilinogen (water soluble) and excreted as stercobilinogen in the stool. The rest is reabsorbed in the terminal ileum and into the liver via enterohepatic circulation and further excretion in bile. Urobilinogen can also be excreted via the kidneys (Fig. 23.2).

GALLSTONES

Note these distinctions:

- Cholelithiasis refers to the presence of gallstones in the gall bladder.
- Choledocholithiasis refers to the clinical situation which occurs when the gallstone passes into the cystic or common bile ducts.

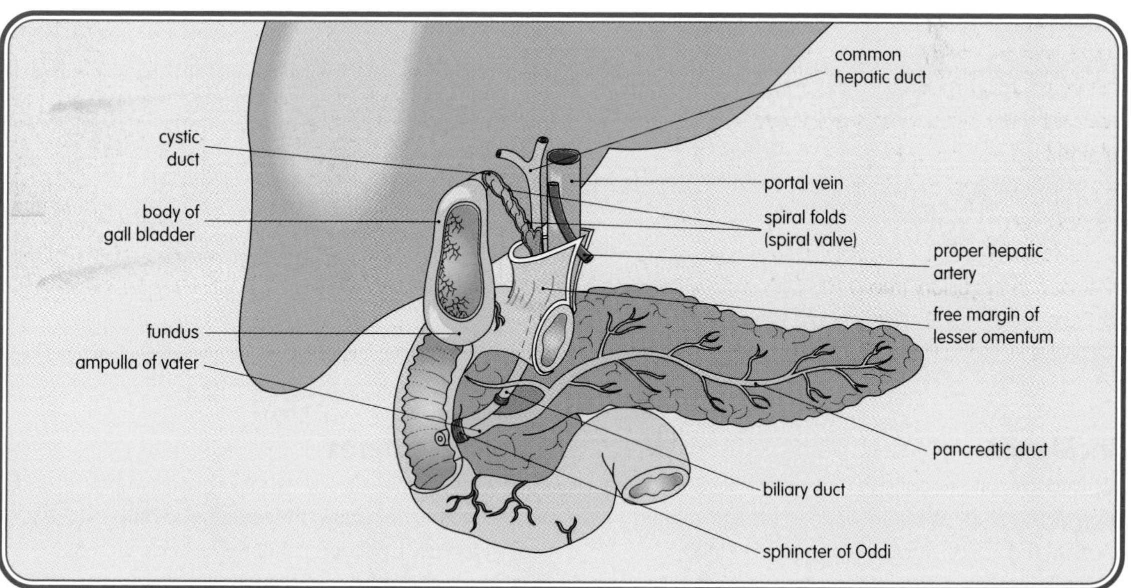

Fig. 23.1 Anatomy of the biliary tract and its relations.

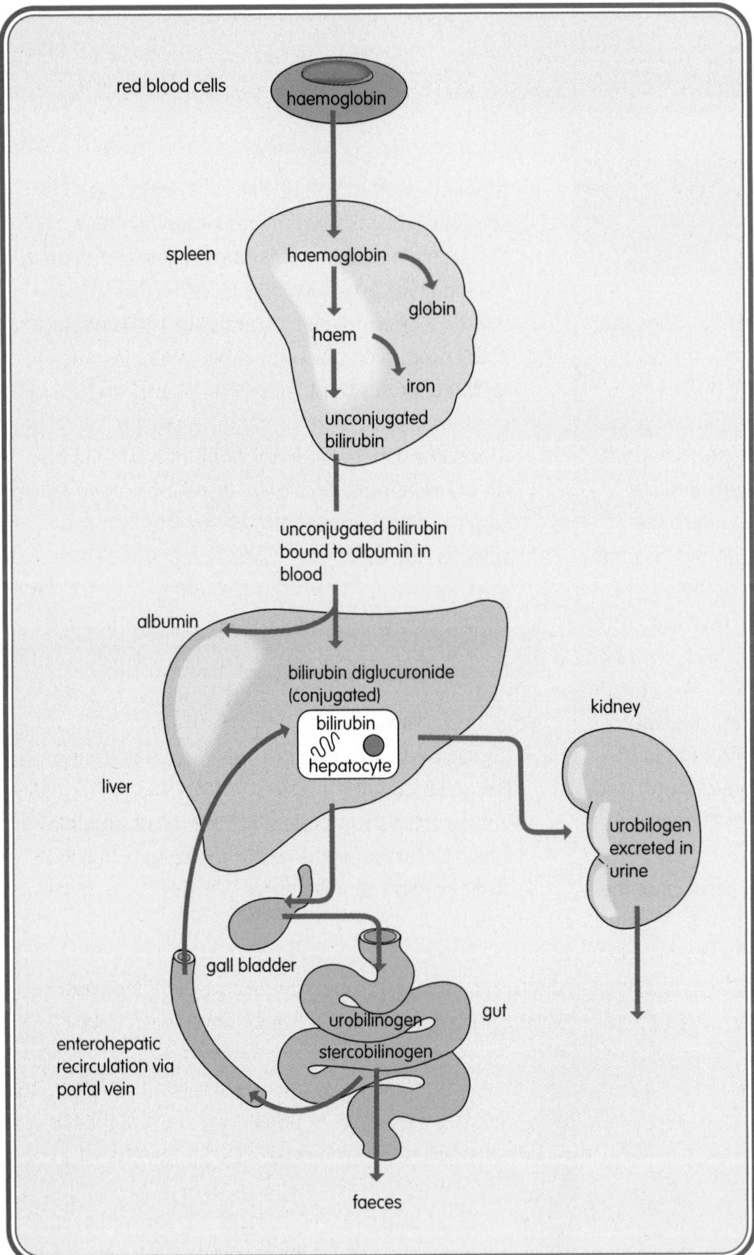

Fig. 23.2 Bilirubin metabolism.

Incidence

Gallstones can be found in approximately 30% of the population in the Western world in an age-related pattern (Fig. 23.3). Rare in Far East and Africa. Underlying dietary factors may be a factor.

Clinical features

Gallstones *per se* do not usually cause symptoms and in the majority of cases, they are found only coincidentally or at autopsies. Symptoms such as flatulence, dyspepsia, and fat intolerance are

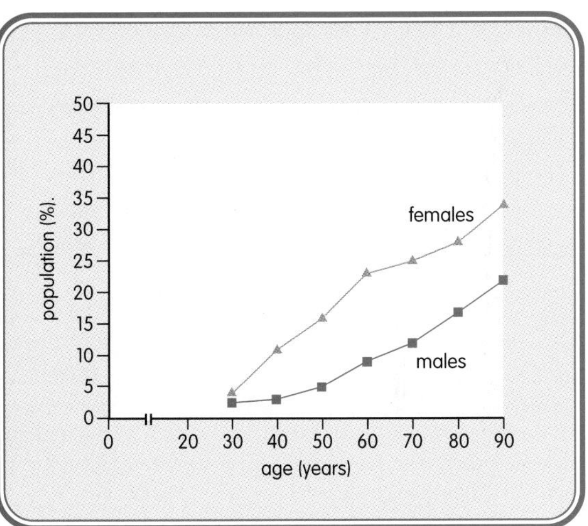

Fig. 23.3 Prevalence of gallstone disease.

commonly attributed to underlying gallstones, but whether there is a true correlation between the two is still debatable.

About 15% of patients with gallstones will require cholecystectomy for symptoms which may be attributable. The following symptoms may occur:

- Biliary colic and cholecystitis account for over 90% of clinical presentations of gallstone disease.
- Cholangitis may occur if bile is infected: features include fever, right upper quadrant pain, nausea and vomiting, and clinical jaundice is common.
- 'Murphy's sign': pain over right upper quadrant on deep inspiration. Localized rebound and guarding is characteristic of cholecystitis.

Diagnosis and investigation

A history of recurrent abdominal pain and history of jaundice with pale stools and dark urine, which resolves may suggest an underlying diagnosis. Investigations to confirm diagnosis should include:

- Full blood count—neutrophilia if acute cholecystitis is present. Biliary colic alone can exist without superimposed infection.
- Liver function test—features of obstructive jaundice, i.e. high bilirubin and alkaline phosphatase.
- Abdominal X-ray—not routinely done because only 10% of gallstones are radio-opaque.
- Ultrasound will demonstrate presence of gallstones, which may not be the cause of clinical symptoms. Additional features such as gall bladder wall thickening, tenderness over visualized gall bladder, or sludge in gall bladder are more diagnostic.
- Radio-isotope scan shows the function of the gall bladder and will demonstrate any blockages in cystic or common bile duct by its delay in bile excretion.
- Endoscopic retrograde cholangiopancreatography (ERCP) will show blockage in the common bile duct which may not be seen ultrasound (Fig. 23.4).

Aetiology and pathogenesis

Three main types of gallstones have been described:

- Mixed stones—70–90% of stones found predominantly contain cholesterol together with bile pigments and calcium. Usually multiple in numbers and in different sizes suggesting development in varying ages.
- Cholesterol stones account for up to 10% of stones, usually solitary, smooth, and pale in colour.
- Pigment stones, rare except in Asia, contain bile pigments (calcium bilirubinate) and are small and multiple. These are sometimes seen in patients with chronic haemolysis, e.g. hereditary spherocytosis, sickle cell disease, etc. due to an increase in bile production.

The exact pathogenesis is unclear, but increased cholesterol intake and bile stasis have been implicated. There is usually a nidus of organic material, often containing bacteria, where precipitation of calcium and cholesterol takes place. This is enhanced by biliary stasis either due to infection or biliary obstruction.

Patients with terminal ileal disease are at an increased risk of developing gallstones. The terminal ileum is responsible for the resorption of bile salts, and

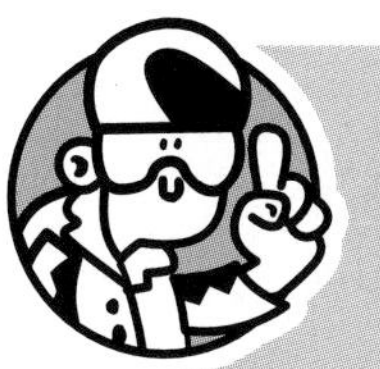

The common bile duct should be <6 mm normally or <8 mm in a patient following cholecystectomy.

a reduction of bile salts in the liver leads to reduced micelle production and, hence, precipitation of cholesterol and formation of cholesterol stones.

Complications

In chronic cholecystitis, the gall bladder is shrunken and features of chronic inflammation are present. However, symptoms of intermittent abdominal pain, nausea, and vomiting can be due to other pathology. If recurrent, attacks of acute cholecystitis can give rise to chronic cholecystitis.

Empyema of the gall bladder means distension with pus, and the patient presents with swinging pyrexia and septicaemia. Risk of perforation and peritonitis is high.

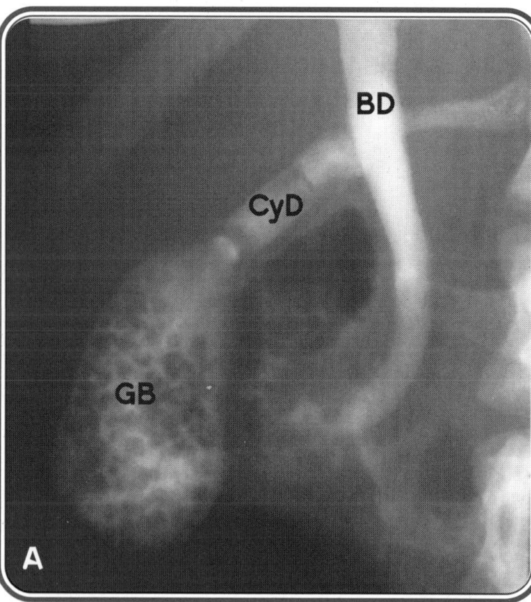

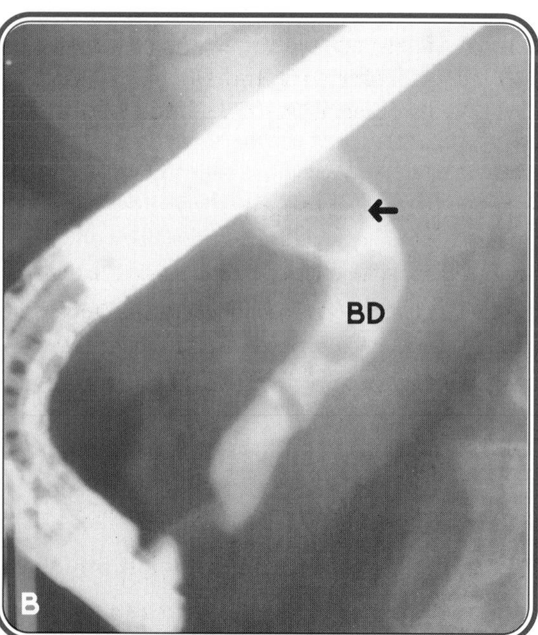

Fig. 23.4 ERCP images. (A) There are multiple small stones in the gall bladder (GB), but the bile duct (BD) is clear. (B) A gallstone measuring 1 cm across can be seen in the middle of the common bile duct (arrow). (C) A gallstone (GS) in the bile duct is being retrieved with the grasping basket following sphincterotomy. (CyD, cystic duct.)

Other complications include:

- Acute pancreatitis—swelling or obstruction at the ampulla of Vater, secondary to gallstones in the common bile duct, is a common cause of acute pancreatitis.
- Ascending cholangitis—result of infection in the common bile duct spreading into intrahepatic ducts.
- Gallstone ileus—erosion of the gall bladder wall by the stone can rarely cause peritonitis and an ileus due to impaction of a large stone in the narrowed ileum can also occur.
- Carcinoma of gall bladder—a rare complication.

Prognosis

Definitive surgery is usually curative, but occasional *in situ* stone formation can occur in common bile duct, causing recurrent symptoms.

Aims and indication for treatment

Asymptomatic patients require no treatment. Symptomatic patients can be treated either medically or surgically. Approximately only 15% of patients have symptoms over a 15-year period.

Treatment

During acute episodes, if there are signs of infection, the following are required:

- Analgesia.
- Intravenous fluids.
- Broad-spectrum antibiotics.

Further intervention is not instituted at this stage unless perforation and generalized peritonitis occur.

Cholecystectomy, open or laparoscopically, is often the treatment of choice, but some patients may not be suitable for a general anaesthetic.

ERCP is the treatment of choice for patients who have choledocholithiasis and are unsuitable for surgery. An endoscope is passed under sedation and contrast is injected to show any stones in the bile duct and gall bladder. A sphincterotomy is usually done to allow passage of further stones once the bile duct is cleared of its obstruction (Fig. 23.4C).

Chenodeoxylate and ursodeoxycolic acid are bile acids that can be taken orally and increase cholesterol solubility in bile. Treatment takes up to 6 months to complete, and recurrence occurs in over 50% of patients once treatment is stopped. This dissolution treatment is rarely used.

TUMOURS OF THE BILIARY TRACT

Carcinoma of gall bladder

Incidence

Predominantly disease of elderly people (>60 years) but may also occur in younger people. There may be an association with pre-existing gallstones, suggesting chronic inflammation as a carcinogenic factor. Gall bladder cancer accounts for <1% of all adenocarcinomas.

Clinical features

Jaundice, right upper quadrant mass, in addition to general malaise and weight loss, are common features. A number of cases are found incidentally on routine cholecystectomy and confirmed on histology

Diagnosis and investigations

Ultrasound is poor at detecting gall bladder carcinomas but will detect metastasis in the liver. The diagnosis is usually made at cholecystectomy for gallstone symptoms.

Prognosis

Due to its late presentation and early local metastasis, patients rarely survive for more than 1 year.

Treatment

Radical resection of the tumour may provide a cure, especially for patients only diagnosed incidentally. Chemotherapy and radiotherapy have unproven benefits.

Cholangiocarcinomas

Incidence

Adenocarcinomas of bile ducts associated with dense fibrous tissue. They can be intrahepatic or extrahepatic. They are uncommon tumours, accounting for only approximately 8–10% of primary liver tumours.

Clinical features

Features differ depending on the type of tumour:

- Extrahepatic tumours present with progressive jaundice similar to sclerosing cholangitis.
- Intrahepatic tumours tend to invade liver parenchyma and present similarly to primary liver tumours and jaundice is rare.

General features such as weight loss, malaise, nausea, and vomiting may be present.

Diagnosis and investigation

Investigations should include:

- Liver function tests indicate cholestatic jaundice with high alkaline phosphatase and bilirubin.
- Ultrasound shows dilated bile ducts if extrahepatic lesions are present, or lesions within the liver parenchyma if intrahepatic, but these features are not specific for cholangiocarcinoma, hence ERCP is required.
- ERCP—the dense fibrous tumour tends to grow along the duct system, producing a shouldered stricture.

Aetiology and pathogenesis

These are unknown, but in the Far East there is an association with infestation by *Clonorchis sinensis*. Up to 20% of patients who have chronic symptomatic primary sclerosing cholangitis develop cholangiocarcinoma.

Chronic inflammation or sepsis may therefore be important factors.

Prognosis

Poor, with survival rarely more than 6 months.

Treatment

Treatment options include:

- Radical resection of extrahepatic tumours can offer a cure, but this is rare.
- Insertion of endoprostheses (stents) during ERCP (see Fig. 17.19) will provide symptomatic relief of jaundice and improve quality of life.

Radiotherapy and chemotherapy are unhelpful.

Ampullary tumours

An adenocarcinoma arising from the ampulla of Vater presents with obstructive jaundice which may or may not be intermittent.

These tumours can be friable and bleed, and present as malaena or anaemia with jaundice.

Diagnosis is made at ERCP and if made early, tumours are amenable to resection with a 60% 5-year survival.

Figure 23.5 shows the pattern of bile duct tumours.

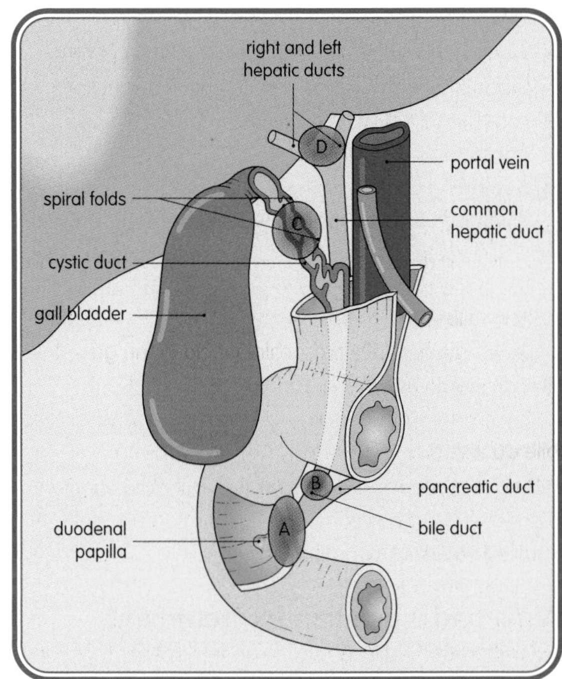

Fig. 23.5 Depiction of tumours involving the bile duct that may then present with jaundice. (A) Ampullary tumour. (B) Carcinoma of the head of the pancreas. (C) Carcinoma of the cystic duct or gallbladder. (D) Cholangiocarcinoma involving the hilum or below.

BENIGN ANATOMICAL BILE DUCT PROBLEMS

Choledochal cyst and other anomalies

Congenital dilatations of the bile duct are known as choledochal cysts. The majority are asymptomatic but can produce jaundice and abdominal pain. Intrahepatic cystic dilatations are known as Caroli's disease and can predispose to cholangitis. Treatment of symptoms initially is with antibiotics, but surgical reconstruction may be required.

Benign stricture of bile duct

A result of damage to bile ducts due to trauma or inflammation (gallstones, ascending cholangitis, or previous gall bladder surgery). Presents as progressive jaundice and can be mistaken for cholangiocarcinoma or sclerosing cholangitis.

Diagnosis is usually made by temporal association with trauma or surgery. Differentiation from tumours can be difficult if the trauma was a long time ago.

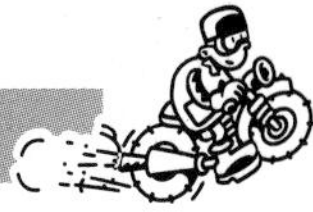

Endoscopic brush cytology or histology may be helpful. Strictures occur in up to 15% patients following liver transplantation. Localized strictures can be treated with stenting or reconstruction surgery.

INFECTIONS OF THE BILIARY TRACT

Usually bile within the biliary tree is sterile. The sphincter of Oddi together with hydrochloric acid in the gastric juice prevents bacteria ascending the tract.

Infection usually occurs only when the integrity of the bile duct sphincter function has been disrupted, e.g. after surgery or by inflammation caused by gallstones.

Cholangitis

Incidence

A potentially serious but common complication of bile stasis secondary to gallstones, bile duct dilatation, or strictures.

Clinical features

In the majority of people the symptoms are:

- Fever.
- Jaundice.
- Right upper quadrant pain.

Septicaemic shock may be a feature in severe cases, especially in elderly people.

Diagnosis and investigation

Investigations to consider:

- Full blood count shows raised neutrophils.
- Liver function tests reveal cholestatic picture, i.e. raised alkaline phosphatase and bilirubin, mild increase in transaminases.
- Blood cultures are positive in over 90% of cases on repeated cultures (usually *E. coli*).
- Ultrasound shows dilatation of bile ducts; liver abscesses can sometimes be seen.

Aetiology and pathogenesis

Commonly an *E. coli* infection secondary to bile stasis. Causes include:

- Gallstones.
- Postcholecystectomy.
- Benign strictures.
- Post-ERCP (especially if a stent is inserted, because stents occlude with time).

Complications

Suppurative cholangitis is a potentially fatal condition that requires urgent drainage either endoscopically or surgically. Patients whose fever and septicaemic shock does not settle with high-dose intravenous antibiotics are at risk of developing this condition.

Treatment

High-dose, broad-spectrum (e.g. cefotaxime and metronidazole) intravenous antibiotics.

Any underlying cause needs to be treated once the infection has been adequately dealt with, e.g. removal of gallstones, blocked endoprosthesis, etc.

Other infections of the biliary tract

These are rarely seen in the Western world and include *Opisthorchis* and *Clonorchis* spp, which are liver flukes that cause ascending cholangitis. There may be a predisposition to cholangiocarcinoma following such an infection. Patients with AIDS following HIV infection can develop sclerosing cholangitis, and it is possible that this could be due to opportunistic infection with *Cryptosporidium parvum* in the GI tract, but its exact association is unclear.

Clonorchis and Opisthorchiasis

Incidence

Clonorchis sinensis and *Opisthorchis felineus* are common flukes found in the Far East that mainly affect animals such as dogs, cats, and pigs.

Clinical features

Patients may remain symptom-free but repeated and prolonged exposure will cause:

- Recurrent jaundice.
- Cholangitis.
- Liver abscess.
- Possibly cholangiocarcinoma.

Diagnosis and investigation

Microscopic examination of faeces or duodenal aspirate is required for diagnosis.

Treatment

Praziquantel is the treatment of choice.

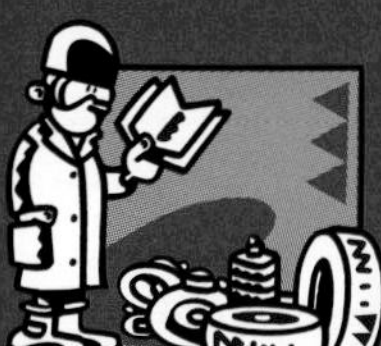

24. Pancreas

ANATOMY, PHYSIOLOGY AND FUNCTION OF THE PANCREAS

The pancreas is a retroperitoneal structure that extends from the second part of the duodenum to the spleen (Fig. 24.1). The pancreatic duct, together with the common bile duct, enter the duodenum at the ampulla of Vater.

The pancreas has two functions, exocrine and endocrine:

- Exocrine secretions include lipase, amylase, and proteases which are responsible for digestion of fat, carbohydrate, and protein, respectively. They are under the control of other gut hormones, such as cholecystokinin, which are released when fatty acids and amino acids enter the duodenum.
- Endocrine secretions are insulin, glucagon, and somatostatin; they are primarily involved in the regulation of glucose storage and use.

ACUTE PANCREATITIS

Incidence

A relatively common condition affecting approximately 1% of the general population.

Clinical features

These include:

- Epigastric pain (typically radiating to the back), nausea, and vomiting are invariably present.
- Local abdominal discoloration, i.e. around the umbilicus (Cullen's sign) or over flanks (Grey–Turner's sign) is rare. It is likely to be due to underlying clotting abnormalites as a result of disseminated intravascular coagulation (DIC).
- Tenderness and guarding, depending on severity.
- Shock may be a feature in severe cases.

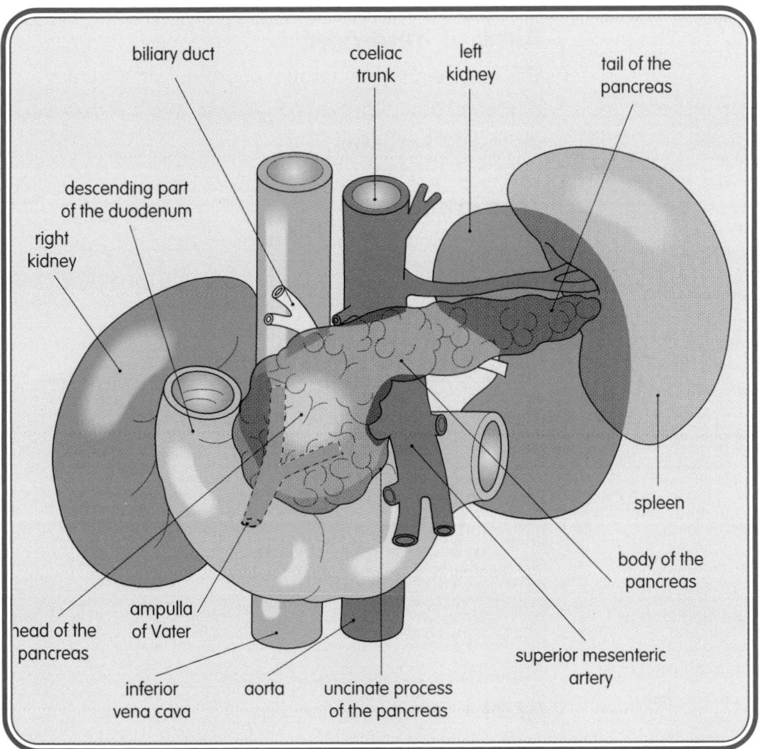

Fig. 24.1 The pancreas and its relations.

Diagnosis and investigation

Investigation should be for those of an acute abdomen, as other conditions may mimic clinical signs and symptoms of acute pancreatitis. Consider the following tests:

- Serum amylase—>1000 units is usually diagnostic.
- Biochemistry—poor prognosis associated with high glucose, high urea, low calcium, and low albumin (Fig. 24.2).
- Arterial gases—hypoxia in severe cases.
- Ultrasound/computed tomography (CT) scans are not routinely done, except if diagnosis is in doubt. Swollen pancreas, ascites, and gallstones can be seen.

Aetiology and pathogenesis

Exact mechanism is unclear, but is thought to be due to autodigestion of proteolytic enzymes in the pancreas, leading to oedema with mild cases and haemorrhagic necrosis in severe cases.

The reflux of bile in the pancreatic duct may contribute to pathogenesis of acute pancreatitis in cases of pre-existing gallstones.

The causes of acute pancreatitis are listed in Fig. 24.3.

Complications

Complications of the disease that can cause a higher mortality can be predicted by certain factors including age, level of amylase, LDH levels, etc. (see Fig. 24.2). Some specific complaints include:

- Adult respiratory distress syndrome (ARDS) is a rare but severe complication of acute pancreatitis which requires artificial ventilation.
- Paralytic ileus is commonly seen.
- Pseudocysts can occur in up to half of patients seen with severe acute pancreatitis. Often no treatment is required because they are usually small and resolve spontaneously. A pseudocyst is a collection of pancreatic fluid in the lesser sac and has no epithelial lining.
- Pancreatic abscesses are due to infection of pancreatic pseudocysts or cysts within the pancreas following acute infection.
- Chronic pancreatitis occurs following repeated attacks of acute pancreatitis, especially secondary to alcohol.
- Metabolic abnormalities such as hypocalcaemia and hyperglycaemia are commonly seen.
- Disseminated intravascular coagulation is often a life-threatening complication.

Prognosis

The mortality rate reaches up to 60% in patients with severe pancreatitis and bad prognostic factors. However, in mild cases, mortality is low (<1%).

Aims of treatment

This is to reduce the amount of proteolytic enzymes produced and hence autodigestion, which is achieved by 'resting' the bowel.

Treatment

Conservative treatment, such as opiate analgesia, intravenous fluid, nasogastric tube, and cessation of all

Poor prognostic criteria in pancreatitis	
Age	>55 years
White blood cell count	>15 x 10 9/L
Blood glucose	>10 mmol/L
Urea	>16 mmol/L
Albumin	<30 g/L
Calcium	<2 mmol/L
AST	>100 IU/L
LDH	>600 IU/L
PaO_2	<8 kPa
Three or more of these factors indicates a poor prognosis (Glasgow scoring system)	

Fig. 24.2 Prognostic criteria of severity in pancreatitis.

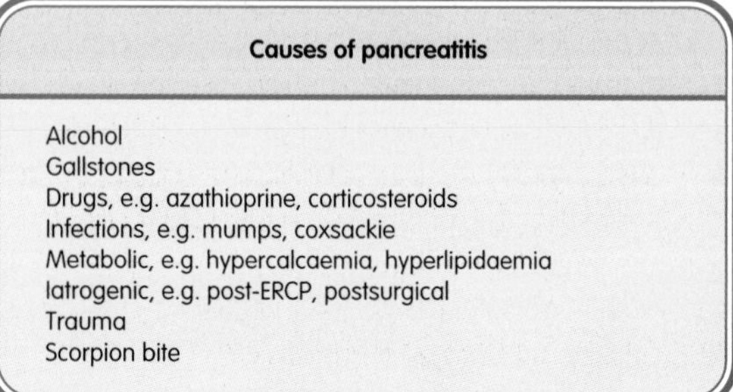

Causes of pancreatitis

Alcohol
Gallstones
Drugs, e.g. azathioprine, corticosteroids
Infections, e.g. mumps, coxsackie
Metabolic, e.g. hypercalcaemia, hyperlipidaemia
Iatrogenic, e.g. post-ERCP, postsurgical
Trauma
Scorpion bite

Fig. 24.3 Causes of pancreatitis.

oral intake, is usually all that is required in mild to moderate cases.

In severe cases, with systemic complications such as disseminated intravascular coagulation and acute respiratory distress syndrome, intensive care unit is usually required. Surgery may be indicated to remove necrotic pancreatic tissues.

CHRONIC PANCREATITIS

Incidence

Usually a result of acute pancreatitis, where there is continuing inflammation with irreversible changes. Alcohol is the most common cause.

Clinical features

These include:

- Chronic abdominal pain over epigastrium, usually radiating to back. Intermittent severe pain can be precipitated by heavy alcohol consumption, similar to that in acute pancreatitis.
- Steatorrhoea occurs due to reduction in pancreatic enzyme activity.
- Diabetes due to destruction of Islet cells.
- Less common presentations include obstructive jaundice and cholangitis.

Diagnosis and investigation

Investigations should include:

- Serum amylase—not usually raised unless an acute attack is present on background of chronic disease.
- Biochemistry—can show high serum glucose due to underlying diabetes.
- Liver function test showing derangement—is a reflection of high alcohol consumption.
- Abdominal X-ray—may reveal calcification of pancreas which is characteristic.
- Abdominal CT—may demonstrate pancreatic swelling or pseudocyst formation.
- Endoscopic retrograde cholangiopancreatography (ERCP)—shows distorted and irregular pancreatic ducts indicating fibrosis (Fig. 24.4).

Aetiology and pathogenesis

The majority of cases are due to high consumption of alcohol. Early changes are due to protein deposition along the pancreatic ducts which lead to duct dilatation. This is followed by acinar atrophy and fibrosis around pancreatic ducts. Calcification of protein plugs occurs.

Damage to the pancreas is long term, but cessation of high alcohol may prevent further damage.

Complications

Unfortunately, complications of chronic pancreatitis are common and include:

- Pain—major complication in patients and some become dependent on opiates for pain relief.
- Malabsorption—due to reduced secretion of pancreatic lipases causing steatorrhoea and fat-soluble vitamin deficiencies.
- Diabetes—often requires insulin treatment as pancreatic function declines.
- Pseudocysts —these are commonly found on ultrasound and cause pain.
- Jaundice—rare, but can occur with ascending cholangitis.
- Portal hypertension occurs occasionally when the portal or splenic vein becomes thrombosed.

Prognosis

Depends on whether the patient is abstaining from alcohol, and in the majority of cases, complete abstinence is rare.

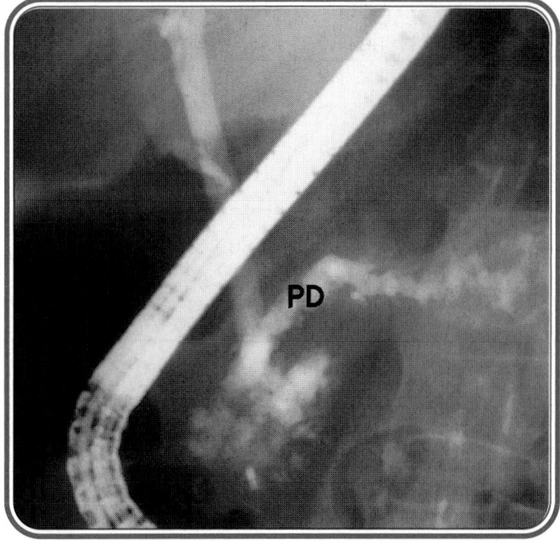

Fig. 24.4 ERCP signs of chronic pancreatitis. The pancreatic duct (PD) is dilated and grossly distorted with ectatic side branches.

In some patients, there are continuing intermittent attacks of acute pancreatitis on a background of chronic pancreatitis. This is known as chronic relapsing pancreatitis.

Treatment

Stop drinking alcohol!

Other treatment options include:

- Pain control usually in some form of opiates with its problem of addiction.
- Pancreatic enzyme supplements are given to improve fat absorption and fat-soluble vitamins.
- Oral hypoglycaemic agents or insulin may be required.
- Surgery, if required, involves removal of pancreatic duct stones with partial pancreatectomy and drainage of ducts into the small bowel. Occasionally, a total pancreatectomy is done. Good result from surgery is variable.
- Coeliac ganglion blockade can provide permanent pain relief, but has no effect on continuing inflammation.

PSEUDOCYSTS

Incidence

Seen following an attack of moderate to severe acute pancreatitis in over 50% of cases. True cysts are those occurring within the pancreas and pseudocysts are those without an epithelial lining, consisting of a collection containing inflammatory fluid and pancreatic enzyme within the lesser sac. They are far more common than true cysts.

Multiple small cysts can also be seen in the pancreas with polycystic disease involving the kidney and liver. This is inherited as an autosomal dominant condition, and the pathology is different to those caused by acute pancreatitis and a more detailed text should be consulted.

Clinical features

Main features are:

- Abdominal pain—occurs especially if the pseudocyst is large, together with nausea and vomiting mimicking unresolved acute pancreatitis.
- Abdominal mass may be palpable over the epigastrium (the cyst will make the aorta more palpable and occasionally is mistaken for an aortic aneurysm).
- Ascites—these can occur due to rupture of the cyst within the peritoneal cavity. Ascitic fluid will have a high concentration of amylase.

Diagnosis and investigation

Failure of improvement after an episode of acute pancreatitis should alert one to the suspicion of pseudocyst formation (Fig. 24.5).

Ultrasound is the investigation of choice, and frequently small cysts can be seen when the patient is asymptomatic.

Aetiology and pathogenesis

Thought to be due to inflammatory exudate produced by the inflamed pancreas collected in the lesser sac. High levels of pancreatic enzyme found in the fluid may indicate extensive damage to the pancreas, causing secretions to leak out. They are more commonly found in severe and chronic pancreatitis.

Complications

Pancreatic abscess is due to infection of the cyst, which can occur spontaneously or as a consequence of repeated aspiration.

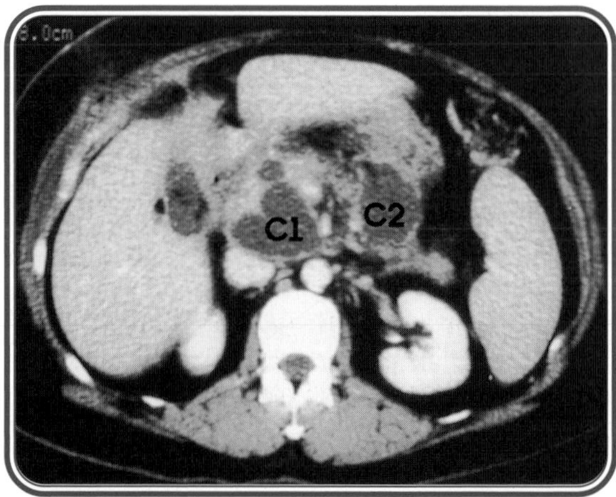

Fig. 24.5 CT scan of pancreatic pseudocyst. A heart-shaped cyst (C1) is seen in the head of the pancreas and a second cyst (C2) is seen near the tail.

Prognosis

Dependent on underlying pathology. Prognosis is poor if pseudocyst is secondary to alcohol-induced chronic pancreatitis, whereas it is excellent if the pancreatitis is due to a treatable cause, e.g. gallstones.

Treatment

No treatment is required for small asymptomatic pseudocysts, as they usually resolve spontaneously. Other treatment includes:

- Aspiration of cyst—usually done under ultrasound guidance and may need to be repeated.
- Surgery if persistent, the cyst can be 'marsupialized' such that fluid will drain into the stomach.

CYSTIC FIBROSIS

Incidence

Affects 1 in 2000 live births.

Clinical features

These include:

- Recurrent chest infections—usually the presenting feature in childhood.
- Steatorrhoea due to pancreatic insufficiency.
- Small bowel obstruction—due to the viscous secretions. Neonates may present with meconium ileus.
- Infertility—females are more likely to conceive. Males are invariably infertile. Delayed puberty is seen in most patients.
- Liver cirrhosis seen in patients who survive into adulthood (see p. 163).

Diagnosis and investigation

Consider the following:

- Sweat test reveals a high sodium concentration.
- Genetic analysis for the recessive gene and the identification of CF protein.
- Pancreatic function tests, e.g. PABA test (see p. 84).

Aetiology and pathogenesis

Due to a gene mutation on the long arm of chromosome 7, resulting in an abnormality of a transmembrane protein known as cystic fibrosis transmembrane conductance regulator (CFTR), which results in production of thick viscous secretions.

Complications

The main complications include malabsorption, especially of fat-soluble vitamins and bronchiectasis and pneumothorax, which are common. Infertility and liver disease occur in adults. Death is usually due to respiratory failure.

Prognosis

Improved over the years and most patients will survive up to mid to late 20s.

Treatment

Treatment of chest infections includes postural drainage as well as antibiotics. Also:

- Enzyme supplements (capsules containing trypsin and lipases, which break down in the duodenum delivering the enzyme).
- Vitamin supplements and high calorie intake.
- Gene therapy has been attempted but early results are disappointing so far.
- Lung transplant is considered in some patients.

TUMOURS OF THE PANCREAS

Carcinoma of pancreas

Incidence

Increases with increasing age and most patients are over 60 years. It is the fourth most common cancer in the UK. More common in males than females.

Clinical features

Signs and symptoms include:

- Weight loss can be substantial.
- Abdominal pain is a common feature usually radiating through to the back and tends to be relieved by sitting forward.
- Jaundice is usually the presenting feature of carcinoma affecting the head of pancreas. Jaundice is obstructive and progressive and is characteristically painless in the early stages.
- Diabetes is thought to be due to insulin resistance, caused by hormones secreted by pancreatic beta cells rather than its destruction.
- Thrombophlebitis migrans is due to a paraneoplastic phenomenon.
- Ascites occurs in the late stages with hepatomegaly due to liver metastasis.

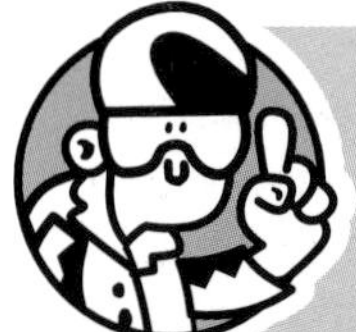

Courvoisier's sign: in carcinoma of the head of the pancreas, a patient presenting with obstructive jaundice can have a palpable dilated gall bladder. This suggests cancer because a dilated gall bladder is not found with gallstone disease due to chronic inflammation of the gall bladder.

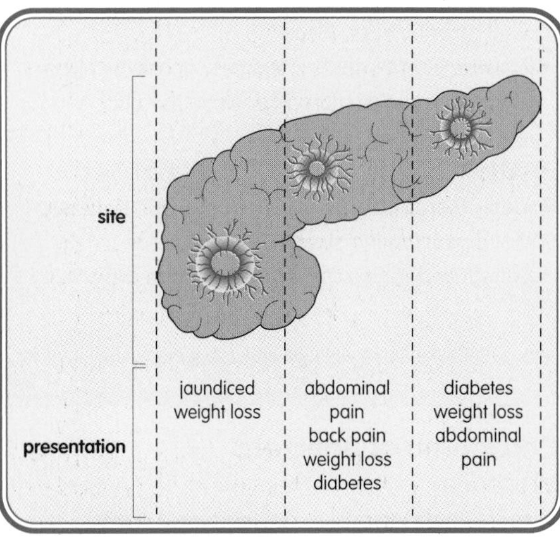

Figure 24.6 shows the sites at which pancreatic tumours occur.

Diagnosis and investigation

Investigations may include:

- ERCP, as part of an investigation for obstructive jaundice, will usually be diagnostic especially of periampullary tumours (Fig. 24.7).
- CT of the abdomen will diagnose most pancreatic tumours, and it is ideally confirmed by biopsy. It will also demonstrate nodal spread at the porta hepatis (Fig. 24.8).

Fig. 24.6 Anatomical sites for pancreatic tumours.

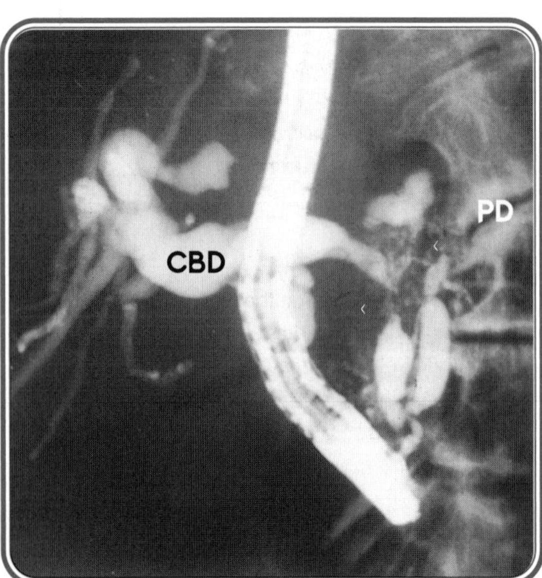

Fig. 24.7 ERCP showing 'double duct stricture' (arrows) in pancreatic carcinoma. (CBD, common bile duct; PD, pancreatic duct.)

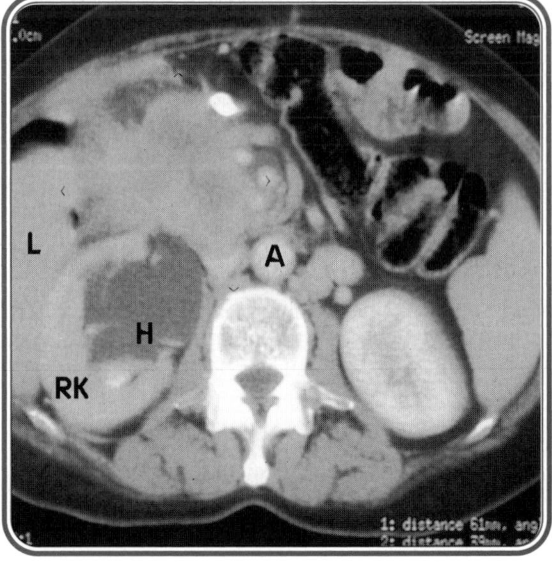

Fig. 24.8 CT scan of pancreatic tumour (arrows) obstructing the right ureter and causing hydronephrosis (H). (A, aorta; L, liver; RK, right kidney.)

- Ultrasound is less sensitive at detecting pancreatic tumours, especially those along the body or the tail of pancreas.

Aetiology and pathogenesis

The aetiology is unknown but smoking and high alcohol consumption have been implicated.

Almost all tumours are due to adenocarcinoma arising from the duct epithelium and around 70% are in the head of the pancreas. The tumours have usually already metastasized to local lymph nodes and the liver by the time of presentation.

Prognosis

Very poor due to its late presentation. The 5-year survival is <5%.

Aims of treatment

This is mainly for palliation because curative treatment is unlikely to be successful due to the nature of the disease.

Treatment

Options include:

- Radical surgical resection provides the only possible chance of a cure, but it is seldom carried out, as most patients are unsuitable for surgery and it carries a high mortality rate. A by-pass operation for the relief of jaundice can be done where the common bile duct is anastomosed to the small bowel as a palliative measure.
- Stent insertion can be achieved endoscopically where a stent is inserted into the narrowed part of the common bile duct to allow free drainage of bile (see Fig. 17.18).
- Analgesia in the form of opiates are indicated, as dependence is not an issue.
- Coeliac axis block may be useful for patients with pain that is not controlled by conventional analgesia.

Endocrine tumours

Incidence

These are rare tumours in the pancreas and can occur with tumours of the pituitary and parathyroid to form a syndrome of multiple endocrine neoplasia (MEN).

Clinical features

Depends on the cell type and the hormone produced.

Gastrinomas (Zollinger–Ellison syndrome)

These arise from the G cells of the pancreas and they secrete gastrin and present as peptic ulceration which is often large and multiple. Perforation and GI haemorrhage is common and diagnosis should be considered in young patients presenting with recurrent peptic ulcer disease.

Diarrhoea due to excess acid production is also common (low pH).

Insulinomas (Islet cell tumours)

Produce insulin and present as episodes of fasting hypoglycaemia, i.e. early morning or late afternoons.

Presentation is often bizarre, hence diagnosis may not be made for years and the patient learns to live with the symptoms, as glucose abolishes the attacks.

Vipomas

This is a rare pancreatic tumour in which vasoactive intestinal peptide (VIP) is produced causing severe secretory diarrhoea, leading to dehydration by stimulating adenyl cyclase to produce intestinal secretions.

Glucagonomas

Tumour of alpha cells that produce glucagon in patients with diabetes mellitus. A characteristic rash (necrolytic migratory erythema) has also been described.

Somatostatinomas

Somatostatin is an inhibitory hormone that produces a reduction in the secretion of insulin, pancreatic enzyme, and bicarbonate, hence produces the clinical syndrome of diabetes mellitus, steatorrhoea, and hypochlorhydria.

Weight loss is also a common feature.

Diagnosis and investigation

This again is dependent on the type of tumour involved and the clinical presentation:

- A CT scan will identify the majority of endocrine tumours in the pancreas.
- Hormone assays—measurement of the specific type of hormone produced will often give the diagnosis. Selective venous sampling from the pancreas will also help to locate the tumour. In cases of insulinoma, measurement is usually made during a 24–48 hour fast when symptoms of hypoglycaemia appear.

Aetiology and pathogenesis

The tumours arise from the APUD cells (amine precursor uptake and decarboxylation), hence their hormonal secretory nature.The MEN type 2 syndrome has an autosomal dominant inheritance.

Prognosis

Gastrinomas are often malignant, hence carry a worse prognosis than insulinoma, which is benign. Overall prognosis will depend on associated MEN syndrome and other tumours involved.

Treatment

Surgical resection of the tumour is required.

Identification of other possible tumours associated with MEN syndrome may be required, and screening of relatives in those with MEN type 2 syndrome (Fig. 24.9).

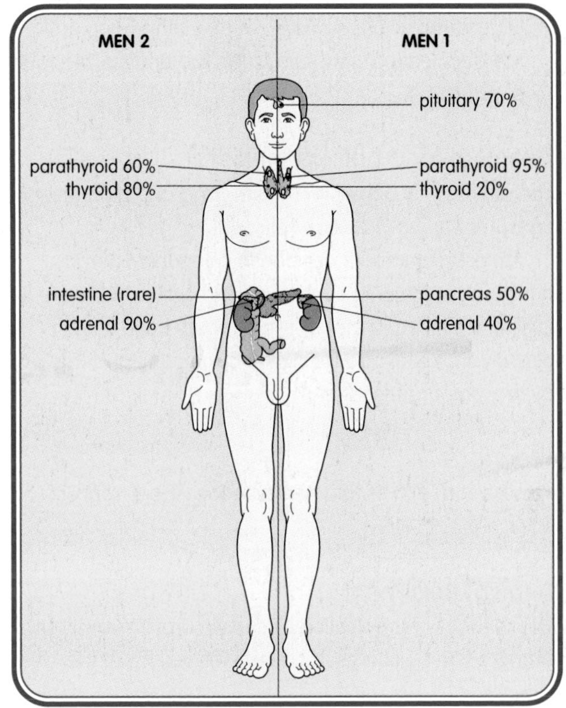

Fig. 24.9 Depiction of MENI and MEN2.

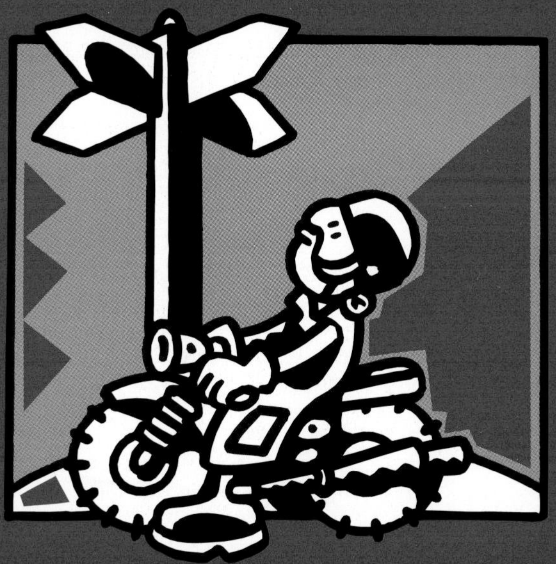

SELF-ASSESSMENT

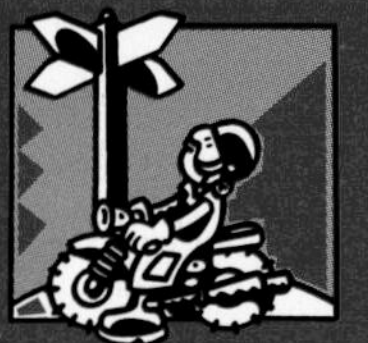

Multiple-choice Questions

Indicate whether each answer is true or false.

1. The following statements are true:

(a) Tylosis is associated with achalasia.
(b) On barium swallow, a 'bird's beak' appearance is suggestive of squamous carcinoma.
(c) Pneumatic dilatation is the treatment of choice for achalasia.
(d) Reduced lower oesophageal sphincter pressure is a common feature of gastro-oesophageal reflux disease .
(e) Oesophageal pH is usually less than 4.

2. The following is true of oesophageal pain:

(a) It can occur in the absence of heartburn.
(b) It can mimic the pain of a myocardial infarction.
(c) It can be relieved by glyceryl trinitrate.
(d) It is usually precipitated by exercise.
(e) It can be caused by candidiasis.

3. The following is true of Barrett's oesophagus:

(a) Columnar epithelium is replaced by squamous epithelium.
(b) It appears in an antegrade (top to bottom) direction.
(c) It is a premalignant condition.
(d) Severe dysplasia is an ominous sign.
(e) It is an indication for surveillance endoscopy.

4. The following is true of postgastrectomy syndromes:

(a) The anaemia can be corrected with ascorbic acid supplements.
(b) The risk of gastric cancer in the long term is increased.
(c) Sweating and palpitations can be due to hypoglycaemia.
(d) Biliary gastritis in the gastric remnant is common.
(e) Diarrhoea is commonly due to bacterial overgrowth.

5. *Helicobacter pylori:*

(a) Causes ulceration in the duodenum.
(b) Causes Barrett's metaplasia in the oesophagus.
(c) Is associated with hypergastrinaemia.
(d) Is often resistant to certain antibiotics.
(e) Can convert urea to ammonia and carbon dioxide.

6. The following is true of neoplastic disease in the stomach:

(a) Maltoma can occasionally respond to antibiotic treatment in combination with a proton pump inhibitor.
(b) Ménétrière's disease is due to metaplasia of the gastric mucosa.
(c) Leiomyoma has a characteristic appearance at endoscopy.
(d) Gastric carcinoma produces abdominal pain that is often worse after eating.
(e) The most common gastric carcinoma is of squamous cell origin.

7. Gastric hypomotility (gastroparesis):

(a) Is commonly associated with diabetes mellitus.
(b) Is a risk factor for gastro-oesophageal reflux disease.
(c) Is a feature of generalized scleroderma (systemic sclerosis).
(d) Occasionally responds to erythromycin.
(e) Is often secondary to duodenal ulcer disease.

8. The following statements are true:

(a) Iron absorption is reduced in hypochlorhydric states.
(b) Vitamin D absorption is often deficient in the presence of gastritis.
(c) Vitamin B_{12} supplements are often necessary following gastrectomy.
(d) Anaemia associated with chronic atrophic gastritis may respond to ascorbic acid supplements.
(e) Intestinal metaplasia in the stomach is a risk factor for gastric carcinoma.

9. The following are features of coeliac disease:

(a) Hypocalcaemia.
(b) Hypercalcaemia.
(c) Normocytic anaemia.
(d) Hypoalbuminaemia.
(e) Positive antiparietal cell antibodies.

10. The following clinical features are associated with coeliac disease:

(a) Anaemia.
(b) Weight loss.
(c) Vomiting.
(d) Diarrhoea.
(e) Jaundice.

11. The following is true of Crohn's disease:

(a) The rectum is always affected.
(b) Commonly affects the terminal ileum.
(c) More commonly occurs in smokers.
(d) Can result in vitamin B_{12} deficiency with a negative Schilling test.
(e) Commonly presents with bloody diarrhoea.

12. The following is true of Crohn's disease:

(a) C-reactive protein mimics inflammatory activity.
(b) Normal albumin indicates remission.
(c) Large bowel barium enema is the most definitive radiological test.
(d) A small bowel biopsy can be helpful in making the diagnosis.
(e) A low blood urea is common.

13. The following is true of giardiasis:

(a) Diarrhoea abates with avoidance of dairy produce.
(b) Diarrhoea abates with avoidance of gluten.
(c) Diarrhoea requires treatment with metronidazole.
(d) Diarrhoea is usually accompanied by vomiting.
(e) Diarrhoea commonly results in vitamin B_{12} deficiency.

14. The following is true of ulcerative colitis:

(a) It commonly presents with pain in the right iliac fossa.
(b) It can be associated with ankylosing spondylitis.
(c) It is a risk factor for toxic dilatation of the colon.
(d) The occurrence of abdominal tenderness is an ominous sign.
(e) It often causes ischiorectal abscesses.

15. The following is true of inflammatory bowel disease:

(a) Increased liver enzymes in the serum usually indicate the complication of carcinoma.
(b) Small bowel barium enema is the best radiological investigation for ulcerative colitis.
(c) It is occasionally complicated by carcinoma of the caecum.
(d) It is commonly associated with thyroiditis.
(e) It is sometimes complicated by iritis.

16. Acholuric jaundice without pain:

(a) Is a common presentation of pancreatic carcinoma.
(b) Is a feature of Gilbert's disease.
(c) Can occur in hereditary spherocytosis.
(d) Is associated with pale-coloured stools.
(e) Is associated with pruritus.

17. The following is true of viral hepatitis:

(a) Hepatitis C commonly presents with jaundice.
(b) Hepatitis E is fatal particularly in pregnant women.
(c) Hepatitis BeAg is a marker of viral replication.
(d) Hepatitis A is a risk factor for hepatoma.
(e) Hepatitis D occurs only in association with hepatitis C.

18. The following is true of risk factors for the development of hepatocellular carcinoma:

(a) Females are at greater risk than males.
(b) Excess iron is a recognized risk factor.
(c) Aflatoxin is a risk factor.
(d) Hepatitis A is a risk factor.
(e) Risk factors generally only operate in the presence of cirrhosis.

19. The following drugs cause jaundice:

(a) Methotrexate.
(b) Flucloxacillin.
(c) Metronidazole.
(d) Isoniazid.
(e) Phenobarbitone.

20. Alcoholic hepatitis:

(a) Recovers rapidly on cessation of drinking.
(b) Is a risk factor for hepatorenal syndrome.
(c) Ascites is a feature.
(d) Coagulopathy is corrected with administration of vitamin K.
(e) Encephalopathy occurs only if infection is present.

21. Haemochromatosis:

(a) Is a genetic defect resulting in copper overload in the liver.
(b) Is a risk factor for the development of hepatoma.
(c) Has an equal sex incidence but presents earlier in males than females.
(d) Is treated by avoiding meat products.
(e) Can cause hypogonadism in the absence of cirrhosis.

22. Primary sclerosing cholangitis:

(a) Occurs predominantly in middle-aged females.
(b) Is a major risk factor for cholangiocarcinoma.
(c) Occurs in 50% patients with ulcerative colitis.
(d) Has been treated with ursodeoxycholic acid.
(e) May require insertion of an endoprosthesis for its treatment.

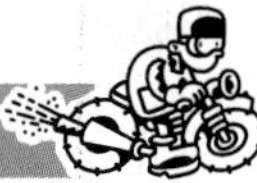

23. Colonic carcinoma:

(a) Most commonly occurs in the right side of the colon.
(b) May present with iron deficiency anaemia in the absence of any gastrointestinal symptoms.
(c) Commonly arises in colonic polyps.
(d) Carries a 5-year survival of less than 10%.
(e) Is the cause of carcinoid syndrome.

---

24. The following GI conditions are associated with microcytic hypochromic anaemia:

(a) Acute duodenal ulceration.
(b) Ankylostoma duodenale.
(c) Terminal ileitis due to Crohn's disease.
(d) Partial gastrectomy.
(e) Carcinoma of caecum.

---

25. The following is true of colon polyps and colon cancer:

(a) The larger the polyp, the greater the risk of carcinoma.
(b) Malignant polyps can be successfully treated by colonoscopy and polypectomy alone.
(c) Hyperplastic polyps have a higher malignant potential than villous polyps.
(d) Polyps are most common in the ascending colon.
(e) Colonic polyps are often recurrent.

---

26. These gastronomic terms are associated with the following gastroenterological conditions:

(a) 'Rice water' diarrhoea with cholera.
(b) 'Anchovy sauce' discharge with amoebic dysentry.
(c) 'Redcurrent jelly' and intussusception.
(d) 'Apple core' lesion and diverticulitis.
(e) 'Coffee grounds' and oesophageal varices.

---

27. The following gastrointestinal diseases are associated with the renal conditions listed:

(a) Crohn's disease and renal amyloidosis.
(b) Hepatitis B and glomerulonephritis.
(c) Gastric ulcer and nephrotic syndrome.
(d) Pancreatic neuroendocrine tumours and polycystic kidney disease.
(e) Liver cysts and glomerulosclerosis.

28. The following is true of breath tests used for investigation of the gastrointestinal tract:

(a) The ^{14}C urea breath test detects *Helicobacter pylori* infection.
(b) The ^{14}C glycocholic acid breath test is used to detect bacterial overgrowth in the colon.
(c) A hydrogen breath test following ingestion of lactulose is used to detect bacterial overgrowth in the small intestine.
(d) A lactose breath test is used to detect disaccharidase deficiency.
(e) A ^{14}C bile salt test can be used to identify bile duct obstruction.

---

29. The following is true of villous atrophy in the small intestine:

(a) If due to coeliac disease, it should recover completely on a gluten-free diet.
(b) It can be caused by tuberculosis.
(c) It can be associated with *Giardi lamblia.*
(d) It can be associated with *Tropheryma whippelei.*
(e) When associated with bacteria, it may cause a rise in serum folate.

---

30. The following autoantibodies are associated with the diseases listed:

(a) Antiendomyseal antibodies are associated with coeliac disease.
(b) Anti-LKM antibodies are associated with Goodpasture syndrome.
(c) Antimitochondrial antibodies are associated with primary biliary cirrhosis.
(d) Antiparietal cell antibodies are associated with Wilson's disease.
(e) Antismooth muscle antibodies are associated with autoimmune chronic active hepatitis.

---

31. The following skin conditions are associated with the named GI diseases:

(a) Dermatitis herpetiformis with coeliac disease.
(b) Pruritus with primary biliary cirrhosis.
(c) Pyoderma gangrenosum with gastric carcinoma.
(d) Bullous pemphigoid with pancreatitis.
(e) Erythema nodosum with Crohn's disease.

---

32. The following statements are true of colitis:

(a) Granulomas are present in collagenous colitis.
(b) Rectal sparing is characteristic of Crohn's colitis.
(c) Caseating granulomas in the terminal ileum are diagnostic of Crohn's disease.
(d) Colitis in a smoker is more likely to be Crohn's than ulcerative colitis.
(e) Pain is a characteristic feature of CMV colitis.

33. The following statements are true in relation to vomiting:

(a) Vomiting occurring 12 hours after a suspicious meal is indicative of Salmonella poisoning.
(b) Vomiting in association with headache is a feature of migraine.
(c) Vomiting associated with weight loss can be indicative of malignant disease.
(d) Vomiting usually precedes the pain of biliary colic.
(e) Vomiting can be a feature of myocardial infarction.

34. The following statements are true of ascites:

(a) A high protein content in ascites is usual in alcoholic liver disease.
(b) Ascites resistant to diuretics is characteristic of hepatic vein thrombosis.
(c) Ascites is sometimes associated with a pleural effusion.
(d) Ascites is a risk factor for bacterial peritonitis.
(e) Ascites due to constrictive pericarditis prevents pulsus paradoxus.

35. Scleroderma can produce the gastrointestinal complications listed:

(a) Diarrhoea due to bacterial overgrowth.
(b) Constipation due to gut hypomotility.
(c) Diarrhoea which is unresponsive to a gluten-free diet.
(d) Gastric ulcer due to chronic gastritis.
(e) Dysphagia due to abnormal peristalsis in the oesophagus.

36. The following statements are true of non-steroidal anti-inflammatory drugs:

(a) They can be given as suppositories to avoid gastrointestinal complications.
(b) They may have a role in the prevention of colon cancer.
(c) They can produce gastric erosions in elderly people causing occult blood loss.
(d) They cause gastric erosions by stimulating gastric acid secretion.
(e) They may exacerbate long-standing ulcerative colitis.

37. Chronic pancreatitis:

(a) Is a cause of diabetes mellitus.
(b) Can result from alcohol ingestion in moderate amounts.
(c) May be hereditary in a minority of cases.
(d) Can be diagnosed by a raised serum amylase.
(e) Is a cause of pancreas divisum.

38. The following is true of pancreatic tumours:

(a) Jaundice occurs only when carcinoma is present in the tail of pancreas.
(b) Presence of diabetes mellitus indicates that the tumour is of neuroendocrine origin.
(c) They are generally unresponsive to chemotherapy.
(d) They characteristically produce back pain when local invasion is present.
(e) They occur with increased frequency in patients with ulcerative colitis.

39. The following is true of haematemesis:

(a) When it occurs in a patient with alcoholic liver disease, it is always due to oesophageal varices.
(b) A visible vessel seen at gastroscopy is a risk factor for further bleeding.
(c) When it occurs in patients over 70 years of age who may have arthritis, usually indicates malignancy.
(d) When it occurs after repeated retching, it is suggestive of an oesophageal tear.
(e) When it is caused by duodenal ulcer, a partial gastrectomy is usually necessary.

40. The following is true of rectal bleeding:

(a) In the absence of haemorrhoids, it is usually due to malignant disease.
(b) It occurs more commonly in Crohn's disease than in ulcerative colitis.
(c) If it occurs in a patient with ulcerative colitis, it usually indicates that carcinoma has developed.
(d) When it is due to diverticular disease, colectomy may be indicated to control it.
(e) It may be caused by ingestion of aspirin.

41. The following drugs can be used for treatment of GORD:

(a) Metronidazole.
(b) Amoxycillin.
(c) Erythromycin.
(d) Metoclopramide.
(e) Omeprazole.

42. The following are risk factors for gastric carcinoma:

(a) Pernicious anaemia.
(b) Coeliac disease.
(c) Partial gastrectomy.
(d) *Helicobacter pylori* infection.
(e) Ménétrière's disease.

43. Which of the following is dependent on bile salts for its absorption:

(a) Vitamin A.
(b) Vitamin B.
(c) Vitamin C.
(d) Vitamin D.
(e) Vitamin K.

44. The following statements are true:

(a) Solitary rectal ulcers are commonly associated with Crohn's disease.
(b) Crypt abscesses are typical of coeliac disease.
(c) Fistula formation can be a feature of Whipple's disease.
(d) Anal fissure predisposes to faecal incontinence.
(e) Right iliac fossa pain is common with diverticular disease.

45. The following are indications for liver biopsy:

(a) Unexplained abnormal liver enzymes.
(b) Pyrexia of unknown origin with normal liver enzymes.
(c) Cirrhosis suspected on an ultrasound scan.
(d) Raised alkaline phosphatase in teenagers with acholuric jaundice.
(e) Abnormal liver enzymes in a patient with epilepsy on phenytoin.

46. The following are true of hepatitis:

(a) Hepatitis B is spread via the faecal–oral route.
(b) A vaccine is available for hepatitis C.
(c) Incubation time for hepatitis A is approximately 2–3 weeks.
(d) Hepatitis B is an RNA virus.
(e) Interferon treatment is required for hepatitis E infection.

47 The following precipitate portasystemic encephalopathy:

(a) Infection.
(b) Diarrhoea.
(c) Gastrointestinal bleeding.
(d) Use of opioid drugs.
(e) Certain antibiotics.

48. The following is a risk factor for the Budd–Chiari syndrome:

(a) Oral contraceptive pill.
(b) Malignancy.
(c) Ascites.
(d) Polycythaemia rubra vera.
(e) Constrictive pericarditis.

49. The following drugs cause cholestatic jaundice:

(a) Rifampicin.
(b) Isoniazid.
(c) Erythromycin.
(d) Halothane.
(e) Paracetamol.

50. The following are true regarding prognostic factors for acute pancreatitis:

(a) A low pAO_2 indicates a poor prognosis.
(b) A high serum GGT has a poor prognosis.
(c) Age of over 55 years usually has a good prognosis.
(d) A low serum albumin indicates a poor prognosis.
(e) Abnormal clotting time has a poor prognosis.

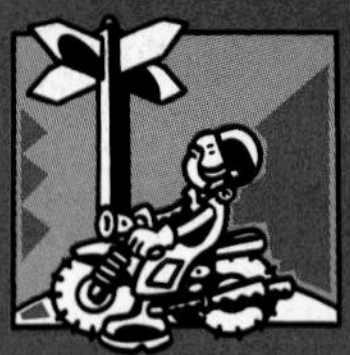

Short-answer Questions

1. A 43-year-old man complains of epigastric pain which is relieved by food. He points to a single site of pain in the epigastrium. What is the most likely diagnosis? His GP gave him a course of treatment and advised him to avoid alcohol while taking the medication. What was the treatment and the rationale for giving it? Why should this patient avoid alcohol?

2. A 40-year-old man presents with shortness of breath and abdominal swelling. He has a history of tuberculosis. What other features would you want to learn from the history? After a surgical procedure, he became asymptomatic. What was the surgical procedure and what investigations led up to it?

3. A 19-year-old student is brought to clinic by her mother who is concerned by her recurrent vomiting. What possible diagnoses would you consider and what physical signs would you look for in support of each of those?

4. A 72-year-old lady is referred by her GP with iron deficiency anaemia. She has no gastrointestinal complaints. On examination you think you can feel a mass in the right iliac fossa. What is the likely diagnosis and how would you investigate? If all investigations are negative, what drug history would be relevant and why?

5. A 43-year-old female presents with painless jaundice and pruritus. Alanine transferase is normal but alkaline phosphatase and gamma glutamyl transferase are 3–5 times the normal upper limit. Discuss how you would investigate this patient. Why is a history of respiratory tract infection for which she received treatment relevant?

6. A 17-year-old boy is referred with a serum bilirubin of 60 mmol/L (N<17); alanine transferase was normal; alkaline phosphatase 145 IU/L (N<125); gamma glutamyl transferase was normal. What is the most likely diagnosis and what is the mechanism of hyperbilirubinaemia in this condition? Why is his alkaline phosphatase raised? List other situations in which alkaline phosphatase may also be elevated in non-hepatological conditions.

7. A 15-year-old girl is brought to casualty vomiting and you notice she is slightly jaundiced. After questioning she admits to taking 20 of her mother's painkillers 2 days earlier because she was upset at school. Discuss your approach to management. What complications can you anticipate for this patient and how would you monitor her progress?

8. A 40-year-old man presents with bloody diarrhoea. List five features that would help you differentiate Crohn's disease from ulcerative colitis.

9. A 40-year-old man has haematemesis and melaena. He has a history of chronic pancreatitis. What are the possible causes of bleeding and how may these be related to his pancreatitis?

10. Describe how hepatic vein thrombosis might present clinically and list three causes.

11. Say what preventive measures could be undertaken to prevent transmission of hepatitis viruses A, B, C, D and E.

12. A 60-year-old man presents with acute pancreatitis. He has had a partial gastrectomy 20 years earlier. What would be the two most likely causes of his pancreatitis and what problems could you anticipate in dealing with him?

13. A 40-year-old man presents with rectal bleeding. In clinic you find he has two small polyps in the rectum. What is the significance of this finding and what further implications does it have for the patient and his family?

14. An 18-year-old male presents with abnormal liver enzymes. He knows that an elder brother died of liver disease in his teenage years. What are the possible causes of his abnormal liver enzymes? What sign would you examine for in his eyes?

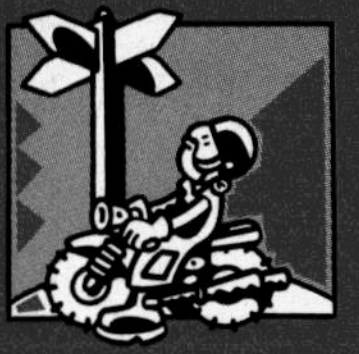

Short-answer Questions

15. An 18-year-old female presents with diarrhoea, weight loss, and anaemia. The following investigations were ordered: small bowel biopsy, small bowel enema, and lactose breath test. Why were these tests done and what would they be expected to show to explain the diarrhoea?

---

16. A 28-year-old man presents with diarrhoea. He has a brother who is known to carry HLA-B27. What conditions would you consider for this man and why?

---

17. A 25-year-old female presents with acute abdominal pain. She has rebound tenderness in the right iliac fossa with tachycardia and hypotension. List five possible diagnoses and give one principal investigation that could 'prove' each?

18. A 65-year-old man presented 3 months ago with obstructive jaundice. A diagnosis of carcinoma in the head of pancreas was made and his jaundice was relieved by endoscopic insertion of a biliary endoprosthesis. Now he returns with jaundice, rigors, pyrexia, and pain in the right upper quadrant. What possibilities would you consider and what investigations and treatment are appropriate?

---

19. A 60-year-old lady presents with chronic abdominal pain. She is found to be constipated. List the causes. Why could it be relevant that she had a parathyroidectomy in the past?

---

20. A 30-year-old female presents with fatigue. Biochemical screening reveals slightly elevated ALT and alkaline phosphatase, serum ferritin is 500 µg/L. All other biochemistry and abdominal ultrasound is normal. She had a blood transfusion 10 years earlier so you consider hepatitis B to be unlikely. What other diagnoses should be considered and what investigations can be undertaken?

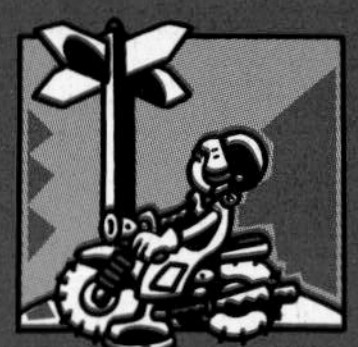

Patient Management Problems

1. A 39-year-old male presents with a 3-month history of dysphagia for solids. He has lost 1 kg in weight as he avoids eating bread and meat. He used to suffer with heartburn but now that you ask, he has not been troubled by it recently. Discuss the differential diagnosis in relation to each of the features in the history. How would you investigate this patient and what findings on investigation would favour one diagnosis over another?

2. A 27-year-old man complains of occasional difficulty with swallowing, 'food seems to stick half-way down'. He has not lost any weight. He has found that he can resolve the problem by regurgitating his food or by standing on his head! What is your differential diagnosis? A barium swallow shows a 'bird's beak' appearance. Discuss your management of this patient.

3. A 15-year-old girl presents with acute-onset abdominal pain localized to the right iliac fossa. She has been vomiting for 24 hours. On examination, she has guarding and rebound tenderness in the right iliac fossa with a tachycardia and pyrexia. What is your differential diagnosis? How you would investigate this patient?

4. A 35-year-old lady presents with a short history of gross abdominal distension and dyspnoea. She denies excessive alcohol ingestion. On examination, she is slightly icteric and has gross abdominal distension with shifting dullness. What is your differential diagnosis? How you would investigate this problem?

5. A 54-year-old female presents with weight loss, hot flushes, and diarrhoea. An abdominal ultrasound showed multiple metastatic deposits in her liver. What is the likely diagnosis? Describe how the symptoms are produced and which investigations are used to confirm the diagnosis.

6. A 16-year-old boy presents with loose pale stools, peripheral oedema, and a vesicular rash. Outline your approach to diagnosis and management.

7. A 43-year-old man presents with central abdominal pain and diarrhoea. List the differential diagnosis and describe how you would investigate him.

8. A 26-year-old female presents with pain in the left iliac fossa and occasional spotting of blood on toilet paper after defecation. What additional features on history would favour a diagnosis of irritable bowel syndrome and how would you differentiate inflammatory bowel disease from this?

9. A 49-year-old man presents with epigastric pain, weight loss, and a microcytic iron deficiency anaemia. Initial investigations include a gastroscopy which reveals a duodenal ulcer. Discuss your further management.

10. Discuss the problems associated with gastrectomy and their management.

1. (a)F, (b)F, (c)T, (d)T, (e)F

2. (a)T, (b)T, (c)T, (d)F, (e)T

3. (a)F, (b)F, (c)T, (d)T, (e)T

4. (a)T, (b)T, (c)T, (d)T, (e)T

5. (a)T, (b)F, (c)T, (d)T, (e)T

6. (a)T, (b)T, (c)T, (d)T, (e)F

7. (a)T, (b)T, (c)T, (d)T, (e)F

8. (a)T, (b)F, (c)T, (d)T, (e)T

9. (a)T, (b)F, (c)F, (d)T, (e)F

10. (a)T, (b)T, (c)F, (d)T, (e)F

11. (a)F, (b)T, (c)T, (d)T, (e)F

12. (a)T, (b)F, (c)F, (d)T, (e)T

13. (a)F, (b)F, (c)T, (d)F, (e)F

14. (a)F, (b)T, (c)T, (d)T, (e)F

15. (a)F, (b)F, (c)T, (d)F, (e)T

16. (a)F, (b)T, (c)T, (d)F, (e)F

17. (a)F, (b)T, (c)T, (d)F, (e)F

18. (a)F, (b)T, (c)T, (d)F, (e)T

19. (a)F, (b)T, (c)F, (d)T, (e)F

20. (a)F, (b)T, (c)T, (d)F, (e)F

21. (a)F, (b)T, (c)T, (d)F, (e)T

22. (a)F, (b)T, (c)F, (d)T, (e)T

23. (a)F, (b)T, (c)T, (d)F, (e)F

24. (a)F, (b)T, (c)T, (d)T, (e)T

25. (a)T, (b)T, (c)F, (d)F, (e)T

26. (a)T, (b)F, (c)T, (d)F, (e)F

27. (a)T, (b)T, (c)F, (d)F, (e)F

28. (a)T, (b)F, (c)T, (d)T, (e)F

29. (a)T, (b)T, (c)T, (d)T, (e)T

30. (a)T, (b)F, (c)T, (d)F, (e)T

31. (a)T, (b)T, (c)F, (d)F, (e)T

32. (a)F, (b)T, (c)F, (d)T, (e)T

33. (a)F, (b)T, (c)T, (d)F, (e)T

34. (a)F, (b)T, (c)T, (d)T, (e)F

35. (a)T, (b)F, (c)T, (d)F, (e)T

36. (a)F, (b)T, (c)T, (d)F, (e)T

37. (a)T, (b)T, (c)T, (d)F, (e)F

38. (a)F, (b)F, (c)T, (d)T, (e)F

39. (a)F, (b)T, (c)F, (d)T, (e)F

40. (a)F, (b)F, (c)F, (d)T, (e)T

41. (a)F, (b)F, (c)F, (d)T, (e)T

42. (a)T, (b)F, (c)T, (d)T, (e)T

43. (a)T, (b)F, (c)F, (d)T, (e)T

44. (a)F, (b)F, (c)F, (d)F, (e)F

45. (a)T, (b)T, (c)T, (d)F, (e)F

46. (a)F, (b)F, (c)T, (d)F, (e)F

47. (a)T, (b)F, (c)T, (d)T, (e)F

48. (a)T, (b)T, (c)F, (d)T, (e)F

49. (a)F, (b)F, (c)T, (d)F, (e)F

50. (a)T, (b)F, (c)F, (d)T, (e)T

209

1. Food often relieves the discomfort of gastritis, duodenitis, or duodenal ulcer disease. Sometimes patients with a duodenal ulcer can point to a specific site. His GP gave him a course of triple therapy for the eradication of *Helicobacter pylori* the aetiological agent for these conditions. This is likely to include a proton pump inhibitor and two antibiotics. Metronidazole is an antibiotic commonly used in many regimens to eradicate *Helicobacter*. This antibiotic has disulfiram-like properties. It inhibits acetaldehyde dehydrogenase so that if the patient were to drink alcohol, this metabolite would build up and causes unpleasant reactions such as nausea, vomiting, and flushing attacks.

2. Tuberculosis could have resulted in constrictive pericarditis which may present with ascites. You would also want to know whether there was any history of alcohol excess to suggest alcoholic liver disease; any history of myocardial ischaemia or renal disease to result in cardiac failure or nephrotic syndrome, respectively; any myeloproliferative disease which might predispose to hepatic vein thrombosis. This man would have had an abdominal ultrasound and an echocardiograph. The surgical procedure might have been a pericardiotomy if constrictive pericarditis were found, or a mesocaval or a mesoatrial shunt procedure if hepatic vein thrombosis were found.

3. The first thing to establish is the nature of the vomiting and to differentiate it from regurgitation which may be due to a congenital oesophageal anomaly. Gastritis should be considered and ingestion of alcohol, drugs or other noxious substances. Anorexia nervosa should be considered if the girl has a distorted body image. Signs to look for are acid burns on the teeth, callosities on the dorsum of the hand, lanugo hair. Also consider thyrotoxicosis and look for exophthalmos, tachycardia, fine tremor and goitre. Cyclical vomiting is a self-limiting functional disorder for which the cause is unknown.

4. A mass in the right iliac fossa in this situation should suggest the possibility of a carcinoma of the caecum which often presents with occult bleeding. Clearly, other causes of GI bleeding should also be considered. If all investigations are normal, then a drug history of taking non-steroidal anti-inflammatory drugs for arthritis is clearly relevant. These can cause gastric erosions and occult GI blood loss.

5. It is reasonable to assume that this is a cholestatic jaundice because the biliary enzymes are raised. The most useful investigation is an abdominal ultrasound to exclude dilated bile ducts—most commonly in this situation due to choledocholithiasis. If the bile ducts are not dilated, all hepatic causes should be considered. In a middle-aged female in particular, primary biliary cirrhosis should be excluded by checking the antimitochondrial antibodies. Antibiotics can cause cholestatic jaundice and may have been given for a respiratory tract infection, in particular co-amoxiclav or flucloxacillin.

6. Check whether he has acholuric jaundice. This is a common age for Gilbert syndrome to present. The normal gamma glutamyl transferase suggests that the raised alkaline phosphatase may not be of hepatic origin. Bones are still actively growing in a 17-year-old, so this level of alkaline phosphatase may be normal in this patient. Isolated hyperbilirubinaemia in this context is most often due to Gilbert syndrome. Haemolytic disease can be excluded by measuring reticulocyte count.

7. The most likely explanation is that her mother's painkillers contained paracetamol. She has probably taken a paracetamol overdose and jaundice characteristically appears about 2 days later. If her hepatic necrosis progresses, she will develop acute liver failure and encephalopthy will ensue. Other complications are acute renal failure, infection, and death. Progress is monitored by careful clinical observation for early signs of encephalopathy (somnolence, irritability). A rising prothrombin time, a high serum creatinine, or the presence of acidosis are bad prognostic signs. N-acetyl cysteine should be given even at this stage of presentation.

8. Crohn's disease is less likely to present with bloody diarrhoea than ulcerative colitis. Mouth ulcers are common in Crohn's because it can occur anywhere in the GI tract. It characteristically affects the terminal ileum or small intestine which are unaffected by ulcerative colitis. The rectum is spared in Crohn's but almost always inflamed in ulcerative colitis. Ulcerative colitis causes superficial ulceration, whereas Crohn's is a transmural disease causing deep ulcers. Histology of ulcerative colitis will show crypt abscesses, Crohn's may show granulomata. Ulcerative colitis occurs more commonly in non-smokers or ex-smokers, Crohn's in smokers. Perianal disease with abscesses or fistulae are more common in Crohn's disease.

9. This man may be bleeding from oesophageal varices, a duodenal ulcer, gastric erosions, or a Mallory–Weiss tear. His chronic pancreatitis may have been caused by alcohol, which may also cause liver disease and cirrhosis, resulting in portal hypertension and oesophageal varices. The other entities may also be caused by alcohol. Chronic pancreatitis may also result in portal vein thrombosis, which could cause non-cirrhotic portal hypertension and bleeding varices.

10. Hepatic vein thrombosis (Budd–Chiari syndrome) usually presents with ascites that is difficult to manage with diuretics; abnormal liver function due to congestion, or even with liver failure. Possible causes include contraceptives, hepatoma, or myeloproliferative disease.

11. Hepatitis A and E are spread by the faecal–oral route. Personal hygiene and public sanitation are very important in retarding their spread. In epidemics, some quarantine measures may be important, especially for immunocompromised people or, in the case of hepatitis E, pregnant women. Hepatitis B, C, and D are spread by contact with contaminated body fluid, particularly blood. Blood products therefore must be screened, and avoid sharing needles or other invasive instruments. Hepatitis B is also commonly transmitted sexually and barrier prophylaxis should be used. Vertical transmission is the most common mode of transmission for hepatitis B. Hepatitis D occurs only in combination with hepatitis B, so the same prophylactic measures should suffice. A vaccine is available for only hepatitis A and B; pooled immunoglobulin is also available for these viruses.

12. The two most common causes of acute pancreatitis are alcohol and gallstones. His gastrectomy may have been the treatment 20 years earlier for peptic ulcer disease associated with alcohol. The prognosis for pancreatitis due to alcohol is not good because many patients will not subsequently abstain from alcohol and continue to suffer recurrent bouts. If alcohol abuse is long-standing, nutritional reserve may be poor making him more susceptible to infection. If gallstones are the cause of this patient's pancreatitis, they will be difficult to treat. Gallstones in the bile duct are most commonly removed endoscopically by retrograde cholangiography (ERCP). This may be difficult or impossible following a partial gastrectomy as the normal duodenal anatomy (and the endoscopic route to the bile duct!) is changed, commonly by inserting a Roux-en-Y intestinal anastomosis. Surgical removal may also prove difficult, as adhesions may have developed because of his previous upper abdominal surgery.

13. Polyps are often multiple and commonly they are villus or tubulovillus in structure. These polyps have the capacity to undergo malignant change and should be removed. This can be achieved endoscopically but it is important to ensure that he has no further polyps in the colon. Polyps have a tendency to recur, and because of their malignant potential, colonscopic surveillance is recommended in this situation. Colonic cancer is often familial; polyps can be as well. If this young patient develops dysplasia or cancer of the colon, consideration may have to be given to screening first degree relatives at an appropriate age.

14. This patient could have abnormal liver enzymes from any cause. In light of his family history, it would be important to exclude chronic hepatitis B in particular, as both boys could have acquired this at birth. Hereditary syndromes of liver disease induce haemochromatosis, Wilson's disease, alpha-one antitrypsin deficiency, certain porphyrias, and cystic fibrosis. Of these, only Wilson's disease is likely to present without other history in the teenage years. Kayser–Fleischer rings are a brown discoloration around the limbus of the cornea in the eye due to copper deposition.

15. Small bowel biopsy was done to exclude coeliac disease (subtotal villous atrophy) and giardiasis. Small bowel enema may identify flocculation due to malabsorption but would also identify strictures or ulcers in the terminal ileum due to Crohn's disease. A lactose tolerance test is done to identify disaccharidase deficiency: blood sugar will only rise following a lactose load if this enzyme is present in the small intestine.

16. HLA-B27 is associated with a group of inflammatory conditions known as the spondylarthritides because they involve arthritis, usually of the spine. They include ankylosing spondylitis, psoriatic arthropathy, and Reiter's disease. All of these conditions are associated with ulcerative colitis. Reiter's disease is an asymmetrical arthritis with urethritis, uveitis, and occasionally, colitis. It is thought to be due to a reaction to *Salmonella* or *Chlamydia*.

17. The clinical signs indicate that this woman may be in shock. You should consider acute appendicitis with perforation or abscess, Crohn's disease, tuberculosis, tubal pregnancy also with rupture, ruptured ovarian cyst, and pyelonephritis. Investigation would include a pregnancy test, abdominal or pelvic ultrasound, mid-stream urine test, small bowel enema, or colonoscopy with ileoscopy and biopsy.

18. This man presents with symptoms of cholangitis. It is likely that the endoprosthesis has become occluded and the biliary tree is infected. It would be appropriate to treat him with antibiotics intravenously initially and then to remove and replace the infected stent.

19. The causes of constipation for this woman should include low residue diet, depression or antidepressants, opioid analgesia, iron tablets, hypothyroidism, and Parkinson's disease. Hyperparathyroidism may cause hypercalaemia which also causes constipation.

20. The high ferritin suggests iron overload or chronic inflammatory disease. Haemochromatosis occurs with an equal sex incidence but is unlikely to manifest in a 30-year-old female with a normal menstrual pattern. Chronic inflammatory disease such as rheumatoid or Crohn's should be considered, although additional history should be available. Hepatitis B is unlikely, as blood products have been screened for this virus in most countries for almost 20 years. Nonetheless, there is a window of infectivity when the screening tests may have been negative and this should be checked. Hepatitis C can cause exactly this kind of clinical picture including the hyperferritinaemia. Hepatitis C virus was identified in 1989 and blood products have been screened only since 1991.

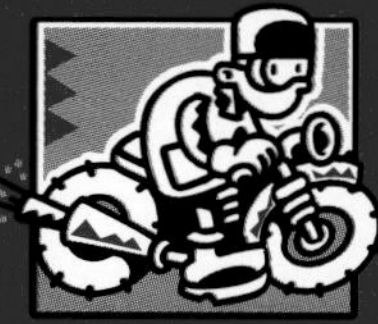

Index

B

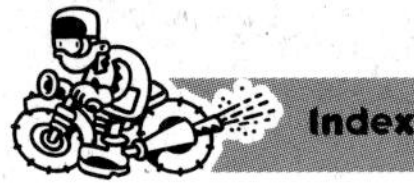

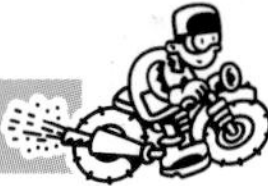

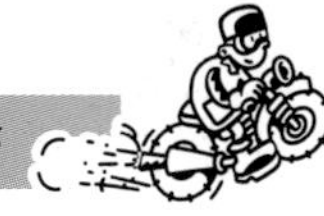

D

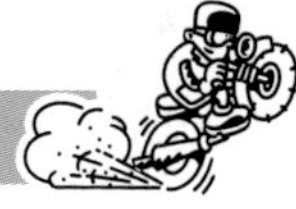

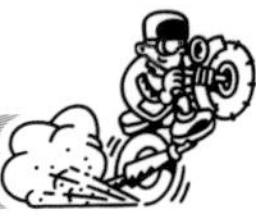

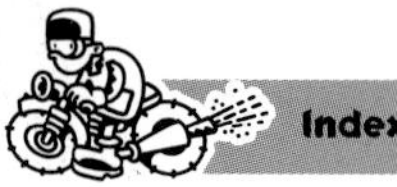

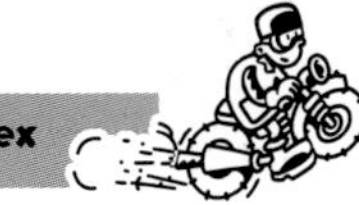

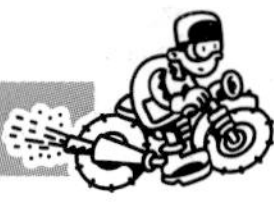

V

W

X

Y

Z